# Contemporary Endoscopic Spine Surgery

# (Volume 1)

# *Cervical Spine*

Edited by

## Kai-Uwe Lewandrowski
*Center For Advanced Spine Care*
*Tucson*
*Arizona*
*USA*

## Jorge Felipe Ramírez León
*Fundación Universitaria Sanitas*
*Clínica Reina Sofía – Clínica Colsanitas*
*Centro de Columna – Cirugía Mínima Invasiva*
*Bogotá, D.C.*
*Colombia*

## Anthony Yeung
*University of New Mexico*
*School of Medicine*
*Albuquerque*
*New Mexico*

# Assistant Editors

## Hyeun-Sung Kim
*Department of Neurosurgery*
*Nanoori Gangnam Hospital*
*Seoul*
*Republic of Korea*

## Xifeng Zhang
*Department of Orthopedics*
*First Medical Center*
*PLA General Hospital*
*Beijing 100853*
*China*

## Gun Choi
*Neurosurgeon and Minimally Invasive Spine Surgeon*
*President Pohang Wooridul Hospital*
*South Korea*

## Stefan Hellinger
*Department of Orthopedic Surgery*
*Arabellaklinik*
*Munich*
*Germany*

## Álvaro Dowling
*Endoscopic Spine Clinic*
*Santiago*
*Chile*

# Contemporary Endoscopic Spine Surgery

*(Volume 1)*

*Cervical Spine*

Editors: Kai-Uwe Lewandrowski, Jorge Felipe Ramírez León and Anthony Yeung

Assistant Editors: Hyeun-Sung Kim, Xifeng Zhang, Gun Choi, Stefan Hellinger and Álvaro Dowling

ISBN (Online): 978-981-4998-63-5

ISBN (Print): 978-981-4998-64-2

ISBN (Paperback): 978-981-4998-65-9

Published by Bentham Science Publishers Pte. Ltd. Singapore. All Rights Reserved.

need for a court order if at any point you breach any terms of this License Agreement. In no event will any delay or failure by Bentham Science Publishers in enforcing your compliance with this License Agreement constitute a waiver of any of its rights.

3. You acknowledge that you have read this License Agreement, and agree to be bound by its terms and conditions. To the extent that any other terms and conditions presented on any website of Bentham Science Publishers conflict with, or are inconsistent with, the terms and conditions set out in this License Agreement, you acknowledge that the terms and conditions set out in this License Agreement shall prevail.

**Bentham Science Publishers Pte. Ltd.**
80 Robinson Road #02-00
Singapore 068898
Singapore
Email: subscriptions@benthamscience.net

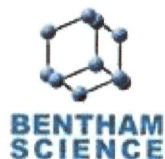

**BENTHAM SCIENCE**

# ENDORSEMENTS

# ISASS

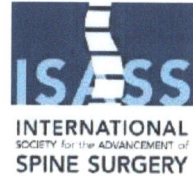

The International Society for the Advancement of Spine Surgery (ISASS; formerly The Spine Arthroplasty Society) has its roots in motion preservation as an alternative to fusion. Since then, it has worked to achieve its mission of acting as a global, scientific and educational society with a surgeon-centered focus. ISASS was organized to provide an independent venue to discuss and address the issues involved with all aspects of basic and clinical science of motion preservation, stabilization, innovative technologies, MIS procedures, biologics, and other fundamental topics to restore and improve motion and function of the spine. ISASS has a robust international membership of orthopedic and neurosurgery spine surgeons and scientists. ISASS is dedicated to advancing evolutionary and innovative spinal techniques and procedures such as endoscopic spine surgery. Every editor of Contemporary Endoscopic Spine Surgery represents ISASS as a member, author, reviewer, or editor of its quarterly circulation – The International Journal of Spine Surgery (IJSS). The contributors of *Contemporary Endoscopic Spinal Surgery* have succeeded in compiling an exhaustive and up-to-date reference text. It is an example of our society's mission pursuit of surgeon education and scientific study. It is my pleasure to endorse this comprehensive text on behalf of ISASS.

**Domagoj Coric**
President
International Society for the Advancement of Spine Surgery (ISASS)
Illinois
USA

# SBC

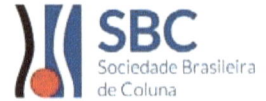

Founded on October 12, 1994, the Brazilian Spine Society (Sociedade Brasileira de Coluna - SBC) is a scientific, non-profit organization whose primary objective is the advancement of spine surgery through basic research and clinical study in orthopedics and neurosurgery. SBC is actively engaged in the accreditation and continued education of spine surgeons in Brazil. It prides itself on bringing the latest high-grade scientific evidence on novel technological advances and therapies to its professional members. SBC pursues this mission with its quarterly circulation Coluna/ Columna and its online courses, including Introduction to Endoscopy. The authors and editors of Contemporary Endoscopic Spine Surgery have put forward a comprehensive reference text essential to SBC's core curriculum of teaching spinal endoscopy to the next generation of surgeons. The presented clinical protocols for the endoscopic treatment of cervical and lumbar spine conditions are vetted and validated by peer-reviewed articles published by its contributors. It is my pleasure to endorse Contemporary Endoscopic Spine Surgery on behalf of the Brazilian Spine Society.

**Cristiano Magalhães Menezes**
President of the Brazilian Spine Society (Sociedade Brasileira de Coluna - SBC)
São Paulo
Brazil

# MISS OF COA

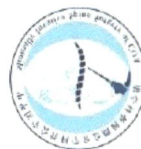

The Minimally Invasive Spine Surgery (MISS) of Chinese Orthopaedic Association (COA) was founded in 2003, which is one of the most special subsidiary societies of Chinese Medical Association, aiming to promote and develop minimally invasive orthopedics especially spine surgeries in China.

The MISS society organizes global discussions and encourages our members to participate international efforts and cooperation to improve surgeon education. With this mission in mind, it is my pleasure to endorse Contemporary Endoscopic Spine Surgery on behalf of the MISS of COA. Many international editors and contributors are from China, who have made great efforts, contributions and dedications to this book. They share with and update readers all over the world about the latest endoscopic spinal surgery techniques. I am confident that *Contemporary Endoscopic Spinal Surgery* can be a textbook for spine surgeons. It should be used as medical school advanced lessons materials for continuing education courses. In sum, it is my pleasure and honor to support it on behalf of the MISS of COA.

**Huilin Yang**
Chairman of MISS of COA
Professor & Chairman of Orthopedic Department
The First Affiliated Hospital of Soochow University
Suzhou
China

# SICCMI

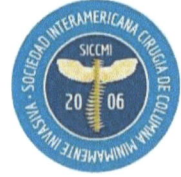

SICCMI (Sociedad Interamericana De Cirugia De Columna Minimamente Invasive) was founded in 2006 with similar objectives pursued by the editors of Contemporary Endoscopic Spine Surgery: the advancement and mainstreaming of minimally invasive spine surgery (MIS). SICMII members joined to implement MIS in all countries of South America, the Caribbean, Central America, and North America. Endoscopic surgery is performed by many of its key opinion leaders at the highest level, some of which have contributed to this multi-volume text. Four of the editors are active SICCMI members in leadership positions. The book contents are exhaustive and comprehensive, encompassing topics of the cervical and lumbar spine and advanced technology applications. Contemporary Endoscopic Spine Surgery will serve as SICCMI's core curriculum and course material for endoscopic surgery of the spine. It is my pleasure to endorse it on behalf of SICCMI.

President of SICCMI
Manuel Rodriguez
President-Elect of SICCMI, Department of Neurosurgery
ABC Medical Center
Ciudad de México, Mexico

# SBMT

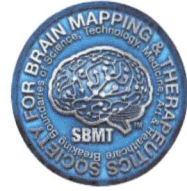

As a nonprofit organization, the Society for Brain Mapping and Therapeutics (SBMT) focuses on improving patient care by translating new technologies into life-saving diagnostic and therapeutic procedures. Contemporary Endoscopic Spine Surgery is a prime example of achieving excellence in education and scientific discovery. Authors and editors from around the globe came together to present the reader with the most up-to-date endoscopic spine surgery protocols and their supporting clinical evidence. SBMT has an active spine section led by productive innovator surgeons – some of which have demonstrated their leadership with their editorial contributions to *Contemporary Endoscopic Spinal Surgery*. The editors have embraced multidisciplinary collaborations across many cultural and geographic barriers. Their effort represents one of the core principles of SBMT's mission: to identify and bridge gaps in modern patient care with technological advances. It is my pleasure to endorse *Contemporary Endoscopic Spinal Surgery* on behalf of SBMT.

**Babak Kateb**
Founding Chairman of the Board of Directors
CEO and Scientific Director of SBMT
Californias
USA

# SILACO

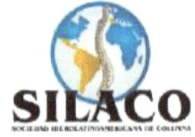

SILICO (Sociedad Ibero Latinoamericana de Columna) had its beginnings in the meetings of the Scoliosis Research Society with the first Hispano-American Congress held in 1991 in Buenos Aires Argentina. Since then, it has morphed into an organization that promotes the study of treatments and prevention of spinal conditions by bringing together spine care professionals from all subspecialties. The scientific activities of our biannual Ibero-Latin American Congress are focused on the promotion of surgeon education to the highest academic standards via international relationships between members from the Americas, Spain and Portugal.

Contemporary Endoscopic Spine Surgery resembles such a collaborative effort where authors worldwide have come together to update the reader on the latest endoscopic spinal surgery techniques.

SILACO has incorporated Contemporary Endoscopic Spine Surgery into its core curriculum and plans on using it as course material for its continuing education courses. It is my pleasure to endorse it on behalf of SILACO.

**Jaime Moyano**
President of SILACO
Editor Revista De Sociedad Ecuatoriana De Ortopedia y Traumatología
de la Sociedad Ecuatoriana De Ortopedia Y Traumatología
Quito, Ecuador

# SOMEEC

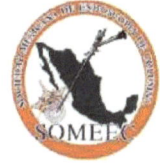

SOMEEC- Sociedad Mexicana de Endoscopia de Columna- is Mexico's prime organization uniting spine surgeons with a diverse training background having a fundamental interest in endoscopic surgery. SOMEEC organizes annual meetings where member surgeons and international faculty update each other on their latest clinical research to promote spine care *via* endoscopic spinal surgery technique. Two of the senior lead editors of *Contemporary Endoscopic Spinal Surgery* have been active international supporters of SOMEEC. I am pleased to endorse their latest three-volume reference text, which will become an integral centerpiece of SOMEEC's continuing medical educational programs.

**Cecilio Quinones**
Past President of the Sociedad Mexicana de Endoscopia de Columnas

# KOSESS

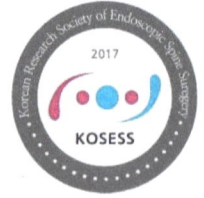

The Korean Research Society of Endoscopic Spine Surgery (KOSESS) was established in 2017. KOSESS was founded to bring endoscopic spine surgeons in the Republic of Korea together to advance the subspecialty of endoscopic spine surgery with high-quality clinical research. It is reflected in *Contemporary Endoscopic Spine Surgery* by the numerous contributions of Korean authors. It is *Contemporary Endoscopic Spine Surgery*. It is my pleasure to endorse it on behalf of KOSESS.

**Hyeun-Sung Kim (Harrison Kim)**
President of the Korean Research Society of the Endoscopic Spine Society
(KOSESS)
Seoul
Republic of Korea

# KOMISS

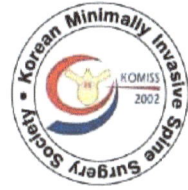

Since its establishment in 2002, the *Korean Minimally Invasive Spinal Surgery Society* (KOMISS) has had a leading role in developing new clinically applicable technologies to advance patient care with less invasive yet more effective therapies. The superiority of minimally invasive spine surgery in Korea is demonstrated by its competitiveness on the world stage at the highest academic level. It is reflected in *Contemporary Endoscopic Spine Surgery* by the numerous Korean authors who have contributed to this timely reference text with their groundbreaking clinical research on endoscopic spine surgery. I am proud of their accomplishments and want to congratulate them on acting as KOMISS ambassadors by carrying the message of Korean excellence in minimally invasive spinal surgery the world over within *Contemporary Endoscopic Spine Surgery*. It is my pleasure to endorse it on behalf of KOMISS.

**Dae Hyun Kim**
President of KOMISS
Seoul
Republic of Korea

# NATIONAL ACADEMY OF MEDICINE OF COLOMBIA

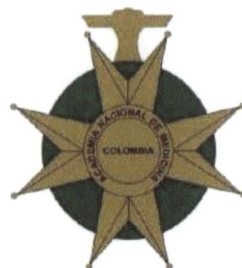

After reviewing the table of content and some representative chapters, I am happy to inform you that the Board of Directors of the National Academy of Medicine of Colombia grants academic endorsement of your book series entitled Contemporary Endoscopy Spine Surgery. Kai-Uwe Lewandrowski, Jorge Felipe Ramírez, and Anthony Yeung produced a text of great interest and scientific impact.

On behalf of the National Academy of Medicine, I would like to express my admiration and respect for your dedication to scientific research that led to this great work's culmination. It meets the high standards required by our National Academy to support such a production spearheaded by one of our most esteemed members - Dr. Jorge Felipe Ramírez.

**Gustavo Landazabal Bernal**
General Secretary
National Academy of Medicine of Colombia
Bogota, Colombia

# IITS

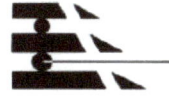

International Intradiscal Therapy Society

The International Intradiscal Therapy Society (IITS) was founded in 1987, initially headquartered in Belgium, Wisconsin, and led by Dr. Eugene Nordby, the first Executive Director of IITS. Members were primarily orthopaedic surgeons, anesthesiologists, radiologists, and rheumatologists dedicated to the treatment, research, and education involving The FDA-approved and validated level I studies that supported intradiscal spinal therapies.

From 2013-2017, the society began operating under International Intradiscal and Transforaminal Therapy Society (IITTSS) to reflect the advancements in endoscopic spine surgery augmenting Intradiscal therapy. The organization wanted to include and reflect the state-of-the-art evolution in intradiscal therapy with advances by intradiscal visualization of pain generators through the endoscope. However, the society reverted to IITS.

IITS now sponsors workshops on intradiscal therapy in conjunction with other International societies when it lost its original pharma support. IITS disseminates a newsletter to provide its membership, other healthcare professionals, and the general public information on the safest and cost-effective techniques to treat conditions such as herniated nucleus pulposus and other intradiscal spinal disorders.

IITS is a 501C3 non-profit organization whose focus is on intradiscal therapy aided by the endoscope as the least invasive, visually-guided treatment for discogenic pain, including extra-discal and complex foraminal decompression and stabilization procedures. The disc has been validated as the primary initial source of common back pain.

Two of the senior lead editors of Contemporary Endoscopic Spinal Surgery have been in active leadership roles in International Spine Organizations as consultants, full and associate professors, and directors. I am pleased to endorse their latest three-volume reference text, which will become integral to IITS' ongoing course programs.

**Anthony Yeung**
Executive Director of IITS
Desert Institute for Spine Care
Phoenix, Arizona
USA

# SLAOT

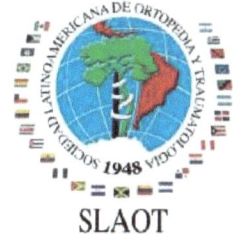

SLAOT

The Sociedad Latinoamericana de Ortopedia y Traumatologia (SLAOT)/ Latin American Society of Orthopaedics and Traumatology is a non-profit, autonomous, scientific organization of orthopaedic surgeons and orthopaedic care professionals. SLAOT has an organization structure that brings together professionals with a diverse scientific interest. It promotes continuous professional development and education at the highest level. *Contemporary Endoscopic Spine Surgery* is of interest to SLAOT because of its illustrative use of cutting-edge technology and discussion of validated clinical endoscopic spinal surgery protocols. It is my pleasure to endorse *Contemporary Endoscopic Spine Surgery* on behalf of SLAOT.

**Horacio Caviglia**
President of SLAOT FEDERACION
USA

# CONTENTS

# PREFACE

Endoscopic surgery of the cervical spine is gaining increasing traction among minimally invasive spinal surgeons. Technology advances with improved miniaturized optical- and surgical access systems have purported expansion of endoscopic minimally invasive spinal surgery techniques into the cervical spine. However, many spine surgeons still hesitate to treat common painful conditions of the cervical spine with endoscopic procedures. The high risk of neurologic- and vascular injury is of concern to many of them. Additionally, damage to the trachea, esophagus, or the recurrent laryngeal nerve may put the patient at significant risk for the deleterious postoperative course. Nevertheless, increased acceptance of endoscopy by traditionally trained spine surgeons in other areas of the spine coupled with more widely available training events and unanswered patient demand has reenergized spine surgeons' interest in the endoscopic platform for the cervical spine.

The editors have come together to develop a multi-authored and clinically focused medical monograph entitled Contemporary Endoscopic Spine Surgery: Cervical Spine to give the reader a most up-to-date snapshot of the current state-of-the-art of cervical spinal endoscopic surgeries. The publication is intended for Orthopedic Spine & Neurosurgeons interested in treating common painful conditions including herniated disc, stenosis, tumor, and infection with minimally invasive endoscopic techniques. A wide array of highly timely and clinically relevant topics have been assembled for this purpose. They range from suitable anesthesia protocols, patient selection algorithms for anterior versus posterior cervical endoscopic decompression, clinical decision-making strategies, indications, and outcomes for endoscopically visualized cervical rhizotomy to more advanced endoscopic techniques, including complex endoscopic decompression techniques for cervical spondylotic myelopathy and other intricate procedures such as pediculotomy, vertebrectomy, and fusion.

The selection of chapters was based on contemporary trends in endoscopic cervical spine surgery. The editors recognize that this trend is based on the need for less costly yet safe and efficient solutions for the cervical spine's common degenerative conditions. Patients and other stakeholders in the ongoing debate on better value-based spine care, including healthcare policymakers and payors, are demanding of spine surgeons less burdensome and less risky treatments with shorter time to recovery, return to work, and social reintegration following spine surgery. Contemporary Endoscopic Spine Surgery: Cervical Spine was written with these goals in mind. The editors hope that the readers will find it an informative knowledge resource they will continue to revert to when implementing a cervical endoscopic spinal surgery program in their practice setting.

**Kai-Uwe Lewandrowski**
Discipline of Anesthesiology
Faculty of Medicine of Ribeirão Preto
São Paulo
Brazil

**Jorge Felipe Ramírez León**
Fundación Universitaria Sanitas
Clínica Reina Sofía – Clínica Colsanitas

Centro de Columna – Cirugía Mínima Invasiva
Bogotá, D.C.
Colombia

**Anthony Yeung**
University of New Mexico
School of Medicine
Albuquerque
New Mexico

**Hyeun-Sung Kim**
Department of Neurosurgery
Nanoori Gangnam Hospital
Seoul
Republic of Korea

**Xifeng Zhang**
Department of Orthopedics
First Medical Center
PLA General Hospital
Beijing 100853
China

**Gun Choi**
Neurosurgeon and Minimally Invasive Spine Surgeon
President Pohang Wooridul Hospital
South Korea

**Stefan Hellinger**
Department of Orthopedic Surgery
Arabellaklinik
Munich
Germany

**Álvaro Dowling**
Endoscopic Spine Clinic
Chile

# List of Contributors

| | |
|---|---|
| **Anthony Yeung** | University of New Mexico School of Medicine, Albuquerque, New Mexico<br>Desert Institute for Spine Care, Phoenix, AZ, USA |
| **Álvaro Dowling** | Endoscopic Spine Clinic, Santiago, Chile<br>Department of Orthopaedic Surgery, USP, Ribeirão Preto, Brazil |
| **Bu Rongqiang** | Department of Orthopedics, First Medical Center, PLA General Hospital, Beijing 100853, China |
| **Carolina Ramírez Martínez** | Minimally Invasive Spine Center for Latinamerican Endoscopic Spine Surgeons, LESS Invasiva Academy, Bogotá, D.C., Colombia |
| **Catherine Ann Cameron** | University of British Columbia, Vancouver, BC & University of New Brunswick, Fredericton, NB, Canada |
| **Cindy Lau** | Independent Scholar based in Hong Kong |
| **Enrique Osorio Fonseca** | Universidad El Bosque, Bogotá, D.C., Colombia |
| **Gabriel Oswaldo Alonso Cuéllar** | Minimally Invasive Spine Center for Latinamerican Endoscopic Spine Surgeons, LESS Invasiva Academy, Bogotá, D.C., Colombia |
| **Hyeun Sung Kim** | Department of Neurosurgery, Nanoori Gangnam Hospital, Seoul, South Korea<br>A President of the Korean Research Society of the Endoscopic Spine Surgery (KOSESS), South Korea<br>A Faculty of the KOrean Minimally Invasive Spine Surgery Society (KOMISS), South Korea<br>A Chairman of the Nanoori Hospital Group Scientific Team, South Korea<br>An Adjunct Professor of the Medical College of the Chosun University, Gwangju, South Korea |
| **Il-Tae Jang** | Department of Neurosurgery, Nanoori Gangnam Hospital, Seoul, Republic of Korea, Beijing 100048, China |
| **Jin-Sung Kim** | Spine Center, Department of Neurosurgery, Seoul St. Mary's Hospital, College of Medicine, The Catholic University of Korea, 222 Banpo Daero, Seocho-gu, Seoul, 137-701, Korea |
| **João Abrão** | Discipline of Anesthesiology, Faculty of Medicine of Ribeirão Preto, University of São Paulo, São Paulo, Brazil |
| **Julia Gillen** | Department of Linguistics and English Language, Lancaster University, Lancaster, UK |
| **Jun-Song Yang** | Department of Spinal Surgery, Hong-Hui Hospital, Medical College of Xi'an Jiaotong University, Xi'an, China |
| **Jorge Felipe Ramírez León** | Minimally Invasive Spine Center for Latinamerican Endoscopic Spine Surgeons, LESS Invasiva Academy, Bogotá, D.C., Colombia<br>Fundación Universitaria Sanitas, Bogotá, D.C., Colombia |
| **José Gabriel Rugeles Ortíz** | Minimally Invasive Spine Center for Latinamerican Endoscopic Spine Surgeons, LESS Invasiva Academy, Bogotá, D.C., Colombia |

| | |
|---|---|
| **Jorge Felipe Ramírez León** | Minimally Invasive Spine Center for Latinamerican Endoscopic Spine Surgeons, Bogotá, D.C., Colombia<br>Universidad El Bosque, Bogotá, D.C., Colombia |
| **José Gabriel Rugeles Ortíz** | Minimally Invasive Spine Center for Latinamerican Endoscopic Spine Surgeons, LESS Invasiva Academy, Bogotá, D.C., Colombia |
| **Jiang Hongzhen** | Minimally Invasive Spinal Surgery, Beijing Yuhe Integrated Traditional Chinese and Western Medicine Rehabilitation Hospital, Beijing 100853, China |
| **Kai-Uwe Lewandrowski** | Center for Advanced Spine Care of Southern Arizona and Surgical Institute of Tucson, Tucson, AZ, USA<br>Department of Orthopaedic Surgery, UNIRIO, Rio de Janeiro, Brazil<br>Department of Orthoapedic Surgery, Fundación Universitaria Sanitas, Bogotá, D.C., Colombia, USA<br>Center for Advanced Spine Care of Southern Arizona and Surgical Institute of Tucson, Tucson, AZ, USA |
| **Lei Chu** | Department of Orthopaedics, the Second Affiliated Hospital, Chongqing Medical University, Chongqing, China |
| **Liang Chen** | Department of Orthopaedics, the Second Affiliated Hospital, Chongqing Medical University, Chongqing, China |
| **Liu Yan-kang** | Shanxi Medical University, Taiyuan 030001, China<br>Center for Advanced Spine Care of Southern Arizona and Surgical Institute of Tucson, Tucson, AZ, USA |
| **Li Dongzhe** | Department of Orthopedics, First Medical Center, PLA General Hospital, Beijing 100853, China |
| **Li Jinlong** | Department of Orthopedics, The Eighth Medical Center, PLA General Hospital, 100091 Beijing, China |
| **Malcolm Pestonji** | Mahatma Gandhi Memorial University of Health Sciences, Navi Mumbai, Kamothe Maharashtra, India |
| **Nicolás Prada Ramírez** | Minimally Invasive Spine Center for Latinamerican Endoscopic Spine Surgeons, LESS Invasiva Academy, Bogotá, D.C., Colombia<br>Colombia Clínica Foscal, Bucaramanga, Colombia |
| **Nora Didkowsky** | Independent Scholar based in Canada and Switzerland |
| **Pang Hung Wu** | Department of Neurosurgery, Nanoori Gangnam Hospital, Seoul, Republic of Korea<br>Departments of Orthopaedic Surgery, National University Health System, Jurong Health Campus, Singapore |
| **Stefan Hellinger** | Department of Orthopedic and Spine Surgery, Arabellaklinik, Munich, Germany |
| **Wang Yipeng** | Department of Orthopedics, The Eighth Medical Center, PLA General Hospital, 100091 Beijing, China |
| **Xi Jiancheng** | Department of Orthopaedic Surgery, UNIRIO, Rio de Janeiro, Brazil |
| **Yan Yu-qiu** | Minimally Invasive Spinal Surgery, Beijing Yuhe Integrated Traditional Chinese and Western Medicine Rehabilitation Hospital, Beijing 100039, China |

**Yuan Heng**            Shanxi Medical University, Taiyuan 030001, China

**Zhong-Liang Deng**     Department of Orthopaedics, the Second Affiliated Hospital, Chongqing Medical University, Chongqing, China

**Zhang Xi-feng**        Department of Orthopedics, First Medical Center, PLA General Hospital, Beijing 100853, China

**Zhang Lei-ming**       Department of Neurosurgery, the Sixth Medical Center, PLA General Hospital, Beijing 100048, China

**Zhu Zexing**           Department of Orthopedics, First Medical Center, PLA General Hospital, Beijing 100853, China

**Zheng Zeze**           Department of Orthopedics, The Eighth Medical Center, PLA General Hospital, 100091 Beijing, China

**CHAPTER 1**

# Cervical Endoscopy: Historical Perspectives, Present & Future

**Kai-Uwe Lewandrowski**[1,2,3,*], **Jin-Sung Kim**[4], **Stefan Hellinger**[5] and **Anthony Yeung**[6,7]

[1] *Center for Advanced Spine Care of Southern Arizona and Surgical Institute of Tucson, Tucson, AZ, USA*

[2] *Department of Orthopaedic Surgery, UNIRIO, Rio de Janeiro, Brazil*

[3] *Department of Orthoapedic Surgery, Fundación Universitaria Sanitas, Bogotá, D.C., Colombia, USA*

[4] *Spine Center, Department of Neurosurgery, Seoul St. Mary's Hospital, College of Medicine, The Catholic University of Korea, 222 Banpo Daero, Seocho-gu, Seoul, 137-701, Korea*

[5] *Department of Orthopedic and Spine Surgery, Arabellaklinik, Munich, Germany*

[6] *University of New Mexico School of Medicine, Albuquerque, New Mexico*

[7] *Desert Institute for Spine Care, Phoenix, AZ, USA*

**Abstract:** Endoscopy of the cervical spine traditionally has been slow to adopt. Initially, spinal endoscopy concentrated on common painful degenerative conditions of the lumbar spine, for which many of the technology breakthroughs were developed. Many of them were validated for defined clinical indications, such as a herniated disc. Stenosis applications followed later as improvements in the endoscopic platform permitted. Cervical spine application of endoscopic surgery commenced around interventional pain management with lasers and radiofrequency to improve their reliability by directly visualizing the painful pathology. Later, anterior cervical discectomies and posterior cervical foraminotomies were performed as endoscopic power burrs, and rongeurs made them possible. The most skilled surgeons moved on to perform anterior and posterior cervical spinal cord decompressions and anterior column reconstructions endoscopically further to take advantage of the potential of this platform so they could transform the traditional surgical treatments from inpatient to outpatient by performing them in a simplified manner in ambulatory surgery centers where better clinical outcomes and higher patient satisfaction could be achieved. In this chapter, the authors strove to briefly illustrate this development by giving credit to the

---

\* **Corresponding author Kai-Uwe Lewandrowski:** Center for Advanced Spine Care of Southern Arizona and Surgical Institute of Tucson, Tucson, AZ, USA, Department of Orthopaedic Surgery, UNIRIO, Rio de Janeiro, Brazil and Department of Orthoapedic Surgery, Fundación Universitaria Sanitas, Bogotá, D.C., Colombia, USA; Tel: +1 520 204-1495; Fax: +1 623 218-1215; E-mail: business@tucsonspine.com

most prominent pioneers of this fast-moving field and by setting the stage for what the reader is about to discover in this most-up-to date publication entitled: *Contemporary Spinal Endoscopy: Cervical Spine.*

**Keywords:** Cervical spine, Decompression, Degeneration, Disc herniation, Endoscopic, Historical considerations, Impingement, Lasers, Minimally invasive, Open, Radiofrequency, Stenosis.

## INTRODUCTION

Endoscopic Spinal Surgery is rapidly becoming more mainstream [1]. Most of the clinical trials published in the last two years have focused on lumbar endoscopy. [1 - 97] Cervical endoscopic surgery is done well by far fewer surgeons, as it requires a more advanced skill level due to the higher risk associated with operating near the spinal cord [9, 44, 46, 48, 98 - 115]. It perhaps is risker than lumbar or even thoracic endoscopic spinal surgery due to potential for life-threatening vascular injury, tracheal- or esophageal perforation, or grave neurological deficits from the spinal cord damage [116 - 119]. However, there is increased activity in that area just within the last year [9, 44, 46, 48, 98 - 104]. For this reason, the editors of Contemporary Endoscopic Spinal Surgery: Cervical Spine have decided to dedicate an entire volume to it as we expected an expansion of clinical indications for cervical endoscopic surgery due to technological advancements [98, 99, 111, 113] and more formalized surgeon postgraduate education programs [5, 9, 120 - 122]. There already is an increasing trend by program directors to include spinal endoscopy into residency- and fellowship programs [122]. Understanding the past, however, and recognizing preceding key opinion leaders for their contributions to the advancement of the cervical spinal endoscopy field is the basis of defining the future in terms of evolving clinical indications, understanding and mitigating risks, incorporating technology advancements into day-to-day clinical practice in a meaningful way [67], so they improve patient outcomes, and safety, and prove to be cost-effective. Therefore, this team of authors came together to help the novice spine surgeon maneuver this fast-moving subspecialty.

## RECYCLED TRENDS

Many historical perspectives have been revisited by repurposing existing technologies in new surgical approaches. Likewise, have we witnessed the resurgence of previously employed surgical techniques that have been applied in the early years of spinal endoscopy. As in the fashion industry, where certain trends reappear in a modernized form by fusing different design elements or materials to create new products and marketing strategies, spine surgeons are similarly susceptible to embracing modern trends in spinal endoscopy in their quest to overcome shortcomings of existing treatment protocols for common degenerative conditions of the cervical spine. Industry recycles existing medical know-how and often modernizes them by technology transfer from other commercial areas, such as the aerospace or the automotive industry, by innovation mechanisms of adoption, miniaturizations, automation, and system integration to develop advanced surgical techniques, instruments-, and equipment of improved performance, reliability, and durability. Innovations widely adopted in other industries are making their way into medical applications [123]. Examples include miniaturized high-definition (HD) video technology with touch-screen displays, high-speed HD recording equipment [124, 125] robotics- [126 - 131] and navigation tools [132 - 134], and 3D heads-up display goggles [9] for surgeons to be worn during surgery to improve eye-hand coordination and many others. Rapid endoscopic spine surgery product development with a myriad of instruments being pushed by an army of salespeople is another area of rapid change that has been playing itself out in the operating room — endoscopes with larger inner working channels, sturdy enough to withstand the abuse of more frequent short sterilization cycles to respond to the rising caseload, motorized shavers, drills, and large Ø rongeurs employed for rapid decompression [24, 31, 37, 38, 48].

## THE CERVICAL ENDOSCOPE OF THE FUTURE

Endoscopes previously rated for 200 to 250 simple discectomy surgeries are now used in more complex and demanding advanced endoscopic procedures of the spine. These include intradiscal therapies with cool lasers [52, 135 - 139] or bipolar radiofrequency [44, 82, 140 - 143] devices for the early stages of the disease and the late stages of the disease where aggressive decompression and reconstructive procedures may be needed for spinal stenosis- and instability related neural element encroachment. Endoscopic placement of spinal implants, such as interbody fusion cages and posterior supplemental fixation with pedicle screw-rod constructs, are other examples of contemporary advancements in endoscopic spinal surgery [51, 60, 63, 77, 80, 92, 144]. This increasing quality and durability demand on spinal endoscopes to work in a large variety of surgical indication scenarios have widened the field of industry competitors with some front-runners pushing clinical product portfolios, reimbursement, and coding agendas. Traditional German endoscopic equipment makers are experiencing competition from China, Korea, and Japan by domestic Asian manufacturers whose technological know-how has now risen to a competitive level at lower manufacturing and acquisition cost with similar quality. In some cases, Asian spinal endoscopy, radiofrequency, and motorized decompression equipment has even advanced beyond what European competitors can put forward mainly because of progressive clinical agendas with broader indications for endoscopic surgery of the cervical spine.

## THE OBJECTIVE

Whether all of these innovations are genuinely impactful and leaps forward to improve patient outcomes at lower cost and are not just vogue trends at an increased cost to patients and the health care system. It is not always obvious and often requires vetting them in the operating room with investigational studies - all of which require clinical testing, resources, and most of all, time. Spine surgeons have little of the latter and, by their very nature, may be innovation aficionados in their quest to overcome shortcomings of existing clinical protocols and technological applications used in the treatment of common degenerative conditions of the spine. The authors of this chapter attempted to put some of these new trends in cervical spinal endoscopy in perspective within the proper historical context by reviewing the contributions of some of the early key players in an attempt to help the aspiring endoscopic spine surgeon to position her-, or himself in the increasingly convoluted field of surgical procedures.

## THE ADOPTION & TRAINING DILEMMA

With spinal endoscopy becoming more mainstream, many North American and European national and international spine surgeons' organizations are struggling with its adoption [100]. They have just begun embracing it by trying to spell out clinical treatment guidelines and figure out how to establish an accredited core curriculum with validated training programs [100]. On the contrary, endoscopic spinal surgery training made it into mainstream core curriculum many years ago, and an informal source of education is less and less relevant in Asia. For the time being, many novice endoscopic spine surgeons in other parts of the world – particularly in North America and Europe - have to rely on industry-sponsored weekend cadaver and other short instructional courses. While some of them are lucky enough to be mentored by veteran key opinion leaders (KOLs), the vast majority - by default - are autodidacts, and primarily self-taught having to go through an endoscopic learning curve that many find out is steeper than with other procedures they are routinely performing [122].

## THE PARADIGM SHIFT

The final goal of spinal surgery is to decompress neural elements and stabilize the unstable spinal motion segments. Traditionally, this required extensive exposure and stripping of soft tissues, which may devitalize and degenerate the very structures whose integrity is paramount to maintaining a healthy spinal motion segment. The jury is still out on stabilization *versus* preservation of motion. On the other hand, spinal endoscopy is supported by sufficient history and validated science to support the concept of treating the predominant pain generator. Problems such as post-laminectomy instability and epidural fibrosis have long been recognized as some of the potential follow-up problems that could arise from traditional open spinal surgery [145 - 147]. Other well-recognized problems include disruption of vascular supply and denervation of paraspinal muscles with resultantly decreased muscle strength and chronic pain syndromes that at least in part arise from extensive spinal exposures [148, 149]. Ten years later, the cumulative rate of development of adjacent level disease in the cervical spine in previously healthy spinal motion segments adjacent to fusions has been reported to be as high as 25% [150 - 152]. This is not a small number, and recognizing this problem has prompted surgeons to look for alternative ways to accomplish the two fundamental goals of each spinal surgical procedure: Neural element decompression and stabilization of unstable motion segments [153].

## THE BENEFITS

From the patient's point of view, reduction of blood loss and surgical time, with rapid recovery and return to work are clear advantages which nowadays are being openly discussed [154 - 156]. With the advent of the internet, social media, blogs, and the overall online availability of educational information, patients have become more educated, curious, at times critical, and hopeful that their specific problem can be solved with less aggressive procedures. To many patients, spinal endoscopy intuitively presents itself as such a solution. From a surgeon's point of view, these advantages are no less critical as they lessen the burden to patients and drive patient satisfaction. Lower blood loss, complications [66], and infection rates [66], faster return to work [11] and social reintegration [157, 158], and less time to narcotic independence [159 - 161], are clinical upsides of spinal endoscopy that can easily be communicated to patients, families, and in due time to hospitals, health insurance companies, and third-party payers, who still frequently deem spinal endoscopy as an experimental procedure.

## THE ACCEPTANCE LAG

Since the publication of the lead editor's Spinal Endoscopy in 2013 [162], several high-grade clinical evidence studies have been published with a large body of literature on spinal endoscopy [85, 163, 164], having emerged out of Asia and China in particular [141]. In North America and Europe, however, spinal endoscopy is still yet to be included in treatment and coverage guidelines despite a substantial increase of peer-reviewed journal articles on the safety, efficacy, and equivalency of endoscopic decompression to other minimally invasive (MIS) and open spinal surgeries. Regional variations [1] of the degree of acceptance and utilization of endoscopic spine surgery in the lumbar spine and changes from the previously dominating transforaminal to the now more popular posterior foraminal- and interlaminar endoscopic decompression [104, 105, 110, 111, 115, 165, 166]. For the cervical spine, the full endoscopic anterior and posterior cervical approach [99, 103, 106, 109, 116, 167, 168] has been employed, but preferences are less clear as fewer surgeons are doing the procedure. The differences in the surgeon's endoscopic approach preference are also reflective of a shift to more complex cervical decompression and reconstructive procedures. Historically being a method developed for simple discectomies, spinal endoscopy is now the most commonly employed minimally invasive spinal surgery technique the world over has found use in a much more extensive range of surgical applications.

## THE HISTORY

The first to report on percutaneous cervical discectomy in 1989 was most likely Tajima *et al.* [169] and Gastambide (1993) [170], independently reported on manually removing the central portion of a cervical disc without removal of the posterior longitudinal ligament under fluoroscopic guidance. This process produced an indirect decompression. Algara *et al.* developed an automated percutaneous cervical discectomy procedure in 1993 [171]. Herman also reported on automated nonendoscopic discectomy one year later [172]. Bonati [173], Sieber (1993) [174], and Hellinger (1994) reported on the utility of laser percutaneous cervical discectomy. Lee *et al.* introduced the combined use of percutaneous manual and laser discectomy popularized the concept of "laser-assisted spinal endoscopy" [175]. This system was based on a straight firing Ho: YAG laser that was introduced through an illuminated and irrigated 3-mm flexible cable. In 1994, Zweifel published experimental laser disc surgery, pointing out that the Ho: YAG laser was the safest yet effective laser for tissue ablation while minimizing thermal damage to surrounding tissues [176].

Another technological break was achieved with the introduction of a 0-degree, 4 mm endoscope with a 1.9 mm working channel (Fig. 1 and Table 1). Surgeons at the Wooridul Spine Hospital in Seoul, South Korea, took advantage of improved endoscopic visualization, and a large working channel [177]. Ahn *et al.* reported that 88.3% of his 111 percutaneous anterior cervical discectomy patients improved at a mean follow up of 49.9 months. Loss of mean disc height was later analyzed in a smaller series of 36 patients and was limited to 11.2% suggesting that sagittal alignment could be maintained without the development of postoperative segmental instability or spontaneous fusion with the use of the percutaneous anterior cervical discectomy procedure [178].

In Latin America, Ramirez *et al.* have employed both lasers and radiofrequency in interventional anterior and posterior cervical procedures to treat axial discogenic neck pain. Some of their clinical results are described in other chapters within this text. The same group of authors recently published their clinical outcomes on anterior endoscopic cervical decompression with discectomy, and foraminotomy is an alternative to open surgical treatment of unrelenting cervical radiculopathy (CR) in patients who have failed non-operative treatment [99]. Their retrospective study of 293 patients found that *Excellent* and *Good* Macnab outcomes in 90.1% of patients at 12 months follow-up with an average VAS score reduction of 5.6. The authors noted complications in 8 patients, who subsequently required additional procedures. Two other patients also had a second procedure without a complication in the immediate postoperative period. Ramirez *et al.* concluded that anterior endoscopic cervical decompression should be considered an alternative to open ACDF because of the comparably low complication- and reoperation rate the authors noted with the procedure.

## LASERS

Lasers have always been very attractive for surgeons when applied in minimally invasive procedures due to the ability to deliver a large amount of energy through a small fiber in a very focused small area. While most of this initial research was done in the lumbar spine, it formed the basis for cervical spine applications and is worthwhile recapping briefly. Peter Ascher employed neodymium:yttrium-aluminum-garnet (Nd: YAG) laser through an 18 gauge needle that was introduced fluoroscopically into the intervertebral disc [179]. He ablated intradiscal tissue in short bursts to avoid heating of adjacent tissues thereby vaporizing tissue that was allowed to escape through the needle. This procedure was ideally suitable for an outpatient setting as the patient was discharged once the needle is withdrawn in the puncture wound was covered with a small Band-Aid. Many subsequent authors demonstrated the utility of different types of lasers including the Ho:YAG which was compared to the Nd:YAG laser in a clinical trial conducted by Quigley *et al.* in 1991 [180]. They concluded that the Ho: YAG laser was the best compromise between the efficacy of absorption and convenience of fiber-optic delivery at that time. In 1990, Davis *et al.* described in 85% success rate in a study on 40 patients who underwent laser discectomy using the potassium-titanyl-phosphate (KTP 532-nm) laser [181]. Only six of the 40 patients required revision with open discectomy procedures because of clinical failures. In 1995, Casper *et al.* [182, 183] described the use of the side-firing Ho: YAG laser which has also been employed later by Yeung *et al.* [184]. At one-year follow-up, Casper *et al.* reported an 84% success rate [182]. In the same year, Siebert *et al.* published on 78% success rate on 100 patients with a mean follow-up of 17 months which were treated with the Nd: YAG laser [185]. The current state-of-the-art has been summarized by Ahn *et al.* in a recent article [186]. While this paper focuses mostly on lumbar spine applications, it is worthwhile to recap the authors' description of laser applications in interventional and minimally invasive spinal surgery in the following three categories: (1) open microscopic laser surgery; (2) percutaneous endoscopic laser surgery; and (3) laser tissue modulation for spinal pain [187]. Ahn *et al.*, encouraged further study of the select clinical indications where efficacy has been demonstrated to substantiate the lack of evidence with randomized clinical trials [187].

Mayer *et al.* were the first to suggest the combined use of an endoscope with laser ablation through an endoscopically introduced fiber for lumbar applications [188]. Large clinical trials followed and were very supportive of the clinical use of lasers for the removal of the herniated disc [188]. Hellinger reported in 1999 on more than 2500 patients whom he treated with the use of the Ascher technique [189]. He stated the success rate of 80% over 13 years. One year later, Yeung *et al.* reported an 84% success rate on more than 500 patients whom he treated with the KTP laser [184]. Deukmedjian *et al.* took these groundbreaking works and applied them to the cervical spine. In his 2012 article, the author describes clinical outcomes with the Cervical Deuk Laser Disc Repair®, which he promoted as a novel full-endoscopic, anterior cervical, trans-discal, motion-preserving, laser-assisted, nonfusion procedure suitable for outpatient applications [190]. As an alternative to ACDF, the author treated symptomatic cervical disc diseases, including herniation, spondylosis, stenosis, and annular tears, which he directly visualized, including the posterior longitudinal ligament, posterior vertebral endplates, annulus, to decompress the cervical neuroforamina, and to remove herniated disc fragments. His study included 142 consecutive adult patients with symptomatic degenerative cervical disc disease with clinical improvements and without postoperative complications. An average volume of herniated disc material of 0.09 ml was removed from the cervical intervertebral disc. Deukmedjian promoted his technique as a nonfusion, motion-preserving outpatient surgery with faster recovery, shorter time to postoperative narcotic independence, and few complications. The method was promoted as particularly attractive since hardware-related problems, pseudoarthrosis, adjacent segment disease, and postoperative dysphagia were not expected. In another prospective follow-up study published in 2013, Deukmedjian studied clinical outcomes on 66 consecutive patients who were candidates for ACDF or cervical disc arthroplasty [191]. Single-level procedures were done on 21 patients, and two adjacent level procedures on another 45 patients, respectively. Postoperatively, patients were evaluated for resolution of headache, neck pain, arm pain, and radicular symptoms. The author reported an average 94.6% success rate. Fifty percent of his patients had 100% resolution of all preoperative cervicogenic symptoms and only 4.5% had less than 80% resolution of preoperative symptoms. This was reflected in the VAS improvements of from 8.7 preoperatively to 0.5 postoperatively (p < 0.001). Again, the author denied any complications. However, one patient (1.5%) had a recurrent disc herniation. There were no significant difference in outcomes (p = 0.774) between patients with a one- or two-level Deuk Laser Disc Repair((R)) procedure. However, the author inidicated that posterior facet syndrome does not respond favorably to this anterior procedures and that it should be ruled out before proceeding with this endoscopic laser procedure.

## RADIOFREQUENCY

High-frequency radiofrequency ablation has found several applications in neurosurgery, endoscopic spine, orthopedic and pain management. High (RF) radio frequency with low temperatures has been employed for tissue dissection (monopolar) and coagulating mode (mono and bipolar). Nowadays, nearly every vendor selling spinal endoscopes also has a radiofrequency probe in the portfolio that is either produced in-house or by a third party. Typically, radiofrequency probes are compatible with the working channel of the spinal endoscope are used for hemostasis, shrinkage or ablative effects in soft tissue to dissect them of a herniated disc. Again, much of the literature emanated from lumbar spine applications. However, the authors are compelled to review some of the prior studies describing radiofrequency- and tissue interactions as they apply to the cervical spine application.

Radiofrequency ablation of tissues is well accepted in other areas such as plastic surgery, oral maxillofacial surgery, and dental procedures. These devices have found their way into spinal surgery for thermal ablation of disc tissue. With further miniaturization and reduced acquisition costs, they nowadays present an attractive alternative to lasers. While the acquisition cost of lasers nowadays may be comparable to the expense of capital equipment purchase of a complete radiofrequency system, radiofrequency is found in most operating rooms. In a routine clinical application in high-turn-over operating rooms radiofrequency with disposable probes is perceived more practical by most and less cumbersome. Besides, lasers may impose additional safety issues for patients, surgeons and supporting staff alike which do not exist with the application of radiofrequency.

Radiofrequency applications specific to the cervical spine were recently described by several authors. Pflum *et al.* described its use during endoscopic anterior cervical diskectomy which was done *via* a working cannula seated in the middle of the disk with small rongeurs through the cannula, followed by a cervical spine arthroscope with a working channel [192]. They removed the endoscope to complete the discectomy with a motorized shaver and radiofrequency probe under fluoroscopic guidance. More recently, its application was demonstrated by Bing *et al.* (2019) in the treatment of cervicogenic headache (CEH) which the authors defined as unilateral posterior head and neck pain [193]. They recommended the use of radiofrequency (RF) ablation of cervical medial branches in patients who did not meet criteria surgical treatment and failed medial branch RF lesion. The authors recommended the use of a diagnostic medial branch block to validate the painful level and to proceed with the endoscopic medial branch neurotomy if medial branch injection provided short-term pain relief. Nowadays, high radiofrequency with low temperatures tissue ablation is useful in spinal endoscopy when controlling bleeding and shrinking tissue to facilitate visualization. The need for a modernized radiofrequency application may arise out of the implementation of advances in endoscopic spinal decompression and reconstructive procedures.

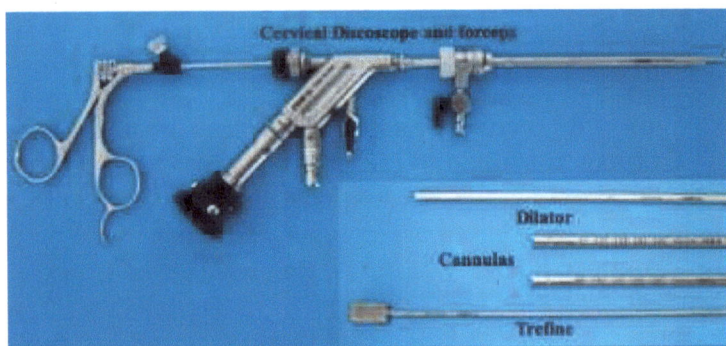

**Fig. (1).** Anterior 0°-degree cervical endoscopic system with instruments (Karl Storz Tuttlingen, Germany).

Choi *et al.* investigated short- and long-term effects of pulsed radiofrequency on cervical radicular pain *via* modulation of the dorsal root ganglion (DRG) in patients with chronic refractory cervical radicular pain in a study of 15 patients [194]. Their patients suffered from chronic radicular pain due to cervical disc herniation or foraminal stenosis refractory to active rehabilitative management, transforaminal cervical epidural steroid injection, and physical therapy. The authors reported a statistically significant reduction of NDI of 8.2% and VAS for arm pain of 2.8 3 months after treatment (p<0.05). Eleven of the 15 patients (77.3%) indicated that they had 50% or more pain relief at the final follow-up without any adverse effects during the peri- and immediate postoperative period. Choi *et al.* concluded that pulsed radiofrequency on the DRG of a painful cervical nerve root might be a minimum of a reasonable short-term intervention for chronic refractory cervical radicular pain. The authors then followed up with a prospective observational long-term cohort study of 112 patients whose charts were analyzed in retrospect after their radicular pain was treated with a cervical transforaminal epidural steroid injection (TFESI) [195]. Twenty-nine patients without relief were treated with additional pulsed radiofrequency ablation of the painful DRG. Clinical outcome measures up to one year postoperatively showed 21 of the 29 patients with improvements. Fifteen of these 21 patients (71.4%) had high satisfaction again, suggesting that the application of pulsed radiofrequency ablation of the DRG in select patients with refractory cervical radicular pain appears to be an effective and relatively safe intervention technique.

## NEW LANDMARK CLINICAL OUTCOME STUDIES

Until recently, randomized prospective trials comparing the traditional open *versus* the endoscopically performed cervical procedures were unavailable. However, some studies stand out that are worth reporting. Ruetten *et al.* conducted a prospective, randomized, controlled study of patients with lateral cervical disc herniations that they surgically treated either in a full-endoscopic posterior or conventional microsurgical anterior technique to see whether the latter can be replaced as the standard procedure for operation of cervical disc herniations with radicular arm pain with the motion-preserving full-endoscopic surgery mainly if the compressive pathology is in the lateral cervical spinal canal [166]. The authors randomly assigned 175 patients with full-endoscopic posterior or microsurgical anterior cervical discectomy. They analyzed the clinical outcomes with the VAS, German version North American Spine Society Instrument, and the Hilibrand Criteria at a two-year follow-up. At the final follow-up, 87.4% of the patients no longer had arm pain, and 9.2% had occasional pain. The authors reported similar clinical outcomes in both groups without a statistically significant difference in the reoperation- or complication rate. However, the authors found advantages with the full-endoscopic technique in postoperative recovery, preservation of mobility, rehabilitation, and less tissue trauma. They concluded that the full-endoscopic posterior foraminotomy is an effective and safe alternative to traditional procedures with similar surgery indications. The authors, followed by another randomized prospective study, were published by the same group of authors comparing surgical outcomes in anterior cervical decompression and fusion (ACDF) with the full-endoscopic anterior cervical discectomy (FECD) in patients suffering from mediolateral soft disc herniations [116]. Employing similar outcome measures, 85.9% of the total of 103 patients with ACDF or FECD no longer had any arm pain at a two-year follow-up. Another 10.1% of patients reported occasional pain. Again, the authors were unable to find any significant clinical differences between the decompression with or without fusion. They recommended the full-endoscopic technique as it afforded similar advantages to the authors reported previously.

**Table 1. Comparison of specifications of the early foraminoscopes 1992 – 1997.**

| Geometric Data & Specs | Karl Storz 1992 (Leu) | Danek Inc. 1992 (Hoodland) | Richard Wolf YESS 1997 (Yeung) |
|---|---|---|---|
| Working Length | 145 mm | 210 mm | 207 mm |
| Outer Ø | 6.0 mm | 6.3 mm | Oval |
| Working Channel Ø | 3.1 mm for 3.5 mm Ø Instruments | 3.6 mm for 3.5 mm Ø Instruments | 2.7 mm for 2.5 mm Ø Instruments |
| Optic | Rod-Lens System | Fiber Optic Cable | Rod-Lens System |
| Two Irrigation Channels | Yes | Yes | Yes |
| Connector For Video Camera | Yes | Yes | Yes |

Yao *et al.* provided 5-year follow-up clinical and radiographic outcomes of 67 patients who underwent ACDF performed *via* the endoscopic approach [196]. Primary clinical outcome measures, including the Japanese Orthopaedic Association (JOA) and VAS, showed 86.6% of patients with excellent results at the final follow-up. The authors assessed anterior intervertebral height (AIH) and the lordosis angle (LDA) as secondary radiographic outcome measures showed that AIH increased, on average, 18.7% from the original height (p < 0.01) with more physiologic LDA as well. In this landmark study of the 67 patients, there was no segmental instability or intra- or postoperative complications, such as dysphagia or injury, to the tracheoesophageal groove's content. The authors reported a fusion rate of 100%. Six-years postoperatively, one patient was revised with an open ACDF for adjacent segment disease. For the surgical indications studied (cervical disc herniation causing cervical myelopathy, or radiculopathy), the authors achieved comparable results as reported with the open technique while exceeding patients' expectations regarding perioperative morbidity, postoperative cosmesis, and recovery.

A recent meta-analysis by Wu *et al.* compared the clinical outcomes, the incidence of complications, and the reoperation rates between full-endoscopic posterior cervical foraminotomy (FE-PCF) and microendoscopic posterior cervical foraminotomy (MI-PCF) for cervical radiculopathy [197]. Their analysis included 26 articles with 2003 patients (FE-PCF, 377; MI-PCF, 1626) and was motivated by the lack of randomized clinical trials or high-quality prospective cohort studies. The authors calculated a pooled clinical success rate of 93.6% (CI: 90.0%-95.9%) for the FE group and 89.9% (CI: 86.6%-92.5%) for the MI group without any statistically significant differences between the groups (p = 0.908). The complication rates were similar without a statistically significant difference (p = 0.128) with 6.1% (CI: 3.2%-11.3%) in the FE group and 3.5% (CI: 2.7%-

4.6%) in the MI group. These complications were transient nerve root palsy in the FE group (12/16, 75.0%) and dural tear in the MI group (20/47, 42.6%). The pooled reoperation rate, the FE group (4.8%, CI: 2.9%-7.8%) and the MI group (5.3%, CI: 3.4%-8.2%), were also not statistically different (p = 0.741). Wu *et al.* admitted that their meta-analysis's reliability was likely limited by a higher degree of bias in the underlying low-quality clinical studies. Based on the available studies, the authors concluded that FE-PCF and MI-PCF could both offer an effective treatment for cervical radiculopathy.

Most recently (2020), Yuan *et al.* compared the clinical efficacy of endoscopic cervical spinal surgery with ACDF in treating cervical spondylotic myelopathy (CSM) in a study of 45 patients [98]. Perioperative data such as surgery time, blood loss and length of stay, and clinical outcome data, including the Japanese Orthopaedic Association (JOA) score before the operation, three months, and one year postop, were analyzed. While the JOA improvement rates in the twenty-two cases in the spinal endoscopy group and twenty-four cases in the ACDF group were no different, there was a significant advantage with endoscopy in terms of shorted mean surgery time, lower intraoperative blood loss and shorter length of stay (p < 0.05). There was no significant difference in the excellent rate (81.8% *vs.* 83.3%) between the spinal endoscopy group and the ACDF group (P>0.05), allowing the authors to conclude that the short-term efficacy of cervical endoscopic surgery and ACDF was equal in the treatment of CSM. This study by Yuan *et al.* is an example of an endoscopy application for the cervical spine's more complex conditions [98].

In 2020, Ahn *et al.*, published results of a prospectively comparative study between percutaneous endoscopic cervical discectomy (PECD) and ACDF by analyzing clinical outcomes of 51 single-level PECD patients to 64 ACDF patients [198]. The authors reported significant improvements in VAS, Neck Disability Index (NDI), and modified Macnab criteria in both groups. Excellent and Good results were obtained in 88.24% and 90.63% in the PECD and ACDF groups. Some patients required revision surgery - 3.92% in the PECD and 1.56% in the ACDF group. Patients in the PECD group showed shorter surgery time, hospital stay, and return to work compared to the ACDF group (p < 0.001). Patients were followed up to five years postoperatively, where there was no significant difference in outcome measures with PCED compared to those with conventional ACDF. The authors concluded that PECD provided the typical benefits of minimally invasive spine surgery and recommended it as an effective alternative to ACDF for treating soft cervical disc herniation.

Du *et al.* compared ACDF outcomes to a motion to a cervical motion-preserving discectomy where the herniated disc was removed through anterior transcorporeal herniotomy (ATH) motivated by the progressive disc collapse often observed following endoscopic transdiscal discectomy [199]. Other authors have also highlighted the problems with the procedure and corroborated its benefits [200 - 202]. The feasibility study by Du *et al.* was performed by the authors to demonstrate the safety and efficacy of the percutaneous full-endoscopic anterior transcorporeal cervical discectomy (PEATCD) and channel repair (CR) for the treatment of cervical disc herniation (CDH). The authors operated on four patients with PEATCD and CR and followed them for at least 22 months, and obtained CT images at one week and three months after postoperatively to assess the healing of the bony access channel. The authors reported no procedure-related complications and significant postoperative VAS and JOA improvements scores. Three of the four patients reported *Excellent* Macnab outcomes, and one patient had a *Good* Macnab outcome. There were no problems related to the migration of the repair implant or collapse of the drilled vertebrae. Three months postoperatively, there was complete healing of the bony access channel. The authors advocated for their method listing less damage to the disc and the more effective preservation of cervical motion at the surgical segment as significant advantages. They concluded that PEATCD is a feasible, safe, and minimally invasive procedure. Deng *et al.* corroborated Du's study's findings by reporting the ability to remove upward or downward migrated disc herniations behind the cervical vertebral body as another advantage of the transcorporeal endoscopic approach to avoid the need for corpectomy [203]. The authors stated that the trajectory to access a migrated cervical herniated disc could be adjusted within the vertebral body, thus, making motion preservation the critical key advantage of the PEATCD procedure. Schubert reported his results with the procedure in a retrospective study of 9 patients and corroborated the advantages found by the other authors [204]. The most extensive clinical research on the percutaneous endoscopic surgery for cervical intervertebral disc herniation was published by Tzaan *et al.*, who studied a total of 107 consecutive patients [205]. Complete 12 months follow-up (ranging from 12 to 60 months; averaging 22.4 months) was available on 86 patients (80%) There were significant VAS and Neck Disability Index improvements (p < 0.001). Excellent and Good Macnab outcome was achieved in 29 (34%) and 49 (57%) patients, respectively. There were two surgical complications – a carotid artery injury in one patient (treated with angiographic stenting), and a postoperative headache in another patient who improved with supportive care. Tzaan *et al.* concluded that the percutaneous endoscopic cervical discectomy procedure is associated with more rapid recovery but carries the risk of significant complications. Careful patient selection and meticulous surgical techniques are essential to render the procedure safe and effective alternative to open cervical discectomy or ACDF.

## CONCLUSION

Endoscopic surgery for common painful degenerative conditions of the cervical spine has gotten some attention with few investigators demonstrating its successful employment for interventional pain management applications, cervical disc herniations, foraminal and central canal stenosis. In terms of its acceptance, it is lagging behind lumbar endoscopy. Still, it is gaining more traction fueled by technology advancements, and more sophisticated endoscopic instruments. These videoendoscopic optical improvements allow for adequate decompression and reconstruction of the cervical spine when indicated. There are several examples illustrated of these more modern endoscopy applications in the cervical spine within this text the authors and editors have put forward in response to the increasing interest and demand for these types of minimally invasive procedures. Its application, however, is riskier than in the lumbar spine because of surgery adjacent to the cervical spinal cord.

## CONSENT FOR PUBLICATION

Not applicable.

## CONFLICT OF INTEREST

This manuscript is not meant for or intended to push any other agenda other than reporting the clinical outcome data following endoscopic spinal decompression. The motive for compiling this clinically relevant information is by no means created and/or correlated to directly enrich anyone due to its publication. The authors are accountable for all aspects of the work in ensuring that questions related to the accuracy or integrity of any part of the work are appropriately investigated and resolved. The first author has no direct or indirect conflicts of interest. The senior author designed and trademarked his inside-out YESS™ technique and receives royalties from the sale of his inventions. Indirect conflicts of interest may exist. Paymnets for honoraria, consultancies to sponsoring organizations are donated to IITS.org, a 501c3 organization.

## ACKNOWLEDGEMENTS

Declared none.

## REFERENCES

[1]   Lewandrowski KU, Soriano-Sánchez JA, Zhang X, *et al.* Regional variations in acceptance, and utilization of minimally invasive spinal surgery techniques among spine surgeons: results of a global survey. J Spine Surg 2020; 6 (Suppl. 1): S260-74.
[http://dx.doi.org/10.21037/jss.2019.09.31] [PMID: 32195433]

[2]   Yeung A, Wei SH. Surgical outcome of workman's comp patients undergoing endoscopic foraminal

decompression for lumbar herniated disc. J Spine Surg 2020; 6 (Suppl. 1): S116-9.
[http://dx.doi.org/10.21037/jss.2019.11.03] [PMID: 32195420]

[3]  Yeung A, Lewandrowski KU. Early and staged endoscopic management of common pain generators in the spine. J Spine Surg 2020; 6 (Suppl. 1): S1-5.
[http://dx.doi.org/10.21037/jss.2019.09.03] [PMID: 32195407]

[4]  Yeung A, Lewandrowski KU. Five-year clinical outcomes with endoscopic transforaminal foraminoplasty for symptomatic degenerative conditions of the lumbar spine: a comparative study of *inside-outversusoutside-in* techniques. J Spine Surg 2020; 6 (Suppl. 1): S66-83.
[http://dx.doi.org/10.21037/jss.2019.06.08] [PMID: 32195417]

[5]  Ransom NA, Gollogly S, Lewandrowski KU, Yeung A. Navigating the learning curve of spinal endoscopy as an established traditionally trained spine surgeon. J Spine Surg 2020; 6 (Suppl. 1): S197-207.
[http://dx.doi.org/10.21037/jss.2019.10.03] [PMID: 32195428]

[6]  Ramírez León JF, Ardila AS, Rugeles Ortíz JG, *et al.* Standalone lordotic endoscopic wedge lumbar interbody fusion (LEW-LIF™) with a threaded cylindrical peek cage: report of two cases. J Spine Surg 2020; 6 (Suppl. 1): S275-84.
[http://dx.doi.org/10.21037/jss.2019.06.09] [PMID: 32195434]

[7]  Qiao G, Feng M, Wang X, *et al.* Revision for endoscopic diskectomy: is lateral lumbar interbody fusion an option? World Neurosurg 2020; 133: e26-30.
[http://dx.doi.org/10.1016/j.wneu.2019.07.226] [PMID: 31398523]

[8]  Mo AZ, Miller PE, Glotzbecker MP, *et al.* The reliability of the aospine thoracolumbar classification system in children: results of a multicenter study. J Pediatr Orthop 2020; 40(5): e352-6.
[http://dx.doi.org/10.1097/BPO.0000000000001521] [PMID: 32032218]

[9]  Lohre R, Wang JC, Lewandrowski KU, Goel DP. Virtual reality in spinal endoscopy: a paradigm shift in education to support spine surgeons. J Spine Surg 2020; 6 (Suppl. 1): S208-23.
[http://dx.doi.org/10.21037/jss.2019.11.16] [PMID: 32195429]

[10]  Lewandrowski KU, Yeung A. Meaningful outcome research to validate endoscopic treatment of common lumbar pain generators with durability analysis. J Spine Surg 2020; 6 (Suppl. 1): S6-S13.
[http://dx.doi.org/10.21037/jss.2019.09.07] [PMID: 32195408]

[11]  Lewandrowski KU, Ransom NA, Yeung A. Return to work and recovery time analysis after outpatient endoscopic lumbar transforaminal decompression surgery. J Spine Surg 2020; 6 (Suppl. 1): S100-15.
[http://dx.doi.org/10.21037/jss.2019.10.01] [PMID: 32195419]

[12]  Lewandrowski KU, Ransom NA, Yeung A. Subsidence induced recurrent radiculopathy after staged two-level standalone endoscopic lumbar interbody fusion with a threaded cylindrical cage: a case report. J Spine Surg 2020; 6 (Suppl. 1): S286-93.
[http://dx.doi.org/10.21037/jss.2019.09.25] [PMID: 32195435]

[13]  Lewandrowski KU, Ransom NA. Five-year clinical outcomes with endoscopic transforaminal outside-in foraminoplasty techniques for symptomatic degenerative conditions of the lumbar spine. J Spine Surg 2020; 6 (Suppl. 1): S54-65.
[http://dx.doi.org/10.21037/jss.2019.07.03] [PMID: 32195416]

[14]  Lewandrowski KU, DE Carvalho PST, DE Carvalho P, Yeung A. Minimal clinically important difference in patient-reported outcome measures with the transforaminal endoscopic decompression for lateral recess and foraminal stenosis. Int J Spine Surg 2020; 14(2): 254-66.
[http://dx.doi.org/10.14444/7034] [PMID: 32355633]

[15]  Lewandrowski KU, Dowling A, de Carvalho P, *et al.* Indication and contraindication of endoscopic transforaminal lumbar decompression. World Neurosurg 2020; 145: 631-42.
[http://dx.doi.org/10.1016/j.wneu.2020.03.076] [PMID: 32201296]

[16]  Lewandrowski KU, Dowling Á, Calderaro AL, *et al.* Dysethesia due to irritation of the dorsal root

ganglion following lumbar transforaminal endoscopy: Analysis of frequency and contributing factors. Clin Neurol Neurosurg 2020; 197: 106073.
[http://dx.doi.org/10.1016/j.clineuro.2020.106073] [PMID: 32683194]

[17]   Lewandrowski KU, de Carvalho PST, Calderaro AL, *et al*. Outcomes with transforaminal endoscopic *versus* percutaneous laser decompression for contained lumbar herniated disc: a survival analysis of treatment benefit. J Spine Surg 2020; 6 (Suppl. 1): S84-99.
[http://dx.doi.org/10.21037/jss.2019.09.13] [PMID: 32195418]

[18]   Lewandrowski KU. The strategies behind "inside-out" and "outside-in" endoscopy of the lumbar spine: treating the pain generator. J Spine Surg 2020; 6 (Suppl. 1): S35-9.
[http://dx.doi.org/10.21037/jss.2019.06.06] [PMID: 32195412]

[19]   Krause KL, Cheaney Ii B, Obayashi JT, Kawamoto A, Than KD. Intraoperative neuromonitoring for one-level lumbar discectomies is low yield and cost-ineffective. J Clin Neurosci 2020; 71: 97-100.
[http://dx.doi.org/10.1016/j.jocn.2019.08.116] [PMID: 31495654]

[20]   Kim JS, Yeung A, Lokanath YK, Lewandrowski KU. Is Asia truly a hotspot of contemporary minimally invasive and endoscopic spinal surgery? J Spine Surg 2020; 6 (Suppl. 1): S224-36.
[http://dx.doi.org/10.21037/jss.2019.12.13] [PMID: 32195430]

[21]   Katzell JL. Risk factors predicting less favorable outcomes in endoscopic lumbar discectomies. J Spine Surg 2020; 6 (Suppl. 1): S155-64.
[http://dx.doi.org/10.21037/jss.2019.11.04] [PMID: 32195424]

[22]   Karhade AV, Bongers MER, Groot OQ, *et al*. Development of machine learning and natural language processing algorithms for preoperative prediction and automated identification of intraoperative vascular injury in anterior lumbar spine surgery. Spine J 2020; S1529-9430(20): 30135-2.
[PMID: 32294557]

[23]   Fujii Y, Yamashita K, Sugiura K, *et al*. Early return to activity after minimally invasive full endoscopic decompression surgery in medical doctors. J Spine Surg 2020; 6 (Suppl. 1): S294-9.
[http://dx.doi.org/10.21037/jss.2019.08.05] [PMID: 32195436]

[24]   Dowling Á, Lewandrowski KU, da Silva FHP, Parra JAA, Portillo DM, Giménez YCP. Patient selection protocols for endoscopic transforaminal, interlaminar, and translaminar decompression of lumbar spinal stenosis. J Spine Surg 2020; 6 (Suppl. 1): S120-32.
[http://dx.doi.org/10.21037/jss.2019.11.07] [PMID: 32195421]

[25]   Brusko GD, Wang MY. Endoscopic Lumbar Interbody Fusion. Neurosurg Clin N Am 2020; 31(1): 17-24.
[http://dx.doi.org/10.1016/j.nec.2019.08.002] [PMID: 31739925]

[26]   Zhang Y, Chong F, Feng C, Wang Y, Zhou Y, Huang B. Comparison of endoscope-assisted and microscope-assisted tubular surgery for lumbar laminectomies and discectomies: minimum 2-year follow-up results. BioMed Res Int 2019; 2019: 5321580.
[http://dx.doi.org/10.1155/2019/5321580] [PMID: 31179327]

[27]   Zhang J, Jin MR, Zhao TX, *et al*. Clinical application of percutaneous transforaminal endoscope-assisted lumbar interbody fusion. Zhongguo Gu Shang 2019; 32(12): 1138-43.
[PMID: 31870074]

[28]   Zhang B, Kong Q, Yang J, Feng P, Ma J, Liu J. Short-term effectiveness of percutaneous endoscopic transforaminal bilateral decompression for severe central lumbar spinal stenosis. Zhongguo Xiu Fu Chong Jian Wai Ke Za Zhi 2019; 33(11): 1399-405.
[PMID: 31650756]

[29]   Yeung AT, Lewandrowski KU. Retrospective analysis of accuracy and positive predictive value of preoperative lumbar MRI grading after successful outcome following outpatient endoscopic decompression for lumbar foraminal and lateral recess stenosis. Clin Neurol Neurosurg 2019; 181: 52.
[http://dx.doi.org/10.1016/j.clineuro.2019.03.011] [PMID: 30986727]

[30]   Yeung A, Wei S-H. Surgical outcome of workman's comp patients undergoing endoscopic foraminal decompression for lumbar herniated disc. J Spine Surg 2020; 6 (Suppl. 1): S116-9.
[http://dx.doi.org/10.21037/jss.2019.11.03] [PMID: 32195420]

[31]   Yeung A, Roberts A, Zhu L, Qi L, Zhang J, Lewandrowski KU. Treatment of soft tissue and bony spinal stenosis by a visualized endoscopic transforaminal technique under local anesthesia. Neurospine 2019; 16(1): 52-62.
[http://dx.doi.org/10.14245/ns.1938038.019] [PMID: 30943707]

[32]   Yang JC. Current problems and challenges for percutaneous endoscopic transforaminal lumbar interbody fusion. Zhonghua Yi Xue Za Zhi 2019; 99(33): 2566-8.
[PMID: 31510713]

[33]   Yang J, Liu C, Hai Y, et al. Percutaneous endoscopic transforaminal lumbar interbody fusion for the treatment of lumbar spinal stenosis: preliminary report of seven cases with 12-month follow-up. BioMed Res Int 2019; 2019: 3091459.
[http://dx.doi.org/10.1155/2019/3091459] [PMID: 31019966]

[34]   Yadav RI, Long L, Yanming C. Comparison of the effectiveness and outcome of microendoscopic and open discectomy in patients suffering from lumbar disc herniation. Medicine (Baltimore) 2019; 98(50): e16627.
[http://dx.doi.org/10.1097/MD.0000000000016627] [PMID: 31852061]

[35]   Xu T, Tian R, Qiao P, Han Z, Shen Q, Jia Y. Application of continuous epidural anesthesia in transforaminal lumbar endoscopic surgery: a prospective randomized controlled trial. J Int Med Res 2019; 47(3): 1146-53.
[http://dx.doi.org/10.1177/0300060518817218] [PMID: 30632428]

[36]   Xiong C, Li T, Kang H, Hu H, Han J, Xu F. Early outcomes of 270-degree spinal canal decompression by using TESSYS-ISEE technique in patients with lumbar spinal stenosis combined with disk herniation. Eur Spine J 2019; 28(1): 78-86.
[http://dx.doi.org/10.1007/s00586-018-5655-4] [PMID: 29909552]

[37]   Xin Z, Huang P, Zheng G, Liao W, Zhang X, Wang Y. Using a percutaneous spinal endoscopy unilateral posterior interlaminar approach to perform bilateral decompression for patients with lumbar lateral recess stenosis. Asian J Surg 2019.
[PMID: 31594687]

[38]   Xin Z, Cai M, Ji W, et al. Percutaneous full-endoscopic bilateral decompression via unilateral posterior approach for lumbar spinal stenosis. Zhongguo Xiu Fu Chong Jian Wai Ke Za Zhi 2019; 33(7): 822-30.
[PMID: 31297998]

[39]   Wasinpongwanich K, Pongpirul K, Lwin KMM, Kesornsak W, Kuansongtham V, Ruetten S. Full-endoscopic interlaminar lumbar discectomy: retrospective review of clinical results and complications in 545 international patients. World Neurosurg 2019; 132: e922-8.
[http://dx.doi.org/10.1016/j.wneu.2019.07.101] [PMID: 31326641]

[40]   Wang Y, Yan Y, Yang J, et al. Outcomes of percutaneous endoscopic trans-articular discectomy for huge central or paracentral lumbar disc herniation. Int Orthop 2019; 43(4): 939-45.
[http://dx.doi.org/10.1007/s00264-018-4210-6] [PMID: 30374637]

[41]   Wang D, Xie W, Cao W, He S, Fan G, Zhang H. A cost-utility analysis of percutaneous endoscopic lumbar discectomy for l5-s1 lumbar disc herniation: transforaminal versus interlaminar. Spine 2019; 44(8): 563-70.
[http://dx.doi.org/10.1097/BRS.0000000000002901] [PMID: 30312274]

[42]   Soo ES, Sourabh C, Ho LS. Posterolateral endoscopic lumbar decompression rotate-to-retract technique for foraminal disc herniation: a technical report. BioMed Res Int 2019; 2019: 5758671.
[http://dx.doi.org/10.1155/2019/5758671] [PMID: 30906777]

[43]  Shi R, Wang F, Hong X, *et al.* Comparison of percutaneous endoscopic lumbar discectomy *versus* microendoscopic discectomy for the treatment of lumbar disc herniation: a meta-analysis. Int Orthop 2019; 43(4): 923-37.
      [http://dx.doi.org/10.1007/s00264-018-4253-8] [PMID: 30547214]

[44]  Sharma SB, Lin GX, Jabri H, Siddappa ND, Kim JS. Biportal endoscopic excision of facetal cyst in the far lateral region of l5s1: 2-dimensional operative video. Oper Neurosurg (Hagerstown) 2020; 18(16): E233.

[45]  Sharma SB, Lin GX, Jabri H, *et al.* Radiographic and clinical outcomes of huge lumbar disc herniations treated by transforaminal endoscopic discectomy. Clin Neurol Neurosurg 2019; 185: 105485.
      [http://dx.doi.org/10.1016/j.clineuro.2019.105485] [PMID: 31421587]

[46]  Ruetten S, Komp M. The trend towards full-endoscopic decompression : current possibilities and limitations in disc herniation and spinal stenosis. Orthopade 2019; 48(1): 69-76.
      [http://dx.doi.org/10.1007/s00132-018-03669-3] [PMID: 30535764]

[47]  Qiao G, Feng M, Wang X, *et al.* Revision for endoscopic discectomy: is lateral lumbar interbody fusion an option? World Neurosurg 2019; 133: e26-30.

[48]  Park SM, Park J, Jang HS, *et al.* Biportal endoscopic *versus* microscopic lumbar decompressive laminectomy in patients with spinal stenosis: a randomized controlled trial. Spine J 2019; 20(2): 156-65.
      [PMID: 31542473]

[49]  Park MK, Park SA, Son SK, Park WW, Choi SH. Correction to: Clinical and radiological outcomes of unilateral biportal endoscopic lumbar interbody fusion (ULIF) compared with conventional posterior lumbar interbody fusion (PLIF): 1-year follow-up. Neurosurg Rev 2019; 42(3): 763.
      [http://dx.doi.org/10.1007/s10143-019-01131-2] [PMID: 31236727]

[50]  Park MK, Park SA, Son SK, Park WW, Choi SH. Clinical and radiological outcomes of unilateral biportal endoscopic lumbar interbody fusion (ULIF) compared with conventional posterior lumbar interbody fusion (PLIF): 1-year follow-up. Neurosurg Rev 2019; 42(3): 753-61.
      [http://dx.doi.org/10.1007/s10143-019-01114-3] [PMID: 31144195]

[51]  Morgenstern C, Yue JJ, Morgenstern R. Full percutaneous transforaminal lumbar interbody fusion using the facet-sparing, trans-kambin approach. Clin Spine Surg 2020; 33(1): 40-5.
      [PMID: 31162179]

[52]  Moon BJ, Yi S, Ha Y, Kim KN, Yoon DH, Shin DA. Clinical efficacy and safety of trans-sacral epiduroscopic laser decompression compared to percutaneous epidural neuroplasty. Pain Res Manag 2019; 2019: 2893460.
      [http://dx.doi.org/10.1155/2019/2893460] [PMID: 30755783]

[53]  Min WK, Kim JE, Choi DJ, Park EJ, Heo J. Clinical and radiological outcomes between biportal endoscopic decompression and microscopic decompression in lumbar spinal stenosis. J Orthop Sci 2020; 25(3): 371-8.
      [PMID: 31255456]

[54]  McGrath LB, White-Dzuro GA, Hofstetter CP. Comparison of clinical outcomes following minimally invasive or lumbar endoscopic unilateral laminotomy for bilateral decompression. J Neurosurg Spine 2019; 1-9.
      [http://dx.doi.org/10.3171/2018.9.SPINE18689] [PMID: 30641853]

[55]  Mahatthanatrakul A, Kotheeranurak V, Lin GX, Hur JW, Chung HJ, Kim JS. Comparative analysis of the intervertebral disc signal and annulus changes between immediate and 1-year postoperative MRI after transforaminal endoscopic lumbar discectomy and annuloplasty. Neuroradiology 2019; 61(4): 411-9.
      [http://dx.doi.org/10.1007/s00234-019-02174-4] [PMID: 30737537]

[56]   Liu W, Li Q, Li Z, Chen L, Tian D, Jing J. Clinical efficacy of percutaneous transforaminal endoscopic discectomy in treating adolescent lumbar disc herniation. Medicine (Baltimore) 2019; 98(9): e14682.
[http://dx.doi.org/10.1097/MD.0000000000014682] [PMID: 30817599]

[57]   Liu KC, Yang SK, Ou BR, *et al.* Using percutaneous endoscopic outside-in technique to treat selected patients with refractory discogenic low back pain. Pain Physician 2019; 22(2): 187-98.
[PMID: 30921984]

[58]   Liu J, Zhang H, Zhang X, He T, Zhao X, Wang Z. Percutaneous endoscopic decompression for lumbar spinal stenosis: protocol for a systematic review and network meta-analysis. Medicine (Baltimore) 2019; 98(20): e15635.
[http://dx.doi.org/10.1097/MD.0000000000015635] [PMID: 31096479]

[59]   Liounakos JI, Wang MY. Lumbar 3-lumbar 5 robotic-assisted endoscopic transforaminal lumbar interbody fusion: 2-dimensional operative video. Oper Neurosurg (Hagerstown) 2020; 19(1): E73-4.

[60]   Ling Q, He E, Zhang H, Lin H, Huang W. A novel narrow surface cage for full endoscopic oblique lateral lumbar interbody fusion: a finite element study. J Orthop Sci 2019; 24(6): 991-8.
[http://dx.doi.org/10.1016/j.jos.2019.08.013] [PMID: 31519402]

[61]   Lin GX, Huang P, Kotheeranurak V, *et al.* A systematic review of unilateral biportal endoscopic spinal surgery: preliminary clinical results and complications. World Neurosurg 2019; 125: 425-32.
[http://dx.doi.org/10.1016/j.wneu.2019.02.038] [PMID: 30797907]

[62]   Li XF, Jin LY, Lv ZD, *et al.* Endoscopic ventral decompression for spinal stenosis with degenerative spondylolisthesis by partially removing posterosuperior margin underneath the slipping vertebral body: technical note and outcome evaluation. World Neurosurg 2019; 126: e517-25.
[http://dx.doi.org/10.1016/j.wneu.2019.02.083] [PMID: 30825627]

[63]   Lewandrowski KU, Ransom NA, Ramírez León JF, Yeung A. The concept for a standalone lordotic endoscopic wedge lumbar interbody fusion: the LEW-LIF. Neurospine 2019; 16(1): 82-95.
[http://dx.doi.org/10.14245/ns.1938046.023] [PMID: 30943710]

[64]   Lewandrowski KU, León JFR, Yeung A. Use of "inside-out" technique for direct visualization of a vacuum vertically unstable intervertebral disc during routine lumbar endoscopic transforaminal decompression-a correlative study of clinical outcomes and the prognostic value of lumbar radiographs. Int J Spine Surg 2019; 13(5): 399-414.
[http://dx.doi.org/10.14444/6055] [PMID: 31741829]

[65]   Lewandrowski KU. Retrospective analysis of accuracy and positive predictive value of preoperative lumbar MRI grading after successful outcome following outpatient endoscopic decompression for lumbar foraminal and lateral recess stenosis. Clin Neurol Neurosurg 2019; 179: 74-80.
[http://dx.doi.org/10.1016/j.clineuro.2019.02.019] [PMID: 30870712]

[66]   Lewandrowski KU. Incidence, management, and cost of complications after transforaminal endoscopic decompression surgery for lumbar foraminal and lateral recess stenosis: a value proposition for outpatient ambulatory surgery. Int J Spine Surg 2019; 13(1): 53-67.
[http://dx.doi.org/10.14444/6008] [PMID: 30805287]

[67]   Lewandrowski K-U, Yeung A. Meaningful outcome research to validate endoscopic treatment of common lumbar pain generators with durability analysis. J Spine Surg 2020; 6 (Suppl. 1): S6-S13.
[http://dx.doi.org/10.21037/jss.2019.09.07] [PMID: 32195408]

[68]   Lewandrowski K-U, Ransom NA, Yeung A. Subsidence induced recurrent radiculopathy after staged two-level standalone endoscopic lumbar interbody fusion with a threaded cylindrical cage: a case report. J Spine Surg 2020; 6 (Suppl. 1): S286-93.
[http://dx.doi.org/10.21037/jss.2019.09.25] [PMID: 32195435]

[69]   Lewandrowski K-U, Ransom NA. Five-year clinical outcomes with endoscopic transforaminal outside-in foraminoplasty techniques for symptomatic degenerative conditions of the lumbar spine. J

Spine Surg 2020; 6 (Suppl. 1): S54-65.
[http://dx.doi.org/10.21037/jss.2019.07.03] [PMID: 32195416]

[70]  Lewandrowski K-U. The strategies behind "inside-out" and "outside-in" endoscopy of the lumbar spine: treating the pain generator. J Spine Surg 2020; 6 (Suppl. 1): S35-9.
[http://dx.doi.org/10.21037/jss.2019.06.06] [PMID: 32195412]

[71]  Lee CW, Yoon KJ, Ha SS. Comparative analysis between three different lumbar decompression techniques (microscopic, tubular, and endoscopic) in lumbar canal and lateral recess stenosis: preliminary report. BioMed Res Int 2019; 2019: 6078469.
[http://dx.doi.org/10.1155/2019/6078469] [PMID: 31019969]

[72]  Korge A, Mehren C, Ruetten S. Minimally invasive decompression techniques for spinal cord stenosis. Orthopade 2019; 48(10): 824-30.

[73]  Kong W, Chen T, Ye S, Wu F, Song Y. Treatment of L5 - S1 intervertebral disc herniation with posterior percutaneous full-endoscopic discectomy by grafting tubes at various positions *via* an interlaminar approach. BMC Surg 2019; 19(1): 124.
[http://dx.doi.org/10.1186/s12893-019-0589-2] [PMID: 31462257]

[74]  Komatsu J, Iwabuchi M, Endo T, Fukuda H, *et al.* Clinical outcomes of lumbar diseases specific test in patients who undergo endoscopy-assisted tubular surgery with lumbar herniated nucleus pulposus: an analysis using the Japanese Orthopaedic Association Back Pain Evaluation Questionnaire (JOABPEQ). Eur J Orthop Surg Traumatol 2019.
[PMID: 31595359]

[75]  Kim JE, Choi DJ, Park EJ. Evaluation of postoperative spinal epidural hematoma after biportal endoscopic spine surgery for single-level lumbar spinal stenosis: clinical and magnetic resonance imaging study. World Neurosurg 2019; 126: e786-92.
[http://dx.doi.org/10.1016/j.wneu.2019.02.150] [PMID: 30878758]

[76]  Katzell JL. Risk factors predicting less favorable outcomes in endoscopic lumbar discectomies. J Spine Surg 2020; 6 (Suppl. 1): S155-64.
[http://dx.doi.org/10.21037/jss.2019.11.04] [PMID: 32195424]

[77]  Kamson S, Lu D, Sampson PD, Zhang Y. Full-endoscopic lumbar fusion outcomes in patients with minimal deformities: a retrospective study of data collected between 2011 and 2015. Pain Physician 2019; 22(1): 75-88.
[http://dx.doi.org/10.36076/ppj/2019.22.75] [PMID: 30700071]

[78]  Houle P, Telfeian AE, Wagner R, Bae J. Interspinous endoscopic lumbar decompression: technical note. AME Case Rep 2019; 3: 40.
[http://dx.doi.org/10.21037/acr.2019.09.07] [PMID: 31728438]

[79]  Heo DH, Sharma S, Park CK. Endoscopic treatment of extraforaminal entrapment of l5 nerve root (far out syndrome) by unilateral biportal endoscopic approach: technical report and preliminary clinical results. Neurospine 2019; 16(1): 130-7.
[http://dx.doi.org/10.14245/ns.1938026.013] [PMID: 30943715]

[80]  Heo DH, Park CK. Clinical results of percutaneous biportal endoscopic lumbar interbody fusion with application of enhanced recovery after surgery. Neurosurg Focus 2019; 46(4): E18.
[http://dx.doi.org/10.3171/2019.1.FOCUS18695] [PMID: 30933919]

[81]  Heo DH, Lee DC, Park CK. Comparative analysis of three types of minimally invasive decompressive surgery for lumbar central stenosis: biportal endoscopy, uniportal endoscopy, and microsurgery. Neurosurg Focus 2019; 46(5): E9.
[http://dx.doi.org/10.3171/2019.2.FOCUS197] [PMID: 31042664]

[82]  Gao K, Yang H, Yang LQ, Hu MQ. Application of intervertebral foramen endoscopy BEIS technique in the lumbar spine surgery failure syndrome over 60 years old. Zhongguo Gu Shang 2019; 32(7): 647-52.
[PMID: 31382724]

[83]   Fujii Y, Yamashita K, Sugiura K, *et al.* Early return to activity after minimally invasive full endoscopic decompression surgery in medical doctors. J Spine Surg 2020; 6 (Suppl. 1): S294-9. [http://dx.doi.org/10.21037/jss.2019.08.05] [PMID: 32195436]

[84]   Duan K, Qin Y, Ye J, *et al.* Percutaneous endoscopic debridement with percutaneous pedicle screw fixation for lumbar pyogenic spondylodiscitis: a preliminary study. Int Orthop 2019; 44: 495-502. [PMID: 31879810]

[85]   Dey PC, Nanda SN. Functional outcome after endoscopic lumbar discectomy by destandau's technique: a prospective study of 614 patients. Asian Spine J 2019; 13(5): 786-92. [http://dx.doi.org/10.31616/asj.2018.0320] [PMID: 31154700]

[86]   Chung J, Kong C, Sun W, Kim D, Kim H, Jeong H. Percutaneous endoscopic lumbar foraminoplasty for lumbar foraminal stenosis of elderly patients with unilateral radiculopathy: radiographic changes in magnetic resonance images. J Neurol Surg A Cent Eur Neurosurg 2019; 80(4): 302-11. [http://dx.doi.org/10.1055/s-0038-1677052] [PMID: 30887488]

[87]   Choi DJ, Kim JE. Efficacy of biportal endoscopic spine surgery for lumbar spinal stenosis. Clin Orthop Surg 2019; 11(1): 82-8. [http://dx.doi.org/10.4055/cios.2019.11.1.82] [PMID: 30838111]

[88]   Cao S, Cui H, Lu Z, *et al.* "Tube in tube" interlaminar endoscopic decompression for the treatment of lumbar spinal stenosis: Technique notes and preliminary clinical outcomes of case series. Medicine (Baltimore) 2019; 98(35): e17021. [http://dx.doi.org/10.1097/MD.0000000000017021] [PMID: 31464962]

[89]   Butler AJ, Alam M, Wiley K, Ghasem A, Rush Iii AJ, Wang JC. Endoscopic lumbar surgery: the state of the art in 2019. Neurospine 2019; 16(1): 15-23. [http://dx.doi.org/10.14245/ns.1938040.020] [PMID: 30943703]

[90]   Barber SM, Nakhla J, Konakondla S, *et al.* Outcomes of endoscopic discectomy compared with open microdiscectomy and tubular microdiscectomy for lumbar disc herniations: a meta-analysis. J Neurosurg Spine 2019; 1-14. [http://dx.doi.org/10.3171/2019.6.SPINE19532] [PMID: 31491760]

[91]   Ao S, Wu J, Tang Y, *et al.* Percutaneous endoscopic lumbar discectomy assisted by o-arm-based navigation improves the learning curve. BioMed Res Int 2019; 2019: 6509409. [http://dx.doi.org/10.1155/2019/6509409] [PMID: 30733964]

[92]   Ahn Y, Youn MS, Heo DH. Endoscopic transforaminal lumbar interbody fusion: a comprehensive review. Expert Rev Med Devices 2019; 16(5): 373-80. [http://dx.doi.org/10.1080/17434440.2019.1610388] [PMID: 31044627]

[93]   Ahn Y, Lee SG, Son S, Keum HJ. Transforaminal endoscopic lumbar discectomy *versus* open lumbar microdiscectomy: a comparative cohort study with a 5-year follow-up. Pain Physician 2019; 22(3): 295-304. [http://dx.doi.org/10.36076/ppj/2019.22.295] [PMID: 31151337]

[94]   Ahn Y, Keum HJ, Lee SG, Lee SW. Transforaminal endoscopic decompression for lumbar lateral recess stenosis: an advanced surgical technique and clinical outcomes. World Neurosurg 2019; 125: e916-24. [http://dx.doi.org/10.1016/j.wneu.2019.01.209] [PMID: 30763754]

[95]   Ahn JS, Lee HJ, Park EJ, *et al.* Multifidus muscle changes after biportal endoscopic spinal surgery: magnetic resonance imaging evaluation. World Neurosurg 2019; 130: e525-34. [http://dx.doi.org/10.1016/j.wneu.2019.06.148] [PMID: 31254694]

[96]   Zhu Y, Zhao Y, Fan G, *et al.* Comparison of 3 anesthetic methods for percutaneous transforaminal endoscopic discectomy: a prospective study. Pain Physician 2018; 21(4): E347-53. [PMID: 30045601]

[97]   Zhou C, Zhang G, Panchal RR, *et al.* Unique complications of percutaneous endoscopic lumbar

discectomy and percutaneous endoscopic interlaminar discectomy. Pain Physician 2018; 21(2): E105-12.
[PMID: 29565953]

[98] Yuan H, Zhang X, Zhang LM, Yan YQ, Liu YK, Lewandrowski KU. Comparative study of curative effect of spinal endoscopic surgery and anterior cervical decompression for cervical spondylotic myelopathy. J Spine Surg 2020; 6 (Suppl. 1): S186-96.
[http://dx.doi.org/10.21037/jss.2019.11.15] [PMID: 32195427]

[99] Ramírez León JF, Rugeles Ortíz JG, Martínez CR, Alonso Cuéllar GO, Lewandrowski KU. Surgical treatment of cervical radiculopathy using an anterior cervical endoscopic decompression. J Spine Surg 2020; 6 (Suppl. 1): S179-85.
[http://dx.doi.org/10.21037/jss.2019.09.24] [PMID: 32195426]

[100] Chung AS, Kimball J, Min E, Wang JC. Endoscopic spine surgery-increasing usage and prominence in mainstream spine surgery and spine societies. J Spine Surg 2020; 6 (Suppl. 1): S14-8.
[http://dx.doi.org/10.21037/jss.2019.09.16] [PMID: 32195409]

[101] Ruetten S, Hahn P, Oezdemir S, Baraliakos X, Godolias G, Komp M. Full-endoscopic uniportal retropharyngeal odontoidectomy for anterior craniocervical infection. Minim Invasive Ther Allied Technol 2019; 28(3): 178-85.
[http://dx.doi.org/10.1080/13645706.2018.1498357] [PMID: 30179052]

[102] Ren J, Li R, Zhu K, *et al.* Biomechanical comparison of percutaneous posterior endoscopic cervical discectomy and anterior cervical decompression and fusion on the treatment of cervical spondylotic radiculopathy. J Orthop Surg Res 2019; 14(1): 71.
[http://dx.doi.org/10.1186/s13018-019-1113-1] [PMID: 30832736]

[103] Oezdemir S, Komp M, Hahn P, Ruetten S. Decompression for cervical disc herniation using the full-endoscopic anterior technique. Oper Orthop Traumatol 2019; 31 (Suppl. 1): 1-10.
[http://dx.doi.org/10.1007/s00064-018-0531-2] [PMID: 29392340]

[104] Lin Y, Rao S, Li Y, Zhao S, Chen B. Posterior percutaneous full-endoscopic cervical laminectomy and decompression for cervical stenosis with myelopathy: a technical note. World Neurosurg 2019; S1878-8750(19): 30051-8.
[http://dx.doi.org/10.1016/j.wneu.2018.12.180] [PMID: 30648610]

[105] Li C, Tang X, Chen S, Meng Y, Zhang W. Clinical application of large channel endoscopic decompression in posterior cervical spine disorders. BMC Musculoskelet Disord 2019; 20(1): 548.
[http://dx.doi.org/10.1186/s12891-019-2920-6] [PMID: 31739780]

[106] Ruetten S, Hahn P, Oezdemir S, *et al.* The full-endoscopic uniportal technique for decompression of the anterior craniocervical junction using the retropharyngeal approach: an anatomical feasibility study in human cadavers and review of the literature. J Neurosurg Spine 2018; 29(6): 615-21.
[http://dx.doi.org/10.3171/2018.4.SPINE171156] [PMID: 30192216]

[107] Ruetten S, Hahn P, Oezdemir S, *et al.* Full-endoscopic uniportal odontoidectomy and decompression of the anterior cervicomedullary junction using the retropharyngeal approach. Spine 2018; 43(15): E911-8.
[http://dx.doi.org/10.1097/BRS.0000000000002561] [PMID: 29438218]

[108] Ruetten S, Hahn P, Oezdemir S, Baraliakos X, Godolias G, Komp M. Surgical treatment of cervical subaxial intraspinal extradural cysts using a full-endoscopic uniportal posterior approach. J Orthop Surg (Hong Kong) 2018; 26(2): 2309499018777665.
[http://dx.doi.org/10.1177/2309499018777665] [PMID: 29793373]

[109] Oezdemir S, Komp M, Hahn P, Ruetten S. Decompression for cervical disc herniation using the full-endoscopic anterior technique - German version. Oper Orthop Traumatol 2018; 30(1): 25-35.
[http://dx.doi.org/10.1007/s00064-017-0528-2] [PMID: 29318336]

[110] Komp M, Oezdemir S, Hahn P, Ruetten S. Full-endoscopic posterior foraminotomy surgery for cervical disc herniations. Oper Orthop Traumatol 2018; 30(1): 13-24.

[http://dx.doi.org/10.1007/s00064-017-0529-1] [PMID: 29318337]

[111]  Wen H, Wang X, Liao W, *et al*. Effective range of percutaneous posterior full-endoscopic paramedian cervical disc herniation discectomy and indications for patient selection. BioMed Res Int 2017; 2017: 3610385.
[http://dx.doi.org/10.1155/2017/3610385] [PMID: 29226132]

[112]  Choi G, Pophale CS, Patel B, Uniyal P. Endoscopic spine surgery. J Korean Neurosurg Soc 2017; 60(5): 485-97.
[http://dx.doi.org/10.3340/jkns.2017.0203.004] [PMID: 28881110]

[113]  Li XC, Zhong CF, Deng GB, Liang RW, Huang CM. Full-endoscopic procedures *versus* traditional discectomy surgery for discectomy: a systematic review and meta-analysis of current global clinical trials. Pain Physician 2016; 19(3): 103-18.
[PMID: 27008284]

[114]  Yoshimoto M, Miyakawa T, Takebayashi T, *et al*. Microendoscopy-assisted muscle-preserving interlaminar decompression for lumbar spinal stenosis: clinical results of consecutive 105 cases with more than 3-year follow-up. Spine 2014; 39(5): E318-25.
[http://dx.doi.org/10.1097/BRS.0000000000000160] [PMID: 24365896]

[115]  Yadav YR, Parihar V, Ratre S, Kher Y, Bhatele PR. Endoscopic decompression of cervical spondylotic myelopathy using posterior approach. Neurol India 2014; 62(6): 640-5.
[http://dx.doi.org/10.4103/0028-3886.149388] [PMID: 25591677]

[116]  Ruetten S, Komp M, Merk H, Godolias G. Full-endoscopic anterior decompression *versus* conventional anterior decompression and fusion in cervical disc herniations. Int Orthop 2009; 33(6): 1677-82.
[http://dx.doi.org/10.1007/s00264-008-0684-y] [PMID: 19015851]

[117]  Haufe SM, Baker RA, Pyne ML. Endoscopic thoracic laminoforaminoplasty for the treatment of thoracic radiculopathy: report of 12 cases. Int J Med Sci 2009; 6(4): 224-6.
[http://dx.doi.org/10.7150/ijms.6.224] [PMID: 19742241]

[118]  Hellinger J. Complications of non-endoscopic percutaneous laser disc decompression and nucleotomy with the neodymium: YAG laser 1064 nm. Photomed Laser Surg 2004; 22(5): 418-22.
[http://dx.doi.org/10.1089/pho.2004.22.418] [PMID: 15671715]

[119]  Fontanella A. Endoscopic microsurgery in herniated cervical discs. Neurol Res 1999; 21(1): 31-8.
[http://dx.doi.org/10.1080/01616412.1999.11740888] [PMID: 10048051]

[120]  Sharif S, Afsar A. Learning curve and minimally invasive spine surgery. World Neurosurg 2018; 119: 472-8.
[http://dx.doi.org/10.1016/j.wneu.2018.06.094] [PMID: 29935319]

[121]  Wang H, Huang B, Li C, *et al*. Learning curve for percutaneous endoscopic lumbar discectomy depending on the surgeon's training level of minimally invasive spine surgery. Clin Neurol Neurosurg 2013; 115(10): 1987-91.
[http://dx.doi.org/10.1016/j.clineuro.2013.06.008] [PMID: 23830496]

[122]  Lewandrowski KU, Soriano-Sánchez JA, Zhang X, *et al*. Surgeon training and clinical implementation of spinal endoscopy in routine practice: results of a global survey. J Spine Surg 2020; 6 (Suppl. 1): S237-48.
[http://dx.doi.org/10.21037/jss.2019.09.32] [PMID: 32195431]

[123]  Boos N. Health care technology assessment and transfer. Eur Spine J 2007; 16(8): 1291-2.
[http://dx.doi.org/10.1007/s00586-007-0440-9] [PMID: 17636348]

[124]  Burkhardt BW, Wilmes M, Sharif S, Oertel JM. The visualization of the surgical field in tubular assisted spine surgery: is there a difference between HD-endoscopy and microscopy? Clin Neurol Neurosurg 2017; 158: 5-11.
[http://dx.doi.org/10.1016/j.clineuro.2017.04.010] [PMID: 28414959]

[125] Siller S, Zoellner C, Fuetsch M, Trabold R, Tonn JC, Zausinger S. A high-definition 3D exoscope as an alternative to the operating microscope in spinal microsurgery. J Neurosurg Spine 2020; 1-10.
[http://dx.doi.org/10.3171/2020.4.SPINE20374] [PMID: 32650307]

[126] Pham MH, Osorio JA, Lehman RA. Navigated spinal robotics in minimally invasive spine surgery, with preoperative and intraoperative workflows: 2-dimensional operative video. Oper Neurosurg (Hagerstown) 2020; 19(4): E422.

[127] Huang J, Li Y, Huang L. Spine surgical robotics: review of the current application and disadvantages for future perspectives. J Robot Surg 2020; 14(1): 11-6.
[http://dx.doi.org/10.1007/s11701-019-00983-6] [PMID: 31243701]

[128] Ahern DP, Gibbons D, Schroeder GD, Vaccaro AR, Butler JS. Image-guidance, robotics, and the future of spine surgery. Clin Spine Surg 2020; 33(5): 179-84.
[PMID: 31425306]

[129] Staub BN, Sadrameli SS. The use of robotics in minimally invasive spine surgery. J Spine Surg 2019; 5 (Suppl. 1): S31-40.
[http://dx.doi.org/10.21037/jss.2019.04.16] [PMID: 31380491]

[130] Galetta MS, Leider JD, Divi SN, Goyal DKC, Schroeder GD. Robotics in spinal surgery. Ann Transl Med 2019; 7 (Suppl. 5): S165.
[http://dx.doi.org/10.21037/atm.2019.07.93] [PMID: 31624731]

[131] Snyder LA. Integrating robotics into a minimally invasive transforaminal interbody fusion workflow. Neurosurg Focus 2018; 45(VideoSuppl 1): V4.
[http://dx.doi.org/10.3171/2018.7.FocusVid.18111]

[132] Crawford N, Johnson N, Theodore N. Ensuring navigation integrity using robotics in spine surgery. J Robot Surg 2020; 14(1): 177-83.
[http://dx.doi.org/10.1007/s11701-019-00963-w] [PMID: 30989617]

[133] Malham GM, Wells-Quinn T. What should my hospital buy next?-guidelines for the acquisition and application of imaging, navigation, and robotics for spine surgery. J Spine Surg 2019; 5(1): 155-65.
[http://dx.doi.org/10.21037/jss.2019.02.04] [PMID: 31032450]

[134] Kochanski RB, Lombardi JM, Laratta JL, Lehman RA, O'Toole JE. Image-guided navigation and robotics in spine surgery. Neurosurgery 2019; 84(6): 1179-89.
[http://dx.doi.org/10.1093/neuros/nyy630] [PMID: 30615160]

[135] Ji GY, Lee J, Lee SW, *et al.* Safety and effectiveness of transforaminal epiduroscopic laser ablation in single level disc disease: a case-control study. Pain Physician 2018; 21(6): E643-50.
[PMID: 30508995]

[136] Lee SH, Kang HS. Percutaneous endoscopic laser annuloplasty for discogenic low back pain. World Neurosurg 2010; 73(3): 198-206.
[http://dx.doi.org/10.1016/j.surneu.2009.01.023] [PMID: 20860958]

[137] Ruetten S, Meyer O, Godolias G. Application of holmium:YAG laser in epiduroscopy: extended practicabilities in the treatment of chronic back pain syndrome. J Clin Laser Med Surg 2002; 20(4): 203-6.
[http://dx.doi.org/10.1089/104454702760230528] [PMID: 12206722]

[138] Chiu JC, Clifford TJ, Greenspan M, Richley RC, Lohman G, Sison RB. Percutaneous microdecompressive endoscopic cervical discectomy with laser thermodiskoplasty. Mt Sinai J Med 2000; 67(4): 278-82.
[PMID: 11021777]

[139] Knight MT, Vajda A, Jakab GV, Awan S. Endoscopic laser foraminoplasty on the lumbar spine--early experience. Minim Invasive Neurosurg 1998; 41(1): 5-9.
[http://dx.doi.org/10.1055/s-2008-1052006] [PMID: 9565957]

[140]   Maeda T, Takamatsu N, Hashimoto A, *et al.* Return to play in professional baseball players following transforaminal endoscopic decompressive spine surgery under local anesthesia. J Spine Surg 2020; 6 (Suppl. 1): S300-6.
[http://dx.doi.org/10.21037/jss.2019.11.09] [PMID: 32195437]

[141]   Pan F, Shen B, Chy SK, *et al.* Transforaminal endoscopic system technique for discogenic low back pain: a prospective Cohort study. Int J Surg 2016; 35: 134-8.
[http://dx.doi.org/10.1016/j.ijsu.2016.09.091] [PMID: 27693825]

[142]   Yeung AT, Gore S. *In-vivo* Endoscopic visualization of patho-anatomy in symptomatic degenerative conditions of the lumbar spine ii: intradiscal, foraminal, and central canal decompression. Surg Technol Int 2011; 21: 299-319.
[PMID: 22505004]

[143]   Haufe SM, Mork AR. Endoscopic facet debridement for the treatment of facet arthritic pain--a novel new technique. Int J Med Sci 2010; 7(3): 120-3.
[http://dx.doi.org/10.7150/ijms.7.120] [PMID: 20567612]

[144]   Yuan C, Wang J, Zhou Y, Pan Y. Endoscopic lumbar discectomy and minimally invasive lumbar interbody fusion: a contrastive review. Wideochir Inne Tech Malo Inwazyjne 2018; 13(4): 429-34.
[http://dx.doi.org/10.5114/wiitm.2018.77744] [PMID: 30524611]

[145]   Caruso R, Pesce A, Martines V, *et al.* Assessing the real benefits of surgery for degenerative lumbar spinal stenosis without instability and spondylolisthesis: a single surgeon experience with a mean 8-year follow-up. J Orthop Traumatol 2018; 19(1): 6.
[http://dx.doi.org/10.1186/s10195-018-0497-8] [PMID: 30171437]

[146]   Law MD Jr, Bernhardt M, White AA III. Cervical spondylotic myelopathy: a review of surgical indications and decision making. Yale J Biol Med 1993; 66(3): 165-77.
[PMID: 8209553]

[147]   Sengupta DK, Herkowitz HN. Lumbar spinal stenosis. Treatment strategies and indications for surgery. Orthop Clin North Am 2003; 34(2): 281-95.
[http://dx.doi.org/10.1016/S0030-5898(02)00069-X] [PMID: 12914268]

[148]   Boswell MV, Shah RV, Everett CR, *et al.* Interventional techniques in the management of chronic spinal pain: evidence-based practice guidelines. Pain Physician 2005; 8(1): 1-47.
[http://dx.doi.org/10.36076/ppj.2006/9/1] [PMID: 16850041]

[149]   Fessler RG, O'Toole JE, Eichholz KM, Perez-Cruet MJ. The development of minimally invasive spine surgery. Neurosurg Clin N Am 2006; 17(4): 401-9.
[http://dx.doi.org/10.1016/j.nec.2006.06.007] [PMID: 17010890]

[150]   Pflugmacher R, Schleicher P, Gumnior S, *et al.* Biomechanical comparison of bioabsorbable cervical spine interbody fusion cages. Spine 2004; 29(16): 1717-22.
[http://dx.doi.org/10.1097/01.BRS.0000134565.17078.4C] [PMID: 15303013]

[151]   Verma K, Gandhi SD, Maltenfort M, *et al.* Rate of adjacent segment disease in cervical disc arthroplasty *versus* single-level fusion: meta-analysis of prospective studies. Spine 2013; 38(26): 2253-7.
[http://dx.doi.org/10.1097/BRS.0000000000000052] [PMID: 24335631]

[152]   Zheng B, Hao D, Guo H, He B. ACDF *vs* TDR for patients with cervical spondylosis - an 8 year follow up study. BMC Surg 2017; 17(1): 113.
[http://dx.doi.org/10.1186/s12893-017-0316-9] [PMID: 29183306]

[153]   Vaishnav AS, Saville P, McAnany S, *et al.* Retrospective review of immediate restoration of lordosis in single-level minimally invasive transforaminal lumbar interbody fusion: a comparison of static and expandable interbody cages. Oper Neurosurg (Hagerstown) 2020; 18(5): 518-23.
[http://dx.doi.org/10.1093/ons/opz240]

[154]   O'Toole JE, Eichholz KM, Fessler RG. Minimally invasive far lateral microendoscopic discectomy for

extraforaminal disc herniation at the lumbosacral junction: cadaveric dissection and technical case report. Spine J 2007; 7(4): 414-21.
[http://dx.doi.org/10.1016/j.spinee.2006.07.008] [PMID: 17630139]

[155] Ortega-Porcayo LA, Leal-López A, Soriano-López ME, *et al.* Assessment of paraspinal muscle atrophy percentage after minimally invasive transforaminal lumbar interbody fusion and unilateral instrumentation using a novel contralateral intact muscle-controlled model. Asian Spine J 2018; 12(2): 256-62.
[http://dx.doi.org/10.4184/asj.2018.12.2.256] [PMID: 29713406]

[156] Skovrlj B, Gilligan J, Cutler HS, Qureshi SA. Minimally invasive procedures on the lumbar spine. World J Clin Cases 2015; 3(1): 1-9.
[http://dx.doi.org/10.12998/wjcc.v3.i1.1] [PMID: 25610845]

[157] Lewandrowski KU. Readmissions after outpatient transforaminal decompression for lumbar foraminal and lateral recess stenosis. Int J Spine Surg 2018; 12(3): 342-51.
[http://dx.doi.org/10.14444/5040] [PMID: 30276091]

[158] Modhia U, Takemoto S, Braid-Forbes MJ, Weber M, Berven SH. Readmission rates after decompression surgery in patients with lumbar spinal stenosis among Medicare beneficiaries. Spine 2013; 38(7): 591-6.
[http://dx.doi.org/10.1097/BRS.0b013e31828628f5] [PMID: 23324923]

[159] Adogwa O, Parker SL, Bydon A, Cheng J, McGirt MJ. Comparative effectiveness of minimally invasive *versus* open transforaminal lumbar interbody fusion: 2-year assessment of narcotic use, return to work, disability, and quality of life. J Spinal Disord Tech 2011; 24(8): 479-84.
[http://dx.doi.org/10.1097/BSD.0b013e3182055cac] [PMID: 21336176]

[160] Drahos GL, Williams L. Addressing the emerging public health crisis of narcotic overdose. Gen Dent 2017; 65(5): 7-9.
[PMID: 28862579]

[161] Wang X, Borgman B, Vertuani S, Nilsson J. A systematic literature review of time to return to work and narcotic use after lumbar spinal fusion using minimal invasive and open surgery techniques. BMC Health Serv Res 2017; 17(1): 446.
[http://dx.doi.org/10.1186/s12913-017-2398-6] [PMID: 28655308]

[162] Lewandrowski KU, Iprenburg M, Lee SH. Endoscopic spinal surgery. 1st ed., KU Lewandrowski. London: Jaypee Brothers Medical Pub 2013.

[163] Casal-Moro R, Castro-Menéndez M, Hernández-Blanco M, Bravo-Ricoy JA, Jorge-Barreiro FJ. Long-term outcome after microendoscopic diskectomy for lumbar disk herniation: a prospective clinical study with a 5-year follow-up. Neurosurgery 2011; 68(6): 1568-75.
[http://dx.doi.org/10.1227/NEU.0b013e31820cd16a] [PMID: 21311384]

[164] Gadjradj PS, van Tulder MW, Dirven CM, Peul WC, Harhangi BS. Clinical outcomes after percutaneous transforaminal endoscopic discectomy for lumbar disc herniation: a prospective case series. Neurosurg Focus 2016; 40(2): E3.
[http://dx.doi.org/10.3171/2015.10.FOCUS15484] [PMID: 26828884]

[165] Ruetten S, Komp M, Merk H, Godolias G. A new full-endoscopic technique for cervical posterior foraminotomy in the treatment of lateral disc herniations using 6.9-mm endoscopes: prospective 2-year results of 87 patients. Minim Invasive Neurosurg 2007; 50(4): 219-26.
[http://dx.doi.org/10.1055/s-2007-985860] [PMID: 17948181]

[166] Ruetten S, Komp M, Merk H, Godolias G. Full-endoscopic cervical posterior foraminotomy for the operation of lateral disc herniations using 5.9-mm endoscopes: a prospective, randomized, controlled study. Spine 2008; 33(9): 940-8.
[http://dx.doi.org/10.1097/BRS.0b013e31816c8b67] [PMID: 18427313]

[167] Hellinger S. The fullendoscopic anterior cervical fusion: a new horizon for selective percutaneous endoscopic cervical decompression. Acta Neurochir Suppl (Wien) 2011; 108: 203-7.

[http://dx.doi.org/10.1007/978-3-211-99370-5_31] [PMID: 21107960]

[168] Lee SH, Lee JH, Choi WC, Jung B, Mehta R. Anterior minimally invasive approaches for the cervical spine. Orthop Clin North Am 2007; 38(3): 327-37.
[http://dx.doi.org/10.1016/j.ocl.2007.02.007] [PMID: 17629981]

[169] Tajima T, Sakamoto H, Yamakawa H. Diskectomy cervical percutanee. Revue Med Orthoped 1989; 17: 7-10.

[170] Gastambide D. Percutaneous cervical discectomy non-automatized SICOT. Seoul, Korea: ISMISS 1993.

[171] Algara M. Automated percutaneous cervical discectomy. 4th Annual Meeting of the European Spine Society. Nantes, France. 1993.

[172] Herman S, Nizard R. La discectomie percutanee au rachis cervical Rachis cervical degenerative et tramatique: expansion scientifique francaise 1993; 6-160.

[173] Bonati A. Percutaneous cervical laser discectomy. International Meeting of Laser Surgery. San Francisco. 1991.

[174] Siebert W. Percutaneous laser discectomy of cervical discs: preliminary clinical results. J Clin Laser Med Surg 1995; 13(3): 205-7.
[http://dx.doi.org/10.1089/clm.1995.13.205] [PMID: 10150647]

[175] Lee SH, Ahn Y, Choi WC, Bhanot A, Shin SW. Immediate pain improvement is a useful predictor of long-term favorable outcome after percutaneous laser disc decompression for cervical disc herniation. Photomed Laser Surg 2006; 24(4): 508-13.
[http://dx.doi.org/10.1089/pho.2006.24.508] [PMID: 16942433]

[176] Jolesz FA, Bleier AR, Jakab P, Ruenzel PW, Huttl K, Jako GJ. MR imaging of laser-tissue interactions. Radiology 1988; 168(1): 249-53.
[http://dx.doi.org/10.1148/radiology.168.1.3380968] [PMID: 3380968]

[177] Ahn Y, Lee SH, Shin SW. Percutaneous endoscopic cervical discectomy: clinical outcome and radiographic changes. Photomed Laser Surg 2005; 23(4): 362-8.
[http://dx.doi.org/10.1089/pho.2005.23.362] [PMID: 16144477]

[178] Ahn Y, Lee SH, Lee SC, Shin SW, Chung SE. Factors predicting excellent outcome of percutaneous cervical discectomy: analysis of 111 consecutive cases. Neuroradiology 2004; 46(5): 378-84.
[http://dx.doi.org/10.1007/s00234-004-1197-z] [PMID: 15103434]

[179] Ascher PW. Status quo and new horizons of laser therapy in neurosurgery. Lasers Surg Med 1985; 5(5): 499-506.
[http://dx.doi.org/10.1002/lsm.1900050509] [PMID: 4068883]

[180] Quigley MR, Maroon JC, Shih T, Elrifai A, Lesiecki ML. Laser discectomy. Comparison of systems. Spine 1994; 19(3): 319-22.
[http://dx.doi.org/10.1097/00007632-199402000-00011] [PMID: 8171364]

[181] Davis JK. Percutaneous discectomy improved with KTP laser. Clin Laser Mon 1990; 8(7): 105-6.
[PMID: 10149820]

[182] Casper GD, Mullins LL, Hartman VL. Laser-assisted disc decompression: a clinical trial of the holmium:YAG laser with side-firing fiber. J Clin Laser Med Surg 1995; 13(1): 27-32.
[http://dx.doi.org/10.1089/clm.1995.13.27] [PMID: 10150570]

[183] Casper GD, Hartman VL, Mullins LL. Percutaneous laser disc decompression with the holmium: YAG laser. J Clin Laser Med Surg 1995; 13(3): 195-203.
[http://dx.doi.org/10.1089/clm.1995.13.195] [PMID: 10150646]

[184] Yeung AT. The evolution of percutaneous spinal endoscopy and discectomy: state of the art. Mt Sinai J Med 2000; 67(4): 327-32.
[PMID: 11021785]

[185]  Siebert WE, Berendsen BT, Tollgaard J. Percutaneous laser disk decompression. Experience since 1989. Orthopade 1996; 25(1): 42-8.
[PMID: 8622845]

[186]  Ahn Y, Lee U. Use of lasers in minimally invasive spine surgery. Expert Rev Med Devices 2018; 15(6): 423-33.
[http://dx.doi.org/10.1080/17434440.2018.1483236] [PMID: 29855205]

[187]  Ahn JS, Lee HJ, Choi DJ, Lee KY, Hwang SJ. Extraforaminal approach of biportal endoscopic spinal surgery: a new endoscopic technique for transforaminal decompression and discectomy. J Neurosurg Spine 2018; 28(5): 492-8.
[http://dx.doi.org/10.3171/2017.8.SPINE17771] [PMID: 29473790]

[188]  Mayer HM, Brock M, Berlien HP, Weber B. Percutaneous endoscopic laser discectomy (PELD). A new surgical technique for non-sequestrated lumbar discs. Acta Neurochir Suppl (Wien) 1992; 54: 53-8.
[http://dx.doi.org/10.1007/978-3-7091-6687-1_7] [PMID: 1595409]

[189]  Hellinger J. Technical aspects of the percutaneous cervical and lumbar laser-disc-decompression and -nucleotomy. Neurol Res 1999; 21(1): 99-102.
[http://dx.doi.org/10.1080/01616412.1999.11740902] [PMID: 10048065]

[190]  Deukmedjian AJ, Cianciabella A, Cutright J, Deukmedjian A. Cervical Deuk Laser Disc Repair(®): A novel, full-endoscopic surgical technique for the treatment of symptomatic cervical disc disease. Surg Neurol Int 2012; 3: 142.
[http://dx.doi.org/10.4103/2152-7806.103884] [PMID: 23230523]

[191]  Deukmedjian AJ, Jason Cutright ST, Augusto Cianciabella PC, Deukmedjian A. Deuk Laser Disc Repair(®) is a safe and effective treatment for symptomatic cervical disc disease. Surg Neurol Int 2013; 4: 68.
[http://dx.doi.org/10.4103/2152-7806.112610] [PMID: 23776754]

[192]  Pflum FA, Selby RM, Vizzone JP. Arthroscopic anterior diskectomy of the cervical spine. Arthroscopy 2008; 24(5): 612-4.
[http://dx.doi.org/10.1016/j.arthro.2007.08.002] [PMID: 18442696]

[193]  Bing N, Tao D, Wei S, Guang L, Hongwei Z. Percutaneous endoscopic c2-c3 medial branches neurotomy for cervicogenic headache. World Neurosurg 2019; 126: 498-501.
[http://dx.doi.org/10.1016/j.wneu.2019.03.072] [PMID: 30885858]

[194]  Choi GS, Ahn SH, Cho YW, Lee DK. Short-term effects of pulsed radiofrequency on chronic refractory cervical radicular pain. Ann Rehabil Med 2011; 35(6): 826-32.
[http://dx.doi.org/10.5535/arm.2011.35.6.826] [PMID: 22506211]

[195]  Choi GS, Ahn SH, Cho YW, Lee DG. Long-term effect of pulsed radiofrequency on chronic cervical radicular pain refractory to repeated transforaminal epidural steroid injections. Pain Med 2012; 13(3): 368-75.
[http://dx.doi.org/10.1111/j.1526-4637.2011.01313.x] [PMID: 22296730]

[196]  Yao N, Wang C, Wang W, Wang L. Full-endoscopic technique for anterior cervical discectomy and interbody fusion: 5-year follow-up results of 67 cases. Eur Spine J 2011; 20(6): 899-904.
[http://dx.doi.org/10.1007/s00586-010-1642-0] [PMID: 21153596]

[197]  Wu PF, Li YW, Wang B, Jiang B, Tu ZM, Lv GH. Posterior cervical foraminotomy *via* Full-endoscopic *versus* microendoscopic approach for radiculopathy: a systematic review and meta-analysis. Pain Physician 2019; 22(1): 41-52.
[PMID: 30700067]

[198]  Ahn Y, Keum HJ, Shin SH. Percutaneous endoscopic cervical discectomy *versus* anterior cervical discectomy and fusion: a comparative cohort study with a five-year follow-up. J Clin Med 2020; 9(2): E371.

[http://dx.doi.org/10.3390/jcm9020371] [PMID: 32013206]

[199]  Du Q, Lei LQ, Cao GR, *et al.* Percutaneous full-endoscopic anterior transcorporeal cervical discectomy and channel repair: a technique note report. BMC Musculoskelet Disord 2019; 20(1): 280.
[http://dx.doi.org/10.1186/s12891-019-2659-0] [PMID: 31182078]

[200]  Kim JS, Eun SS, Prada N, Choi G, Lee SH. Modified transcorporeal anterior cervical microforaminotomy assisted by O-arm-based navigation: a technical case report. Eur Spine J 2011; 20 (Suppl. 2): S147-52.
[http://dx.doi.org/10.1007/s00586-010-1454-2] [PMID: 20490870]

[201]  Choi G, Lee SH, Bhanot A, Chae YS, Jung B, Lee S. Modified transcorporeal anterior cervical microforaminotomy for cervical radiculopathy: a technical note and early results. Eur Spine J 2007; 16(9): 1387-93.
[http://dx.doi.org/10.1007/s00586-006-0286-6] [PMID: 17203272]

[202]  Choi G, Arbatti NJ, Modi HN, *et al.* Transcorporeal tunnel approach for unilateral cervical radiculopathy: a 2-year follow-up review and results. Minim Invasive Neurosurg 2010; 53(3): 127-31.
[http://dx.doi.org/10.1055/s-0030-1249681] [PMID: 20809454]

[203]  Deng ZL, Chu L, Chen L, Yang JS. Anterior transcorporeal approach of percutaneous endoscopic cervical discectomy for disc herniation at the C4-C5 levels: a technical note. Spine J 2016; 16(5): 659-66.
[http://dx.doi.org/10.1016/j.spinee.2016.01.187] [PMID: 26850173]

[204]  Schubert M, Merk S. Retrospective evaluation of efficiency and safety of an anterior percutaneous approach for cervical discectomy. Asian Spine J 2014; 8(4): 412-20.
[http://dx.doi.org/10.4184/asj.2014.8.4.412] [PMID: 25187857]

[205]  Tzaan WC. Anterior percutaneous endoscopic cervical discectomy for cervical intervertebral disc herniation: outcome, complications, and technique. J Spinal Disord Tech 2011; 24(7): 421-31.
[http://dx.doi.org/10.1097/BSD.0b013e31820ef328] [PMID: 21430567]

# CHAPTER 2

# Anesthesia for Minimally Invasive Surgery of the Cervical Spine

**João Abrão¹, Kai-Uwe Lewandrowski²,³,⁴ and Álvaro Dowling⁵,⁶**

¹ *Discipline of Anesthesiology, Faculty of Medicine of Ribeirão Preto, University of São Paulo, São Paulo, Brazil*

² *Center for Advanced Spine Care of Southern Arizona and Surgical Institute of Tucson, Tucson, AZ, USA*

³ *Department of Orthopaedic Surgery, UNIRIO, Rio de Janeiro, Brazil*

⁴ *Department of Orthoapedic Surgery, Fundación Universitaria Sanitas, Bogotá, D.C., Colombia, USA*

⁵ *Endoscopic Spine Clinic, Santiago, Chile*

⁶ *Department of Orthopaedic Surgery, USP, Ribeirão Preto, Brazil*

**Abstract:** Anesthesia for the outpatient ambulatory surgery center has to be tailored to the surgery. The length of surgery, the trauma of painful dissection, and the amount of blood loss have to be considered. Outpatient spine surgery is characterized by shorter simplified versions of their inpatient counterparts carried out in a hospital setting. Many outpatient spine surgeries are minimally invasive through small incisions with less blood loss, tissue disruption, and, more importantly, less painful stimulus during surgery. These modern spine surgery versions also apply local anesthesia strategically to diminish the need for deep anesthesia. In some scenarios, the surgeon may wish to speak to the sedated yet awake patient to lower the risk of injury to neural structures when performing the more dangerous portions of the endoscopic decompression surgery. The need to communicate with the patient is undoubtedly of high relevance in the cervical spine, which requires the anesthesiologist to tailor the management of the patient's anesthesia to the surgeons' needs. The monitored anesthesia care (MAC), where sedation is achieved with various sedatives and narcotics, is most appropriate for outpatient endoscopic cervical spinal surgeries. These surgeries may be performed with the patient in supine (anterior cervical surgery) or in a prone position (posterior cervical surgery). Patients in the prone position may pose additional problems maintaining adequate ventilation and sedation while keeping the patient comfortable enough to tolerate the procedure and yet still communicating with the surgeon. In other scenarios or different surgeon preferences communicating with the patient during an outpatient endoscopic cervical surgery may not be required. A Laryngeal Mask Airway (LMA) may be more appropriate with the patient in a prone position. This chapter describes

---

* **Corresponding author Álvaro Dowling:** Orthopaedic Spine Surgeon, Director of Endoscopic Spine Clinic, Santiago, Chile, Visiting Professor, Department of Orthopaedic Surgery, USP, Ribeirão Preto, Brazil; Tel: +56 9 6227 1201; E-mail: alrodomo@gmail.com

modern MAC concepts, airway management in the supine and prone position, and sedatives as it applies to cervical endoscopic spinal surgery in an ambulatory surgery center.

**Keywords:** Balanced Anesthesia, Cervical Spine Endoscopy, Monitored Anesthesia Care.

## INTRODUCTION

Open spine surgery is increasingly replaced by Minimally Invasive Spine Surgery (MISS). Nowadays, MISS is the technique of choice in treating common degenerative conditions of the cervical spine [1 - 3]. The main indication for MISS is the cervical herniated intervertebral disc [1 - 6]. The minimal tissue trauma, reduced blood loss, decreased postoperative pain, and a diminished need for deep anesthesia have been recognized as significant advantages [5, 7, 8]. Many patients experience a much shorter length of inpatient stay [9]. In endoscopic spine surgery, light sedation monitored anesthesia care is the critical element in allowing patients to discharge early from the recovery room or the ambulatory surgery center (ASC) [9, 10].

In this chapter, the authors attempt to describe their methodology of providing anesthesia tailored to the outpatient endoscopic cervical decompression surgery, where patients need minimal amounts of sedatives and narcotics to feel comfortable throughout different stages of the cervical endoscopy. The surgeon also heavily relies on the patient's verbalization ability during the procedure. The awake patient able to speak during operation with the surgeon is the most reliable and best monitoring of the patient's neurological function during this delicate and potentially dangerous procedure. Surgeons and anesthesiologists need to communicate closely to tailor the anesthesia to support the surgeon's needs so the cervical surgery can be executed safely, efficiently, and timely. This chapter is as much about this communication between surgeon and anesthesiologist as it is about the actual anesthesia protocols described herein.

## ANESTHESIA STRATEGIES

In general, recovery from anesthesia and surgery is faster when patients can be sent home with higher patient satisfaction. Considering the authors intend to demystify the belief that spinal surgery is a complicated procedure, we stipulate that the patient should not be admitted to a hospital. However, there are several concerns with this stipulation. First, the majority of cervical spine endoscopies are posterior procedures. They seem preferred by most endoscopic spine surgeons for greater versatility, simplicity, and less risk to the vital structures in the neck. Posterior procedures are done, though, with the patient in the prone position. Most anesthesiologists prefer endotracheal intubation and general anesthesia to secure the airway. While endotracheal intubation with general anesthesia is helpful in quickly correcting intraoperative respiratory depression or even maintain the patient's mechanical ventilation should the patient cease to breathe spontaneously under overzealous use of sedation or anesthesia, it certainly prolongs the postoperative recovery. Second, general anesthesia may lead to other postoperative problems, including prolonged wakeup, urinary retention with the need for catheterization in the recovery room, cardiopulmonary compromise, constipation, *etc.* Hence, posterior and anterior endoscopic cervical spine surgeries are preferably carried out in an ambulatory surgery center with local anesthesia with sedation. Endoscopic surgery in awake patients minimizes the risk of neural injury. Moreover, this monitored anesthesia care streamlines wake up and recovery. It improves workflow. The authors' experience is that general anesthesia is unnecessary for many patients who undergo ambulatory surgeries. Still, it may be advisable in some patients with medical comorbidities requiring complex endoscopic decompression. This team of authors typically decides for conscious sedation under monitored anesthesia care (MAC) whenever possible [10, 11]. To achieve the right sedation level and comfort in the patient undergoing cervical endoscopy, the anesthesiologist has to perceive and anticipate situations where the patient may feel severe pain and needs to be responsive and cooperative. Since the surgeon may concentrate on the operation, the anesthesiologists should also assess his monitors' stimulation level.

## SEDATION

There are many scales to quantify the sedation grade. The most popular amongst anesthesiologists is the Ramsay Sedation Scale (Table **1**) [12-17]. Following this scale, our target is level 3. The patient can still recognize the manipulation of the spinal nerve by touch while reasonably being able to tolerate the pain and even follow commands. The ventilation is adequate at this level, and typically only a supplementary oxygen nasal cannula is needed. Sometimes after introducing the dilators to place the endoscopic working cannula, the surgeon wants to check the neurological status by asking the patient to move his feet. Ramsay stage 3 is the ideal sedation level to accomplish cooperation from the patient. The question of the perfect sedative is of particular significance. The properties of such a perfect sedative are listed in Table **2**. All the pharmacokinetics and pharmacodynamic characteristics have to be considered when choosing a drug for the MAC.

**Table 1. Ramsay Sedation Scale.**

| Definition | Score |
|---|---|
| Patient is anxious and agitated or restless, or both | 1 |

(Table 1) cont.....

| | |
|---|---|
| Patient is cooperative, oriented and calm | 2 |
| Patient responds to commands only | 3 |
| Patient exhibits brisk response to light glabellar tap or loud auditory stimulus | 4 |
| Patient exhibits a sluggish response to light glabellar tap or loud auditory stimulus | 5 |
| Patient exhibits no response | 6 |

**Table 2. The Ideal Sedative.**

| |
|---|
| Fast onset and end of action |
| Minimal respiratory depression |
| No effect on cardiovascular function |
| Inactive or lacking metabolites |
| Non-dependent elimination of liver and |
| No interaction with other drugs |
| Do not cause pain upon injection |
| Failure to produce tolerance or withdraw syndrome |
| Must produce amnesia |
| Be economical |

## ANESTHESIA FOR CERVICAL ENDOSCOPY IN AMBULATORY SURGERY CENTER (ASC)

Simplified anesthesia with sedation and local anesthesia in ASC may potentially produce an unpleasant situation for the patient. Therefore, the painful portion of the procedure should be communicated to the anesthesiologist to make adjustments in the protocol, thus, making it tolerable and more comfortable to the patient. The patient needs to be monitored for decreased consciousness since the sedation is a continuous process encompassing anxiolysis and deep state nociception [12]. The goal of MAC for cervical endoscopy is a short time onset of sedation followed by a rapid recovery. Ideally, the chosen sedatives do not cause any adverse hemodynamics, respiratory depression, and metabolic upsets. Some of the most commonly used sedative drugs are midazolam, propofol, ketamine, dexmedetomidine, remifentanil, and fentanyl. A newer benzodiazepine, remimazolam, is under investigation in phase three clinical trials. By default, the anesthesiologist often supervises the comfortable position of the patient on the operating table. It is relevant to position the patient in such a way that allows the best ventilation. A relaxed environment in the prone position on a lordotic frame or chest rolls is of particular importance. The surgeon should use local anesthesia to anesthetize the entire surgical access corridor and the surgical site. The concurrent use of long-acting local anesthetic may diminish painful stimulus during surgery and control postoperative pain, and avoid a dysphoric wake in the recovery room.

## SEDATIVES

### Benzodiazepines

Diazepam, midazolam, and lorazepam are frequently used benzodiazepines [13 - 16]. All of them have active metabolites and can provoke agitation in older people. Today, the only one that should be used in ambulatory anesthesia is midazolam, although in low doses [17 - 20]. Benzodiazepines are metabolism liver dependent and, for safety reasons, have to be avoided in patients with low hepatic function. The new benzodiazepine, remimazolam, undergoes rapid metabolism by plasma and tissue esterases. Its metabolism is therefore independent of the liver or kidneys.

Midazolam has a relatively long half-life - t1/2ke0. On average, the drug achieves the same concentration in the brain as in the plasma in 9 min [21]. The anesthetist has to consider this pharmacokinetic dynamic when a second dose is used to avoid complications such as hypoventilation, airway obstruction, hypoxia, and hypotension [12].

### Propofol

Intravenous propofol is the drug commonly used in short-duration procedures because of its rapid onset and offsets time [22 - 24]. The pain on injection can be easily overcome by adding a small amount of lidocaine. Propofol has a narrow therapeutic window. Patients may quickly go into hypotension and respiratory depression at plasma concentrations similar to those needed for ambulatory surgery sedation [25]. Hypotension may quickly develop because of its vasodilative properties [22]. Intravenous volume replenishment and vigilant monitoring of the patient's vital signs are critical when using propofol. When the patient is prone with a nasal oxygen cannula, the intravenous propofol dose should not be higher than the recommended 1mg/kg IV. The constant infusion can be established at about 50 µg/kg/min [26].

The propofol concentration in the plasma should be maintained at 1 µg/mL when using the target-controlled infusion (TCI) technology. However, variations may be necessary depending on the respiratory drive. The anesthesiologist should always use his clinical judgment when assessing the patients' anxiety and level of pain control and sedation while safely providing comfort during the endoscopic procedure on the cervical spine. The latter is of particular importance when recognizing the patients' ability to metabolize sedatives and narcotics rapidly.

Specific attention should be taken to a narcotic-naive patient who may be easily profoundly sedated.

## Dexmedetomidine

Dexmedetomidine is an α-2-adrenoceptor agonist with sedative, anxiolytic, sympatholytic, and analgesic-sparing effects while causing minimal depression of respiratory function (Fig. **1**) [27 - 30]. Hemodynamic effects include transient hypertension, bradycardia, and hypotension [27]. Dexmedetomidine exerts its hypnotic action by activating alfa-2 receptors in the locus coeruleus, inducing unconsciousness similar to natural sleep, and the patient remains easily arousable and cooperative [28]. Dexmedetomidine is rapidly distributed and is mainly hepatic metabolized into inactive metabolites [31]. Typically, during intravenous infusion, one uses an induction dose of 1µg/kg for 10 min and a maintenance dose of 0.5 µg/kg /h. This dose can be adjusted by the patient's response, up to 1 µg/kg /h [28]. When administering MAC, dexmedetomidine may be effectively used for maintaining the patient's baseline sedation. Complementary propofol and remifentanil may be employed as needed during the more painful parts of the endoscopic cervical decompression surgery [28]. Judicious application of local anesthesia with 1% lidocaine by the surgeon may also significantly improve patient comfort and decrease systemic drug application.

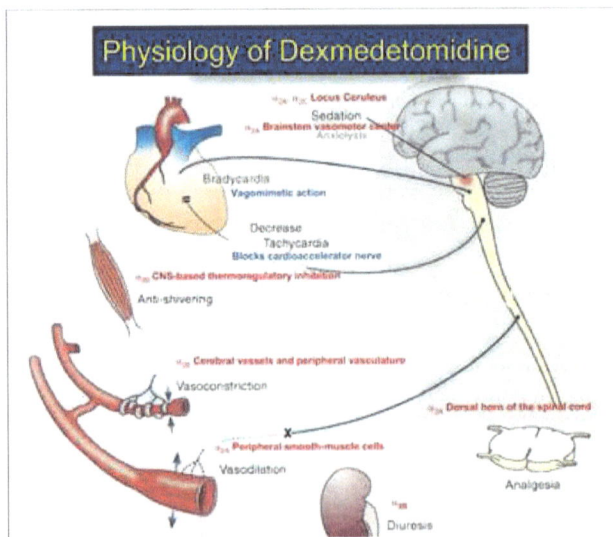

**Fig. (1).** This figure was kindly authorized by Jesse B. Hall, Professor of Medicine, Anesthesia & Critical Care at the University of Chicago.

## Remifentanil

Remifentanil is a μ-receptor agonist short-acting synthetic opioid. It is hydrolyzed by plasma and tissue esterases and does not accumulate with a prolonged infusion. Its half-life is +/- 4 min [32 - 36]. The combination of drugs with potent respiratory depressant properties can lead to a rapid respiratory compromise. In conjunction with propofol, remifentanil is administered at 0,05 μg/kg /min [33]. Remifentanil can be easily titrated due to its short half-life (t1/2ke0) of 1.3 minutes [35]. This rapid pharmacokinetic and pharmacodynamic profile makes remifentanil uniquely suitable for fast onset- and offset scenarios [32]. Remifentanil has a small central volume of distribution. Therefore, it is not practical in bolus application and should only be employed by pump infusion. It is highly suitable for outpatient spine surgery [37].

## Ketamine

Ketamine has a carbon chiral with S(+) and R(-) enantiomers. The former is four times as potent as the latter. The racemic mixture is only available in the United States. In South America, on the other hand, the S(+) Ketamine, named dextroketamine, is in use. It has found little use as a mono-anesthetic because of postoperative hallucinations. Therefore, it is typically is used in conjunction with other drugs with sedative effects [38 - 44]. Ketamine provides a high level of analgesia without respiratory depression [41], making it useful in patients undergoing prone posterior cervical endoscopy. Analgesia can be achieved at minimal doses of 0.2-0.5 mg/kg. Employing ketamin is of genuine interest when the patient is obese, asthmatic, or has sleep apnea. The mixture of propofol and ketamine, known as ketofol, is widely used [24, 45]. The ratio customarily used for these two drugs is 1:1 to 1:10. [9] Recovery times of patients treated with ketofol may be longer than those of patients receiving propofol and fentanyl [39]. The use of ketamine is helpful for better analgesia, which in low doses may be safely employed during cervical endoscopy in the prone position.

## DISCUSSION

Simplified anterior and posterior minimally invasive cervical spine procedures such as foraminotomies, laminotomies, or partial laminectomies are conducive to outpatient ambulatory surgery center settings. Neurectomy procedures, including mechanical, thermal, or radiofrequency rhizotomies, are other examples of applying the endoscopic spinal surgery platform to treat axial neck- instead of radicular arm pain. The most suitable anesthesia protocol may vary by anterior or posterior approach. If local anesthesia is employed, less systemic sedation and analgesia are required. Intubation may need to be avoided if the surgeon desires to communicate with the patient during surgery. A face mask or nasal cannula for continuous oxygenation of the patient may be preferred. If necessary, a laryngeal mask airway (LMA) may be a valuable adjunct to ventilation to avoid obstruction, mainly if the patient is in a prone position and is under general anesthesia. A secure airway with endotracheal intubation may be the best choice in asthmatic patients or those who suffer from chronic obstructive pulmonary disease (COPD), cardiopulmonary disease, diabetes, or obesity. As outlined in the various sedatives review, their pharmacokinetics and dynamics may quickly take a patient from cooperative and responsive (Ramsay stage 2 to 3) to respond sluggishly or be entirely unresponsive to a stimulus (Ramsay Stage 5 and 6). Therefore, combining sedatives and anesthetics tailored to endoscopic cervical decompression procedures is the preferred course of action.

Combination multimodal sedation combines the advantages of several medications. One example is ketofol. The combination preparation of ketamine and propofol has excellent analgesic effects without suppressing respiration. Remifentanil is also quite suitable for outpatient cervical spine surgery because of its rapid onset and offset of action. It may be cost-prohibitive in some surgery centers. Therefore, fentanyl may be an alternative to remifentanil but has a much longer half-life. Dexmedetomidine is a newer analgesic drug with minimal depression of respiratory function. 27-30 However, it has been known to cause transient hypertension, bradycardia, and hypotension. Most anesthesiologists adhere to what they know best – a simple combination regimen of fentanyl and propofol – a time-proven and cost-effective solution to outpatient endoscopic sedation requirements cervical decompression surgery. In patients in whom an LMA has been placed, even light inhalation anesthesia with sevoflurane could be considered at a fresh gas flow rate of 1 L/min in adults. The recommended mean maximum concentrations in the anesthesia circuit are approximately 20 ppm (0.002%) with soda-lime and 30 ppm (0.003%) with Baralyme.

In summary, balanced anesthesia tailored to the patients needs to undergo minimally invasive cervical spine surgery. Many of the procedures can be done under local anesthesia and sedation, allowing communication between surgeon and patient to assure preservation of neurological function during the operation. The bare minimum anesthesia protocols should be worked out between surgeon and anesthesiologist to facilitate rapid wake-up and discharge of patients from the postoperative recovery unit. Suppose cooperation by the patient is not needed. In that case, this team of authors recommends the deliberate use of LMA or endotracheal intubation with general anesthesia. It secures the airway and enhances ventilation while diminishing airway obstruction problems. Patient comfort during awake cervical endoscopy requires satisfactory analgesia and sedation. Anesthesiologist-surgeon teams that worked together consistently for a long time typically achieve the best patient satisfaction with the anesthesia. This chapter recommends that such joint anesthesia –surgery protocols are written out and communicated to all relevant staff members involved in the patient's perioperative care. Such protocols will likely guarantee consistent clinical outcomes with high patient satisfaction.

## CONCLUSIONS

MAC in an ambulatory surgery center is best suited for anterior and posterior endoscopic cervical decompressions. Intubation of the patient is generally not required. An LMA with general anesthesia may suffice in many patients. Short and straightforward procedures may even be carried out under local anesthesia with sedation and a nasal oxygen cannula or a face mask. Typically, these airway management strategies work for patients placed in the supine or prone position. Outpatient endoscopic surgeries on the cervical spine are usually short and suitable for patients with complex medical comorbidities. For those patients in whom intubation may be preferred, admission to the hospital may be more appropriate if the patient requires longer recovery or ventilation. Surgeon and anesthesia teams should avoid complacency in selecting patients for outpatient cervical spine surgery. Every patient should be screened by trained staff by employing a robust preoperative checklist to avoid surgery cancellation.

## CONSENT FOR PUBLICATION

Not applicable.

## CONFLICT OF INTEREST

The authors declare no conflict of interest, financial or otherwise.

## ACKNOWLEDGEMENTS

Declared none.

## REFERENCES

[1]    Adamson TE. The impact of minimally invasive cervical spine surgery. Invited submission from the Joint Section Meeting on Disorders of the Spine and Peripheral Nerves, March 2004. J Neurosurg Spine 2004; 1(1): 43-6.
       [http://dx.doi.org/10.3171/spi.2004.1.1.0043] [PMID: 15291019]

[2]    Skovrlj B, Qureshi SA. Minimally invasive cervical spine surgery. J Neurosurg Sci 2017; 61(3): 325-34.
       [http://dx.doi.org/10.23736/S0390-5616.16.03906-0] [PMID: 27787486]

[3]    Rubino F, Deutsch H, Pamoukian V, Zhu JF, King WA, Gagner M. Minimally invasive spine surgery: an animal model for endoscopic approach to the anterior cervical and upper thoracic spine. J Laparoendosc Adv Surg Tech A 2000; 10(6): 309-13.
       [http://dx.doi.org/10.1089/lap.2000.10.309] [PMID: 11132909]

[4]     Fessler RG, O'Toole JE, Eichholz KM, Perez-Cruet MJ. The development of minimally invasive spine surgery. Neurosurg Clin N Am 2006; 17(4): 401-9.
[http://dx.doi.org/10.1016/j.nec.2006.06.007] [PMID: 17010890]

[5]     McClelland S III, Goldstein JA. Minimally Invasive *versus* Open Spine Surgery: What Does the Best Evidence Tell Us? J Neurosci Rural Pract 2017; 8(2): 194-8.
[http://dx.doi.org/10.4103/jnrp.jnrp_472_16] [PMID: 28479791]

[6]     Patel PD, Canseco JA, Houlihan N, Gabay A, Grasso G, Vaccaro AR. Overview of Minimally Invasive Spine Surgery. World Neurosurg 2020; 142: 43-56.
[http://dx.doi.org/10.1016/j.wneu.2020.06.043] [PMID: 32544619]

[7]     Klingler JH, Sircar R, Scheiwe C, *et al.* Comparative Study of C-arms for Intraoperative 3-dimensional Imaging and Navigation in Minimally Invasive Spine Surgery Part I: Applicability and Image Quality. Clin Spine Surg 2017; 30(6): 276-84.
[http://dx.doi.org/10.1097/BSD.0000000000000186] [PMID: 28632551]

[8]     Afolabi A, Weir TB, Usmani MF, *et al.* Comparison of percutaneous minimally invasive *versus* open posterior spine surgery for fixation of thoracolumbar fractures: A retrospective matched cohort analysis. J Orthop 2019; 18: 185-90.
[http://dx.doi.org/10.1016/j.jor.2019.11.047] [PMID: 32042224]

[9]     Ghisi D, Fanelli A, Tosi M, Nuzzi M, Fanelli G. Monitored anesthesia care. Minerva Anestesiol 2005; 71(9): 533-8.
[PMID: 16166913]

[10]    Berkenstadt H, Perel A, Hadani M, Unofrievich I, Ram Z. Monitored anesthesia care using remifentanil and propofol for awake craniotomy. J Neurosurg Anesthesiol 2001; 13(3): 246-9.
[http://dx.doi.org/10.1097/00008506-200107000-00013] [PMID: 11426102]

[11]    Pergolizzi JV Jr, Gan TJ, Plavin S, Labhsetwar S, Taylor R. Perspectives on the role of fospropofol in the monitored anesthesia care setting. Anesthesiol Res Pract 2011; 2011: 458920.
[http://dx.doi.org/10.1155/2011/458920] [PMID: 21541247]

[12]    Barends CRM, Absalom AR, Struys MMRF. Drug selection for ambulatory procedural sedation. Curr Opin Anaesthesiol 2018; 31(6): 673-8.
[http://dx.doi.org/10.1097/ACO.0000000000000652] [PMID: 30124543]

[13]    García-Pedrajas F, Monedero P. Benzodiazepines in anesthesiology. Clinical applications (II). Rev Esp Anestesiol Reanim 1992; 39(2): 126-31.
[PMID: 1350685]

[14]    Riefkohl R, Cole NM, Cox EB. The effectiveness of benzodiazepines and narcotics in outpatient surgery. Aesthetic Plast Surg 1984; 8(4): 227-30.
[http://dx.doi.org/10.1007/BF01570708] [PMID: 6532165]

[15]    Loeffler PM. Oral benzodiazepines and conscious sedation: a review. J Oral Maxillofac Surg 1992; 50(9): 989-97.
[http://dx.doi.org/10.1016/0278-2391(92)90061-4] [PMID: 1354722]

[16]    Lepresle E, Debras C. Use of benzodiazepines in anesthesia and resuscitation. Encephale 1983; 9(4) (Suppl. 2): 267B-71B.
[PMID: 6144523]

[17]    Lewis BS, Shlien RD, Wayne JD, Knight RJ, Aldoroty RA. Diazepam *versus* midazolam (versed) in outpatient colonoscopy: a double-blind randomized study. Gastrointest Endosc 1989; 35(1): 33-6.
[http://dx.doi.org/10.1016/S0016-5107(89)72682-1] [PMID: 2920882]

[18]    Avramov MN, Smith I, White PF. Interactions between midazolam and remifentanil during monitored anesthesia care. Anesthesiology 1996; 85(6): 1283-9.
[http://dx.doi.org/10.1097/00000542-199612000-00009] [PMID: 8968175]

[19]   Taylor E, Ghouri AF, White PF. Midazolam in combination with propofol for sedation during local anesthesia. J Clin Anesth 1992; 4(3): 213-6.
[http://dx.doi.org/10.1016/0952-8180(92)90068-C] [PMID: 1610577]

[20]   Gold MI, Watkins WD, Sung YF, *et al.* Remifentanil *versus* remifentanil/midazolam for ambulatory surgery during monitored anesthesia care. Anesthesiology 1997; 87(1): 51-7.
[http://dx.doi.org/10.1097/00000542-199707000-00007] [PMID: 9232133]

[21]   Gelfman SS, Gracely RH, Driscoll EJ, Wirdzek PR, Sweet JB, Butler DP. Conscious sedation with intravenous drugs: a study of amnesia. J Oral Surg 1978; 36(3): 191-7.
[PMID: 272450]

[22]   Kwak HJ, Kim JY, Kim YB, Chae YJ, Kim JY. The optimum bolus dose of remifentanil to facilitate laryngeal mask airway insertion with a single standard dose of propofol at induction in children. Anaesthesia 2008; 63(9): 954-8.
[http://dx.doi.org/10.1111/j.1365-2044.2008.05544.x] [PMID: 18557970]

[23]   Hertzog JH, Campbell JK, Dalton HJ, Hauser GJ. Propofol anesthesia for invasive procedures in ambulatory and hospitalized children: experience in the pediatric intensive care unit. Pediatrics 1999; 103(3): E30.
[http://dx.doi.org/10.1542/peds.103.3.e30] [PMID: 10049986]

[24]   Frey K, Sukhani R, Pawlowski J, Pappas AL, Mikat-Stevens M, Slogoff S. Propofol *versus* propofol-ketamine sedation for retrobulbar nerve block: comparison of sedation quality, intraocular pressure changes, and recovery profiles. Anesth Analg 1999; 89(2): 317-21.
[PMID: 10439740]

[25]   Klein SM, Hauser GJ, Anderson BD, *et al.* Comparison of intermittent *versus* continuous infusion of propofol for elective oncology procedures in children. Pediatr Crit Care Med 2003; 4(1): 78-82.
[http://dx.doi.org/10.1097/00130478-200301000-00016] [PMID: 12656549]

[26]   Sukhani R, Lurie J, Jabamoni R. Propofol for ambulatory gynecologic laparoscopy: does omission of nitrous oxide alter postoperative emetic sequelae and recovery? Anesth Analg 1994; 78(5): 831-5.
[http://dx.doi.org/10.1213/00000539-199405000-00002] [PMID: 8160978]

[27]   Uusalo P, Guillaume S, Siren S, *et al.* Pharmacokinetics and sedative effects of intranasal dexmedetomidine in ambulatory pediatric patients. Anesth Analg 2020; 130(4): 949-57.
[http://dx.doi.org/10.1213/ANE.0000000000004264] [PMID: 31206433]

[28]   Kumari A, Singh AP, Vidhan J, Gupta R, Dhawan J, Kaur J. The sedative and propofol-sparing effect of dexmedetomidine and midazolam as premedicants in minor gynecological day care surgeries: a randomized placebo-controlled study. Anesth Essays Res 2018; 12(2): 423-7.
[http://dx.doi.org/10.4103/aer.AER_8_18] [PMID: 29962610]

[29]   Long K, Ruiz J, Kee S, *et al.* Effect of adjunctive dexmedetomidine on postoperative intravenous opioid administration in patients undergoing thyroidectomy in an ambulatory setting. J Clin Anesth 2016; 35: 361-4.
[http://dx.doi.org/10.1016/j.jclinane.2016.08.036] [PMID: 27871557]

[30]   Das A, Dutta S, Chattopadhyay S, *et al.* Pain relief after ambulatory hand surgery: a comparison between dexmedetomidine and clonidine as adjuvant in axillary brachial plexus block: A prospective, double-blinded, randomized controlled study. Saudi J Anaesth 2016; 10(1): 6-12.
[http://dx.doi.org/10.4103/1658-354X.169443] [PMID: 26955303]

[31]   Weerink MAS, Struys MMRF, Hannivoort LN, Barends CRM, Absalom AR, Colin P. Clinical pharmacokinetics and pharmacodynamics of dexmedetomidine. Clin Pharmacokinet 2017; 56(8): 893-913.
[http://dx.doi.org/10.1007/s40262-017-0507-7] [PMID: 28105598]

[32]   Wu JX, Assel M, Vickers A, *et al.* Impact of intraoperative remifentanil on postoperative pain and opioid use in thyroid surgery. J Surg Oncol 2019; 120(8): 1456-61.

[http://dx.doi.org/10.1002/jso.25746] [PMID: 31680250]

[33]   Torun AC, Yilmaz MZ, Ozkan N, Ustun B, Koksal E, Kaya C. Sedative-analgesic activity of remifentanil and effects of preoperative anxiety on perceived pain in outpatient mandibular third molar surgery. Int J Oral Maxillofac Implants 2017; 46(3): 379-84.
[http://dx.doi.org/10.1016/j.ijom.2016.11.005] [PMID: 27956057]

[34]   Sklika E, Kalimeris K, Perrea D, Stavropoulos N, Kostopanagiotou G, Matsota P. Remifentanil *Vs* fentanyl during day case dental surgery in people with special needs: a comparative, pilot study of their effect on stress response and postoperative pain. Middle East J Anaesthesiol 2016; 23(5): 509-15.
[PMID: 27487636]

[35]   Sclar DA. Remifentanil, fentanyl, or the combination in surgical procedures in the United States: predictors of use in patients with organ impairment or obesity. Clin Drug Investig 2015; 35(1): 53-9.
[http://dx.doi.org/10.1007/s40261-014-0251-9] [PMID: 25471739]

[36]   Hara R, Hirota K, Sato M, *et al.* The impact of remifentanil on incidence and severity of postoperative nausea and vomiting in a university hospital-based ambulatory surgery center: a retrospective observation study. Korean J Anesthesiol 2013; 65(2): 142-6.
[http://dx.doi.org/10.4097/kjae.2013.65.2.142] [PMID: 24023997]

[37]   Chillemi S, Sinardi D, Marino A, Mantarro G, Campisi R. The use of remifentanil for bloodless surgical field during vertebral disc resection. Minerva Anestesiol 2002; 68(9): 645-9.
[PMID: 12370680]

[38]   Garg K, Grewal G, Grewal A, *et al.* Hemodynamic responses with different dose of ketamine and propofol in day care gynecological surgeries. J Clin Diagn Res 2013; 7(11): 2548-50.
[http://dx.doi.org/10.7860/JCDR/2013/6860.3607] [PMID: 24392397]

[39]   Kramer KJ, Ganzberg S, Prior S, Rashid RG. Comparison of propofol-remifentanil *versus* propofol-ketamine deep sedation for third molar surgery. Anesth Prog 2012; 59(3): 107-17.
[http://dx.doi.org/10.2344/12-00001.1] [PMID: 23050750]

[40]   Cillo JE Jr. Analysis of propofol and low-dose ketamine admixtures for adult outpatient dentoalveolar surgery: a prospective, randomized, positive-controlled clinical trial. J Oral Maxillofac Surg 2012; 70(3): 537-46.
[http://dx.doi.org/10.1016/j.joms.2011.08.036] [PMID: 22177821]

[41]   Aydin ON, Ugur B, Ozgun S, Eyigör H, Copcu O. Pain prevention with intraoperative ketamine in outpatient children undergoing tonsillectomy or tonsillectomy and adenotomy. J Clin Anesth 2007; 19(2): 115-9.
[http://dx.doi.org/10.1016/j.jclinane.2006.06.003] [PMID: 17379123]

[42]   White M, de Graaff P, Renshof B, van Kan E, Dzoljic M. Pharmacokinetics of S(+) ketamine derived from target controlled infusion. Br J Anaesth 2006; 96(3): 330-4.
[http://dx.doi.org/10.1093/bja/aei316] [PMID: 16415315]

[43]   Dalsasso M, Tresin P, Innocente F, Veronese S, Ori C. Low-dose ketamine with clonidine and midazolam for adult day care surgery. Eur J Anaesthesiol 2005; 22(1): 67-8.
[http://dx.doi.org/10.1097/00003643-200501000-00014] [PMID: 15816577]

[44]   Ersek RA. Dissociative anesthesia for safety's sake: ketamine and diazepam--a 35-year personal experience. Plast Reconstr Surg 2004; 113(7): 1955-9.
[http://dx.doi.org/10.1097/01.PRS.0000122402.52595.10] [PMID: 15253183]

[45]   Badrinath S, Avramov MN, Shadrick M, Witt TR, Ivankovich AD. The use of a ketamine-propofol combination during monitored anesthesia care. Anesth Analg 2000; 90(4): 858-62.
[http://dx.doi.org/10.1213/00000539-200004000-00016] [PMID: 10735789]

CHAPTER 3

# Algorithms to Choose Between Anterior and Posterior Cervical Endoscopy

**Álvaro Dowling**[1,2], **Kai-Uwe Lewandrowski**[3,4,5,*] and **Helton Delfino**[6]

*¹ Endoscopic Spine Clinic, Santiago, Chile*

*² Department of Orthopaedic Surgery, USP, Ribeirão Preto, Brazil*

*³ Center for Advanced Spine Care of Southern Arizona and Surgical Institute of Tucson, Tucson, AZ, USA*

*⁴ Department of Orthopaedic Surgery, UNIRIO, Rio de Janeiro, Brazil*

*⁵ Department of Orthoapedic Surgery, Fundación Universitaria Sanitas, Bogotá, D.C., Colombia, USA*

*⁶ Department of Orthopaedic and Anesthesiology, Ribeirão Preto Medical School, University of São Paulo, São Paulo, Brazil*

**Abstract:** Full endoscopic surgery of the cervical spine has gained more popularity, raising the question of its indications, patient selection criteria, and the appropriate choice of the various anterior and posterior techniques. In this chapter, the authors attempt to delineate the criteria for selecting patients for the different full endoscopic surgical techniques for the cervical spine's common painful degenerative conditions. The authors review the common forms of surgical pathology, including foraminal, lateral- and central canal stenosis, and distinguish between radiculopathy and myelopathy. They introduce algorithms for the full endoscopic treatment of these conditions by relying on validated classification systems for cervical disc herniations and their associated appearance on advanced imaging studies, including magnetic resonance imaging and computed tomography. Moreover, the authors review the risks, contraindications, and limitations of the various anterior and posterior full endoscopic surgery techniques related to the current technology standards.

**Keywords:** Anterior and posterior approaches, Cervical foraminal and central stenosis, Cervical herniated disc, Full endoscopy, Indications, Iimitations.

* **Corresponding author Kai-Uwe Lewandrowski:** Center for Advanced Spine Care of Southern Arizona and Surgical Institute of Tucson, Tucson, AZ, USA, Department of Orthopaedic Surgery, UNIRIO, Rio de Janeiro, Brazil and Department of Orthoapedic Surgery, Fundación Universitaria Sanitas, Bogotá, D.C., Colombia, USA; Tel: +1 520 204-1495; Fax: +1 623 218-1215; E-mail: business@tucsonspine.com

Kai-Uwe Lewandrowski, Jorge Felipe Ramírez León, Anthony Yeung, Hyeun-Sung Kim, Xifeng Zhang, Gun Choi, Stefan Hellinger and Álvaro Dowling (Eds.)

## INTRODUCTION

Innovative technology and techniques have revolutionized the minimally invasive spine (MIS) surgery of the lumbar spine [1 - 12]. Cervical pathologies present with different anatomical problems, indications, and risks [13 - 17]. MIS applications have gained some traction in posterior cervical spine surgeries [18 - 22], but endoscopic surgery has taken longer to garner support in the cervical spine [23 - 29]. The smaller working space, proximity to vital structures, and the potentially high-risk nature of operating on compressive pathology affecting the spinal cord and the exiting nerve roots [15, 17]. Anterior cervical approaches can be complicated by injury to the great vessels, dysphagia, and phonation problems [13]. Posterior approaches can result in severe postoperative neck pain from muscular dissection and delayed iatrogenic deformities and instability [30, 31]. Consideration of fusion and non-fusion procedures also play a critical role in surgical decision making of MIS cervical MIS options [32 - 35]. Despite these potential problems, advances in MIS surgery for common cervical pathologies have gained traction in recently with many peer-reviewed articles having been published within the last year alone [21, 23, 25, 36 - 44].

Anterior endoscopic approaches have been employed to treat soft hernias, axillary stenosis due to uncovertebral hypertrophy, and central decompression and fusion for endstage degenerative disc disease, instability, and spinal cord compression [38, 39, 42, 44 - 46]. Posterior endoscopic approaches were practical for decompressive laminotomy and foraminotomy in treating lateral cervical canal stenosis and paramedial hernias [27, 43, 46, 47]. Advances in spinal instrumentation have permitted to replace traditional lateral mass screw and rod constructs with percutaneous facet screws, further facilitating the application of MIS techniques in the cervical spine [48, 49]. Advanced surgeon training and refined skill level, as well as enhanced understanding of the indications and outcomes with endoscopic cervical spinal surgery, have let to an increase in these procedures, as reflected by the number of recent peer-reviewed publications being on the rise [50]. In the following, we describe an algorithm for the best choice of these novel endoscopic surgery techniques to treat the cervical spine's common degenerative conditions. Classification of the compressive pathology to be treated is an appropriate way to build an algorithm for the optimum choice of anterior *versus* posterior full endoscopic approach to the cervical spine. However, as with most surgical procedures, algorithms, while complying with many evidence-based concepts, it is becoming more critical to depend on not just on safety, cost-effectiveness, and the concept, but as a surgical procedure, the surgeon factor and the surgical skill of each individual surgeon is the big variable that cannot be defined by algorithms. Therefore, the authors of this chapter ask the prospective endoscopic spine surgeon take their own training and skill level into account when attempting to perform these full endoscopic procedures in the cervical spine.

## HERNIATED DISC

The level and the location of the herniated disc in the disease cervical motion segment is a-critical consideration. Secondary considerations relate to whether the disc herniation is soft or calcified as different endoscopic instruments and procedural steps may be required for these calcified herniations. The retraction of cervical nerve roots and the spinal cord may be less practical and is best avoided. The inability to retract these sensitive neural elements dictates surgical exposure and approaches in particular with central disc herniations at the C4/5 level, where the risk for the neurological deficit is the highest – patients may develop a postoperative C5 nerve palsy, which is by far the most commonly reported neurological complication with cervical spine surgery in general [45]. In comparison, a paramedian disc herniation may be decompressed by both approaches. Absolute and relative contraindications to spinal endoscopy applications in the cervical spine may exist in some individual or particular situations. For example, the anterior approach may be contraindicated in collapsed disc spaces where the disc height is less than 4 mm, making the introduction of the endoscopic working cannula virtually impossible with most current systems. Another example is a large anterior vertebral osteophyte or discal calcification. Also, cases involving substantial craniocaudal disc sequestration may be a complete contraindication to anterior cervical endoscopic discectomy (ACED) because of a high likelihood of causing iatrogenic injury to the spinal cord. This team of authors routinely employs the criteria of the Odom classification of cervical herniated disc when stratifying patients for endoscopic discectomyy surgery (Table **1**) [51 - 54] Examplary intraoperative images of PECD and AECD are shown in Fig. (**1**).

Table 1.  Types of cervical disc herniations ad defined by the Odom classification [54].

| Odom Classification | |
| --- | --- |
| **Type I** | Unilateral soft disc protrusion with nerve root compression |
| **Type II** | Foraminal spur or hard disc with nerve root compression |
| **Type III** | Medial soft disc protrusion with spinal root compression |
| **Type IV** | Transverse ridge or cervical spondylosis with spinal cord compression |

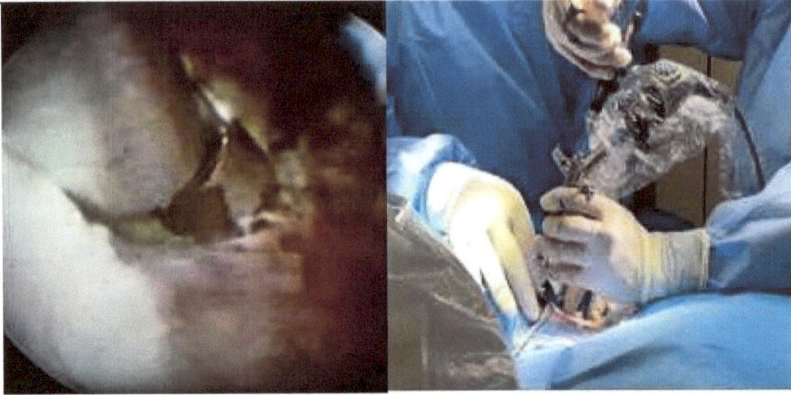

Fig. (1). a) shown is an Intraoperative view through the cervical spinal endoscope during posterior endoscopic cervical discectomy (PECD) and b) an intraoperative photograph during anterior endoscopic cervical discectomy (AECD).

Yang *et al.* published the first comparative study between the anterior and posterior approaches for full-endoscopic cervical discectomy (FECD) in the treatment of cervical intervertebral disc herniation (CIVDH) [46]. These authors reported clinical results of 84 consecutive patients with symptomatic CIVDH who underwent FECD using the anterior or posterior approach between the years of 2010-2012.

Their patients had a disc height higher than 4 mm and exclusively underwent single-level fusion. No foraminal stenosis without hernia was included. The clinical outcomes were equally favorable with both approaches. The authors reported a decreased postoperative vertical height of the operated cervical motion segment, particularly in the patients' anterior approach. This observation was attributed to a higher quantity of disc tissue being removed with the anterior transdiscal approach. None of the posterior approach patients experienced kyphosis or instability.

## ALGORITHM FOR HERNIATED DISC

Patient selection is crucially important when selecting patients for endoscopic cervical decompression and discectomy surgery. As a result of their combined clinical experience and consensus discussion amongst each other taking current clincial and technology standards into account, the authors recommend the discision algorithm shown in Fig. (2) for determining the most appropriate surgical approach and surgical treatment.

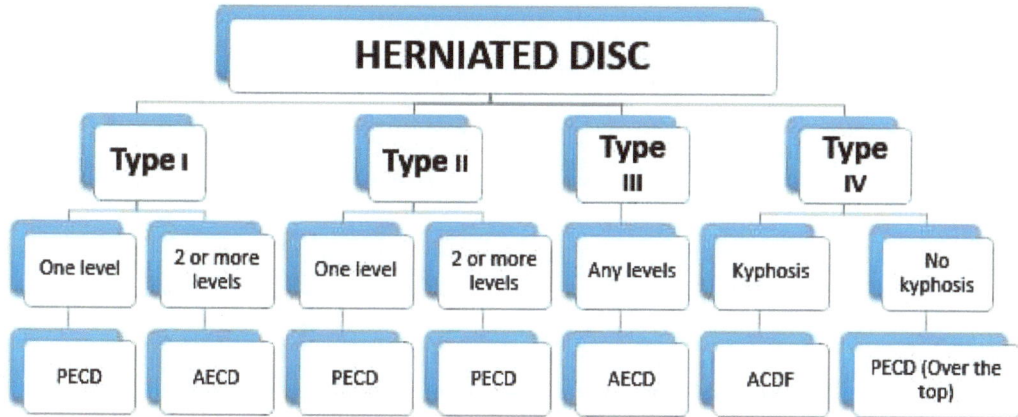

**Fig. (2).** Decision algorithm for selecting patients with symptomatic cervical herniated disc for anterior or posterior endoscopic *versus* traditional anterior cervical discectomy and fusion surgery employing the Odom classification of cervical herniated disc: PECD – posterior endoscopic cervical discectomy, AECD – anterior endoscopic cervical discectomy, ACDF – anterior cervical discectomy and fusion.

## ALGORITHM FOR FORAMINAL STENOSIS

Approximately 20% of degenerative cervical conditions requiring surgical intervention are due to foraminal stenosis. Treatment decisions are determined predominantly by the individual surgeon's preference and skill level. The authors' preferred surgical treatment for foraminal stenosis is to use PECF because it can be performed under local anesthesia and sedation with continuous neurological monitoring and monitored anesthesia care (MAC) protocols. When treating patients with foraminal stenosis at the C4-C5 levels, our surgical protocol calls for extension of the decompression laterally to resect part of the pedicle. This partial pediculoectomy is intended to minimize injury to the C5 nerve root. Preoperative imaging studies should be carefully reviewed for any anatomical anomalies to avoid surprises during surgery. Generally, this chapter's authors prefer posterior endoscopic cervical foraminotomy (PECF) for unilateral radiculopathy with arm pain unless there is a concomitant central disc hernia or biforaminal stenosis or kyphosis. In those patients with these problems, the anterior endoscopic approach is preferred.

Cervical monoradiculopathy symptoms is in the authors opinion the preferred indication for PECF. For example, recurrent mono-radicular symptoms with unilateral or bilateral neck, shoulder, and arm pain due to cage subsidence following ACDF. Recently, the reoperation rates after index ACDF were reported as part of several prospective randomized FDA trials for cervical total disc arthroplasty, where ACDF served as a control arm. These five trails reported the ACDF reoperation rate within two years of the index procedure of 9.02%. Occasionally, diabetic [56] or smoker [57] patients have a painless motor radiculopathy syndrome. Because this focal anteriorly located pathology - graded 2ª according to the modified Kim classification (Fig. **3**) - does not cause relevant compression of the sensory and nociceptive dorsal nerve root or spinal ganglion, and produces an isolated motor deficits can occur without concomitant pain or sensory deficits [55, 58].

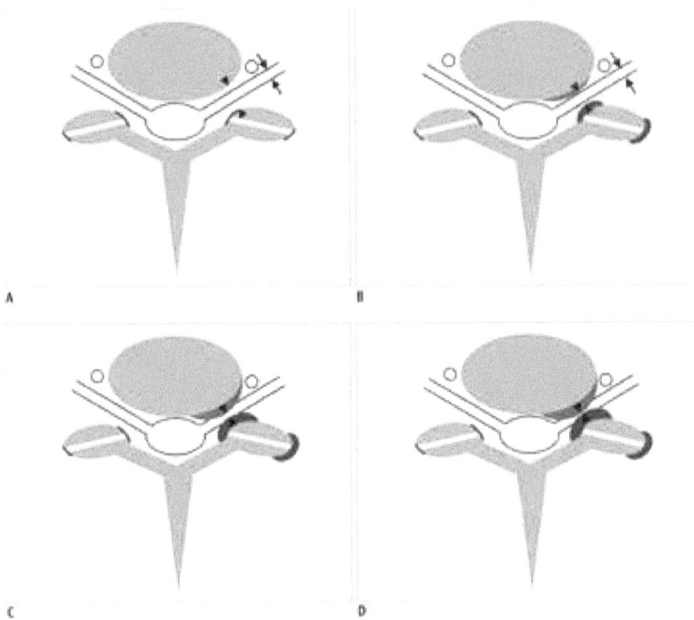

**Fig. (3).** "**A, B**. Grade 0, normal-absence of neural foraminal stenosis with narrowest width of neural foramen (arrowheads) more than extraforaminal nerve root (black arrows). A shows no narrowing of neural foramen, and **B** shows mild narrowing. **C**. Grade 1, non-severe cervical neural foraminal stenosis, including narrowest width of neural foramen (arrowheads) same or less than (but more than 50% of) extraforaminal nerve root width. **D**. Grade 2, severe cervical neural foraminal stenosis, including narrowest width of neural foramen (arrowheads) same or less than 50% of extraforaminal nerve root width." Reproduced and cited from Kim *et al.* [55].

This isolated ventral nerve root compression was overwhelmingly identified in 98.0% of all cases and was strongly associated with the clinical syndrome of painless severe paresis of the respective nerve root [59]. The causative ventral pathology can easily be classified on MRI as a highly characteristic imaging pattern making MRI and CT the diagnostic tool of choice for this rare clinical syndrome. Overall, 4% of all patients with an indication for surgical decompression of the cervical nerve roots due to degenerative diseases were found to have this rare form of radiculopathy [59]. If this problem occurs at C4/5 – arguably, the most high-risk level for neurological injury – PECF could, in the authors' opinion, still be considered because the exiting C5 nerve root could be retracted sufficiently after a partial dorsal pediculolectomy and removal of the anterior osteophyte without undue risk of neurological injury. The algorithm for foraminal stenosis is summarized in Fig. (**4**).

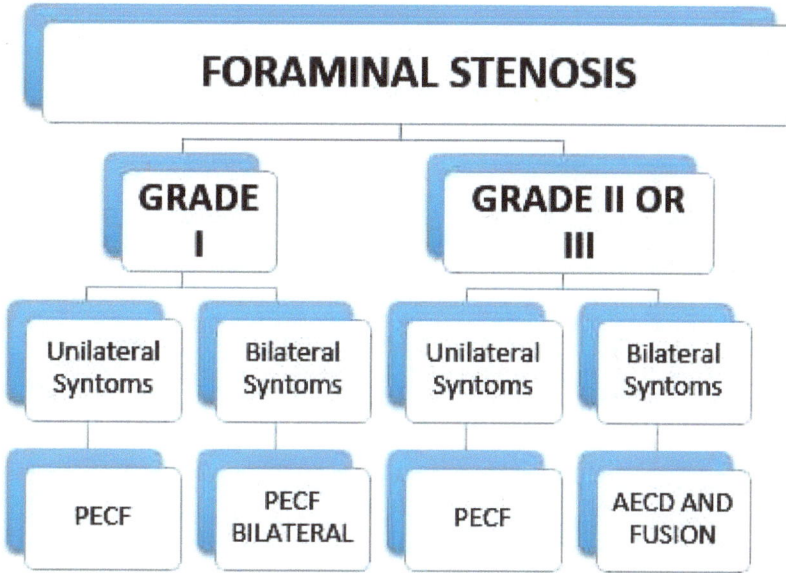

**Fig. (4).** Decision algorithm for selecting patients with symptomatic cervical foraminal stenosis for posterior endoscopic endoscopic cervical discectomy (PECD) *versus* anterior endoscopic cervical discectomy (AECD) and anterior cervical discectomy and fusion (ACDF) surgery employing Kim's classification of cervical foraminal stenosis.

## ALGORITHM FOR CENTRAL CERVICAL STENOSIS

The indications for full endoscopic surgery for central cervical stenosis was less clearly defined until recently. Few publications outline the success of the full endoscopic technique when applied in patients suffering from symptomatic central cervical stenosis [28, 60 - 63]. One study employed full endoscopy in conjunction with MED-type tubular retractors and reported satisfactory clincial outcomes in the patients studied. good results [62].

Generally, the central cervical canal stenosis should be approached from the side of where the compressive pathology is located. For example, infolding hypertrophied ligamentum flavum should be approached with posterior full endoscopic technique. A centrally located cervical disc herniation or end-stage degenerative disc-osteophyte complex, or ossified posterior longitudinal ligament should be addressed employing an anterior full endoscopic technique [64]. Fusion with interbody cages should be considered in patients with kyphosis (Fig. **5**). There are several limitations for both techniques which makes the choice of procedure highly dependent on the surgeon's experience and skill level.

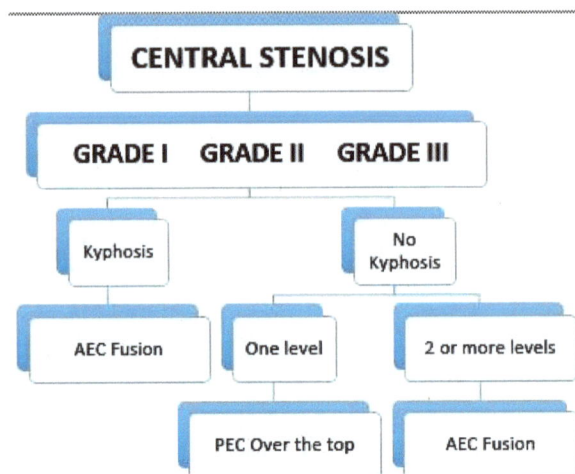

**Fig. (5).** Decision algorithm for selecting patients with symptomatic central cervical stenosis depending on the presence of kyphosis and number of levels involved. Severity of stenosis is secondary. AEC - Anterior endoscopic cervical, PEC – posterior endoscopic cervical.

One of the potential limitations of the PECD technique with the current technology is that it is mostly only practical when applied to one level. While multilevel PECD full endoscopic decompressions are theoretically conceivable, the authors observed that it prolongs operative times substantially and increases the amount of irrigation fluid trapped in the posterior cervical musculature.

Typically, after a one-level full endoscopic PECD, enough time has passed beyond which M.A.C. anesthesia under monitored sedation (preferred by A.D.) in the prone position becomes too uncomfortable for the patient, or the postoperative wound swelling from entrapped irrigation fluid is at a point where it takes away from the ambulatory nature of the procedure. The two senior endoscopic spine surgeon authors of this chapter (A.D. and K.U.L.) perform most of their surgeries in an ambulatory surgery center (A.S.C.).

The question of the most appropriate choice of anesthesia for these full-endoscopic surgeries in the cervical spine has been discussed at length in another chapter in this text, and the authors would refer the reader to this reading when considering treatment of central cervical stenosis. Therefore, such procedure-related limitations and time constraints may play out differently in the hands of highly-skilled or novice endoscopic spine surgeons when scheduling patients for single- or multilevel full endoscopic surgery from anterior or posterior approach (Figs. **6** and **7**).

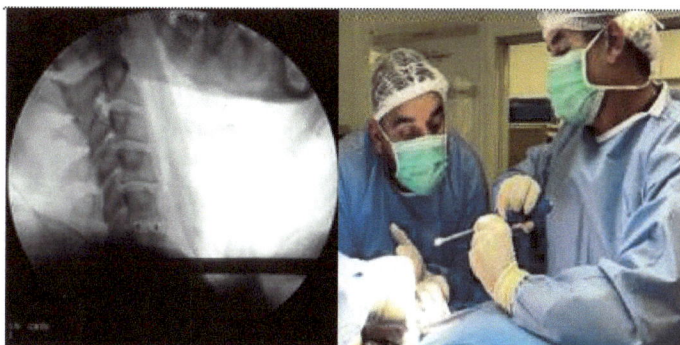

**Fig. (6).** Anterior endoscopic cervical discectomy (AECD) with fusion at the C5/6 level and C6/7 AECD without fusion under monitored anesthesia care with secation with the patient in supine position and a nasal cannula without intubation.

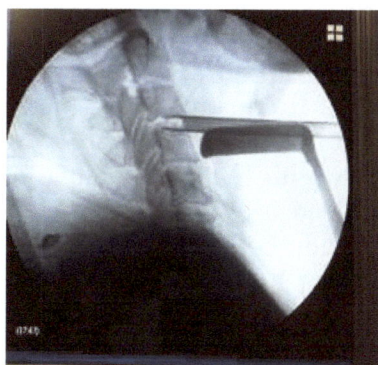

**Fig. (7).** Mini-open AECD at C2/3 where the approach was done through a small less than 2 cm skin incision, digital dissection, placement of an endoscopic working cannular after serial dilation. Initially, the authors utilized this technique during the endoscopically assisted anterior cervical decompression surgeries before transitioning to the full endoscopic technique.

There may be specific case scenarios where anterior alone or combined anterior and posterior approach techniques may be considered. However, combined anterior and posterior approaches are typically impractical in an ASC. They should be staged and scheduled on different days since these surgeries require an entirely different setup in the prone or supine position in the operating room. Performing these procedures in the same sitting goes against the high turnover in ASC and may pose an additional undue risk for neurologically injured patients. Therefore, the authors do not perform these combined procedures but stage them when deemed indicated to allow the patient to recover from one procedure's insult before commencing the other.

## THE IMPACT OF TECHNOLOGY ADVANCES

In the last decade, there also has been a transition endoscopically assisted to full endoscopy surgery of the cervical spine. Instead of using the endoscope through a MED-type tubular retractor [65], the cervical spinal endoscope is directly introduced through a much smaller endoscopic working cannula, which further reduced the surgical trauma but may also impact the choice of PECD *versus* AECD based on the available endoscopic equipment at the disposal of the operating endoscopic spine surgeon. Having access to power burrs, drills, Kerrison rongeurs, chisels, and other custom endoscopic instrument designed to perform specific maneuvers during the PECD and AECD procedures certainly speeds up the decompression and may change how surgeons indicate full endoscopic spine surgeries in their patients and how they choose anterior *versus* posterior or combined endoscopic approaches. The authors expect that such technology advances affording more efficient decompression or reconstruction of more complex spinal pathology with associated instability or deformity will likely impact the future direction of this ultra-minimally invasive procedure. The senior endoscopic spine surgeons (A.D. and K.U.L.) have transitioned their endoscopic cervical spine surgery program from employing a small less than 2 cm anterior cervical incision, digital dissection with the little finger, palpation of the anterior cervical spine, serial dilation with the placement of a small tubular retractor through which they introduced a spinal endoscope to execute the actual discectomy surgery, to a full endoscopic procedure with the use of an endoscopic working cannula. Other authors beautifully describe the procedural technique steps of this full endoscopic AECD in their respective chapters of this text.

## DISCUSSION

Recent technology advances may add to the confusion as to how to efficiently employ full endoscopic spinal surgery in the cervical spine. Particularly, for the novice spine surgeon navigating this seemingly disorganized field may be difficult. There is a relative lack of articles on full endoscopic cervical spine surgery, even in the most recent literature [66]. However, a few landmark studies comparing the various anterior and posterior full endoscopic surgery techniques to traditional open and other forms of MIS surgeries have been published [22, 36, 67 - 69]. However, full endoscopic surgery of the cervical spine is far from mainstream, and it continues to be practiced by few. Potential reasons include the high skill level required to safely execute the surgery, the high-risk nature compared to lumbar endoscopy, and the lack of clarity on its surgical indications. The authors of this chapter set out to remedy the latter problem.

As with any painful spinal pathology, the location, extent of neural compression, and the structural nature of the compressive pathology – whether soft herniation, or hard calcified disc herniation, a central or foraminal osteophyte complex, a thickened or infolding ligamentum flacum, or an ossified posterior longtudinal ligament – must be considered. In the case of cervical disc herniations requiring decompression, the surgeon should be aware of each individual patients specific anatomy and classifiy the location of the associated central and foraminal stenosis carefully. Classification systems provided by Odom *et al.* [51 - 53, 70] and Kim *et al.* [55, 58, 71] have proven useful in the authors day-to-day routine clincial practice. Anatomical considerations including higher risk of surgery at the C4/5 level with injury to the C5 nerve root should be taken into account.

In this chapter, the authors presented several algorithms for cervical herniated disc, as well as stenosis in the foramen, lateral, and central canal (Figs. **2** - **4**). Over the years, we have made several observations worth discussing within the framework of this chapter. For example, soft central cervical disc herniations may best be treated with AECD. The procedure is fast and more efficient, especially in patients with end-stage degenerative disc disease who may be a candidate for fusion because of vertical collapse or kyphotic deformity. Fusion may be considered as an adjunct to AECD at each surgeon's discretion. AECD is undoubtedly a more straightforward procedure than ACDF and appears more appropriate for the ASC setting. We always choose AECD in cases of central soft herniations. These types of patients are also generally suitable for MAC in the outpatient spine surgery center. The simplicity of this percutaneous approach and minimal dissection required to reach the anterior cervical spine by employing serial dilation and placement of a percutaneous endoscopic working cannula make AECD highly suitable for an outpatient full endoscopic cervical spine surgery program. Depending on available equipment and each surgeon's skill level, surgeons may decide to avoid degenerative cervical disc spaces that have collapsed to less than 4 mm of residual anterior disc height. However, this experienced team of authors has found no difference in the degree of difficulty or clinical outcomes with the AECD. Perhaps systematic clinical investigations with longer follow-up could provide higher-grade clinical evidence in the future. Few surgeons perform AECD, making it difficult to conduct more sophisticated studies beyond the scope of a single site or single surgeon retrospective analysis to produce higher-grade clinical evidence.

In cases of symptomatic myelopathy central stenosis, patients often require more extensive decompression. Cervical myelopathy can typically present with gait disturbance, motor weakness, loss of hand dexterity, bowel or bladder dysfunction, and paresthesia [72 - 77]. In 2018, Jian Shen *et al.* published eighteen patients who underwent fully endoscopic posterior cervical bilateral laminotomy and decompression *via* a unilateral approach [69]. The authors operated on one to three levels with an average surgery time of 72 minutes. They had no surgery-related complications. Muscle weakness and sensory deficit significantly improved in all patients. The gait improved in 15 patients. Analysis of the modified score of the Japanese Orthopaedic Association (mJOA) scores also improved at a statistically significant level. The same team of authors suggested other approaches [69]. In 2019, Qian Du *et al.* published a novel application of the transcorporeal AECD technique on a limited series of 4 patients to reduce disc height-associated full-endoscopic AECD [23]. Others had reported the utility of this approach previously [78 - 82]. The authors reported decreased vertical collapse rates after AECD and recommended channel repair criteria [83]. Including vertical collapse analysis into the algorithms provided herein was beyond this chapter's scope but may become relevant in the future as the full endoscopic cervical surgery gains more traction and case numbers increase.

Preliminary results with the full endoscopic technique are encouraging especially because nowadays there are spinal endoscopes with large working channels that allow us to use more effective decompression instruments. On the flipside of these advanced motorized power instruments is the danger of injury the cervical nerve roots and spinal cord due to vibration or torque of the high-speed motorized instrument. Nonetheless, there is no question that these modern endoscopes with large working channels are an advance of the now outdated endoscopically assisted tubular retractor surgery described above. From todays perspective, some of these endoscopically assisted techniques that used to involve microsurgical dissection at times to assist during the initial steps of the procedure seem utterly outdated particularly when it comes to the quality of the videoendoscopic visualization of the anterior cervical spine, the interior of the disc space, cervical nerve roots and spinal cord and its vascular supply. The irrigated full endoscopic surgery provides excellent highly magnified views of the compressive pathology and the remaining surgical anatomy while maintaining hemostasis due to the lavage effect under minimal hydrostatic pressure.

## CONCLUSIONS

Both AECD and PECD are useful modern full endoscopic minimally invasive surgery techniques. The contemporary literature suggests that in skilled hands, favorable clinical outcomes can be achieved with both techniques. However, there are some limitations to be considered. While most clinically relevant compressive pathology in the cervical spine may be addressed with the PECD through the posterior approach, the procedure is not entirely practical in an outpatient setting under MAC anesthesia for more than one level. Multilevel procedures are not recommended at least to the novice surgeon. Additional contraindications may arise in patients with instability or excessive deformity or focal kyphosis about the surgical level. Clinical outcomes in patients with these conditions should be further studied. Anterior pathology, such as OPLL, may not be reached with the PECD approach. AECD is most suitable for predominantly anterior pathology.

Multilevel decompressions with the addition of fusion, if indicated, are feasible. The authors recommend employing their proposed algorithms to stratify patients with foraminal, central, anterior, and posterior pathology for the cervical spine's full endoscopic surgery.

## CONSENT FOR PUBLICATION

Not applicable.

## CONFLICT OF INTEREST

The author declares no conflict of interest, financial or otherwise.

## ACKNOWLEDGEMENTS

Declared none.

## REFERENCES

[1]     Gao K, Yang H, Yang LQ, Hu MQ. Application of intervertebral foramen endoscopy BEIS technique in the lumbar spine surgery failure syndrome over 60 years old. Zhongguo Gu Shang 2019; 32(7): 647-52.
        [PMID: 31382724]

[2]     Heo DH, Lee DC, Park CK. Comparative analysis of three types of minimally invasive decompressive surgery for lumbar central stenosis: biportal endoscopy, uniportal endoscopy, and microsurgery. Neurosurg Focus 2019; 46(5): E9.
        [http://dx.doi.org/10.3171/2019.2.FOCUS197] [PMID: 31042664]

[3]     Ishimoto Y, Yamada H, Curtis E, *et al.* Spinal endoscopy for delayed-onset lumbar radiculopathy resulting from foraminal stenosis after osteoporotic vertebral fracture: a case report of a new surgical strategy. Case Rep Orthop 2018; 2018: 1593021.
        [http://dx.doi.org/10.1155/2018/1593021] [PMID: 30498611]

[4]     Kim HS, Adsul N, Kapoor A, *et al.* A mobile outside-in technique of transforaminal lumbar endoscopy for lumbar disc herniations. J Vis Exp 2018; 138: 57999.

[5]     Kim JE, Choi DJ. Unilateral biportal endoscopic decompression by 30° endoscopy in lumbar spinal stenosis: technical note and preliminary report. J Orthop 2018; 15(2): 366-71.
        [http://dx.doi.org/10.1016/j.jor.2018.01.039] [PMID: 29881155]

[6]     Komatsu J, Iwabuchi M, Endo T, *et al.* Clinical outcomes of lumbar diseases specific test in patients who undergo endoscopy-assisted tubular surgery with lumbar herniated nucleus pulposus: an analysis using the Japanese Orthopaedic Association Back Pain Evaluation Questionnaire (JOABPEQ). Eur J Orthop Surg Traumatol 2019; 30(2): 207-13.
        [PMID: 31595359]

[7]     Leu H, Schreiber A. Percutaneous nucleotomy with disk endoscopy--a minimally invasive therapy in non-sequestrated intervertebral disk hernia. Schweiz Rundsch Med Prax 1991; 80(14): 364-8.
        [PMID: 2034933]

[8]     Lewandrowski K-U. The strategies behind "inside-out" and "outside-in" endoscopy of the lumbar spine: treating the pain generator. J Spine Surg 2020; 6 (Suppl. 1): S35-9.
        [http://dx.doi.org/10.21037/jss.2019.06.06] [PMID: 32195412]

[9]     Song H, Hu W, Liu Z, Hao Y, Zhang X. Percutaneous endoscopic interlaminar discectomy of L5-S1

disc herniation: a comparison between intermittent endoscopy technique and full endoscopy technique. J Orthop Surg Res 2017; 12(1): 162.
[http://dx.doi.org/10.1186/s13018-017-0662-4] [PMID: 29084558]

[10] Xin Z, Huang P, Zheng G, Liao W, Zhang X, Wang Y. Using a percutaneous spinal endoscopy unilateral posterior interlaminar approach to perform bilateral decompression for patients with lumbar lateral recess stenosis. Asian J Surg 2020; 43(5): 593-602.
[PMID: 31594687]

[11] Yeung AT. The evolution of percutaneous spinal endoscopy and discectomy: state of the art. Mt Sinai J Med 2000; 67(4): 327-32.
[PMID: 11021785]

[12] Yoshimoto M, Miyakawa T, Takebayashi T, *et al.* Microendoscopy-assisted muscle-preserving interlaminar decompression for lumbar spinal stenosis: clinical results of consecutive 105 cases with more than 3-year follow-up. Spine 2014; 39(5): E318-25.
[http://dx.doi.org/10.1097/BRS.0000000000000160] [PMID: 24365896]

[13] Arshi A, Wang C, Park HY, *et al.* Ambulatory anterior cervical discectomy and fusion is associated with a higher risk of revision surgery and perioperative complications: an analysis of a large nationwide database. Spine J 2018; 18(7): 1180-7.
[http://dx.doi.org/10.1016/j.spinee.2017.11.012] [PMID: 29155340]

[14] Engel A, Rappard G, King W, Kennedy DJ. Standards division of the international spine intervention society. The effectiveness and risks of fluoroscopically-guided cervical medial branch thermal radiofrequency neurotomy: a systematic review with comprehensive analysis of the published data. Pain Med 2016; 17(4): 658-69.
[http://dx.doi.org/10.1111/pme.12928] [PMID: 26359589]

[15] Narain AS, Hijji FY, Haws BE, *et al.* Risk factors for medical and surgical complications after 1--level anterior cervical discectomy and fusion procedures. Int J Spine Surg 2020; 14(3): 286-93.
[http://dx.doi.org/10.14444/7038] [PMID: 32699749]

[16] Quarrington RD, Jones CF, Tcherveniakov P, *et al.* Traumatic subaxial cervical facet subluxation and dislocation: epidemiology, radiographic analyses, and risk factors for spinal cord injury. Spine J 2018; 18(3): 387-98.
[http://dx.doi.org/10.1016/j.spinee.2017.07.175] [PMID: 28739474]

[17] Yew AY, Nguyen MT, Hsu WK, Patel AA. Quantitative risk factor analysis of postoperative dysphagia after Anterior Cervical Discectomy and Fusion (ACDF) using the eating assessment tool-10 (EAT-10). Spine 2019; 44(2): E82-8.
[http://dx.doi.org/10.1097/BRS.0000000000002770] [PMID: 29965886]

[18] Adamson TE. Microendoscopic posterior cervical laminoforaminotomy for unilateral radiculopathy: results of a new technique in 100 cases. J Neurosurg 2001; 95(1) (Suppl.): 51-7.
[PMID: 11453432]

[19] Benedetti A, Carbonin C, Colombo F. Extended posterior cervical rhizotomy for severe spastic syndromes with dyskinesias. Appl Neurophysiol 1977-1978; 40(1): 41-7.
[PMID: 666311]

[20] Fang W, Huang L, Feng F, *et al.* Anterior cervical discectomy and fusion *versus* posterior cervical foraminotomy for the treatment of single-level unilateral cervical radiculopathy: a meta-analysis. J Orthop Surg Res 2020; 15(1): 202.
[http://dx.doi.org/10.1186/s13018-020-01723-5] [PMID: 32487109]

[21] Li C, Tang X, Chen S, Meng Y, Zhang W. Clinical application of large channel endoscopic decompression in posterior cervical spine disorders. BMC Musculoskelet Disord 2019; 20(1): 548.
[http://dx.doi.org/10.1186/s12891-019-2920-6] [PMID: 31739780]

[22] Yuchi CX, Sun G, Chen C, *et al.* Comparison of the biomechanical changes after percutaneous full-endoscopic anterior cervical discectomy *versus* posterior cervical foraminotomy at C5-C6: a finite

element-based study. World Neurosurg 2019; 128: e905-11.
[http://dx.doi.org/10.1016/j.wneu.2019.05.025] [PMID: 31096026]

[23]   Du Q, Lei LQ, Cao GR, *et al.* Percutaneous full-endoscopic anterior transcorporeal cervical discectomy and channel repair: a technique note report. BMC Musculoskelet Disord 2019; 20(1): 280.
[http://dx.doi.org/10.1186/s12891-019-2659-0] [PMID: 31182078]

[24]   Fontanella A. Endoscopic microsurgery in herniated cervical discs. Neurol Res 1999; 21(1): 31-8.
[http://dx.doi.org/10.1080/01616412.1999.11740888] [PMID: 10048051]

[25]   Oezdemir S, Komp M, Hahn P, Ruetten S. Decompression for cervical disc herniation using the full-endoscopic anterior technique. Oper Orthop Traumatol 2019; 31 (Suppl. 1): 1-10.
[http://dx.doi.org/10.1007/s00064-018-0531-2] [PMID: 29392340]

[26]   Ruetten S, Komp M, Merk H, Godolias G. A new full-endoscopic technique for cervical posterior foraminotomy in the treatment of lateral disc herniations using 6.9-mm endoscopes: prospective 2-year results of 87 patients. Minim Invasive Neurosurg 2007; 50(4): 219-26.
[http://dx.doi.org/10.1055/s-2007-985860] [PMID: 17948181]

[27]   Ruetten S, Komp M, Merk H, Godolias G. Full-endoscopic cervical posterior foraminotomy for the operation of lateral disc herniations using 5.9-mm endoscopes: a prospective, randomized, controlled study. Spine 2008; 33(9): 940-8.
[http://dx.doi.org/10.1097/BRS.0b013e31816c8b67] [PMID: 18427313]

[28]   Yabuki S, Kikuchi S. Endoscopic surgery for cervical myelopathy due to calcification of the ligamentum flavum. J Spinal Disord Tech 2008; 21(7): 518-23.
[http://dx.doi.org/10.1097/BSD.0b013e31815a6151] [PMID: 18836365]

[29]   Yadav YR, Parihar V, Ratre S, Kher Y, Bhatele PR. Endoscopic decompression of cervical spondylotic myelopathy using posterior approach. Neurol India 2014; 62(6): 640-5.
[http://dx.doi.org/10.4103/0028-3886.149388] [PMID: 25591677]

[30]   Hussain I, Schmidt FA, Kirnaz S, Wipplinger C, Schwartz TH, Härtl R. MIS approaches in the cervical spine. J Spine Surg 2019; 5 (Suppl. 1): S74-83.
[http://dx.doi.org/10.21037/jss.2019.04.21] [PMID: 31380495]

[31]   Minamide A, Yoshida M, Simpson AK, *et al.* Microendoscopic laminotomy *versus* conventional laminoplasty for cervical spondylotic myelopathy: 5-year follow-up study. J Neurosurg Spine 2017; 27(4): 403-9.
[http://dx.doi.org/10.3171/2017.2.SPINE16939] [PMID: 28708041]

[32]   Hillard VH, Apfelbaum RI. Surgical management of cervical myelopathy: indications and techniques for multilevel cervical discectomy. Spine J 2006; 6(6) (Suppl.): 242S-51S.
[http://dx.doi.org/10.1016/j.spinee.2006.05.005] [PMID: 17097544]

[33]   Komotar RJ, Mocco J, Kaiser MG. Surgical management of cervical myelopathy: indications and techniques for laminectomy and fusion. Spine J 2006; 6(6) (Suppl.): 252S-67S.
[http://dx.doi.org/10.1016/j.spinee.2006.04.029] [PMID: 17097545]

[34]   König SA, Spetzger U. Surgical management of cervical spondylotic myelopathy - indications for anterior, posterior or combined procedures for decompression and stabilisation. Acta Neurochir (Wien) 2014; 156(2): 253-8.
[http://dx.doi.org/10.1007/s00701-013-1955-y] [PMID: 24292777]

[35]   Broekema AE, Kuijlen JM, Lesman-Leegte GA, *et al.* FACET study group investigators. Study protocol for a randomised controlled multicentre study: the Foraminotomy ACDF cost-effectiveness trial (FACET) in patients with cervical radiculopathy. BMJ Open 2017; 7(1): e012829.
[http://dx.doi.org/10.1136/bmjopen-2016-012829] [PMID: 28057652]

[36]   Yuan H, Zhang X, Zhang LM, Yan YQ, Liu YK, Lewandrowski KU. Comparative study of curative effect of spinal endoscopic surgery and anterior cervical decompression for cervical spondylotic myelopathy. J Spine Surg 2020; 6 (Suppl. 1): S186-96.

[http://dx.doi.org/10.21037/jss.2019.11.15] [PMID: 32195427]

[37]   Yang JS, Chu L, Chen H, Liu P, Hao DJ. Comment on "effective range of percutaneous posterior full-endoscopic paramedian cervical disc herniation discectomy and indications for patient selection". BioMed Res Int 2020; 2020: 3548194.
[http://dx.doi.org/10.1155/2020/3548194] [PMID: 32337243]

[38]   Yang J, Chu L, Deng Z, *et al.* Clinical study of single-level cervical disc herniation treated by full-endoscopic decompression *via* anterior transcorporeal approach. Zhongguo Xiu Fu Chong Jian Wai Ke Za Zhi 2020; 34(5): 543-9.
[PMID: 32410418]

[39]   Yu KX, Chu L, Yang JS, *et al.* Anterior transcorporeal approach to percutaneous endoscopic cervical diskectomy for single-level cervical intervertebral disk herniation: case series with 2-year follow-up. World Neurosurg 2019; 122: e1345-53.
[http://dx.doi.org/10.1016/j.wneu.2018.11.045] [PMID: 30448574]

[40]   Yu KX, Chu L, Chen L, Shi L, Deng ZL. A novel posterior trench approach involving percutaneous endoscopic cervical discectomy for central cervical intervertebral disc herniation. Clin Spine Surg 2019; 32(1): 10-7.
[http://dx.doi.org/10.1097/BSD.0000000000000680] [PMID: 29979215]

[41]   Xiao CM, Yu KX, Deng R, *et al.* Modified K-Hole percutaneous endoscopic surgery for cervical foraminal stenosis: partial pediculectomy approach. Pain Physician 2019; 22(5): E407-16.
[PMID: 31561650]

[42]   Ruetten S, Hahn P, Oezdemir S, Baraliakos X, Godolias G, Komp M. Full-endoscopic uniportal retropharyngeal odontoidectomy for anterior craniocervical infection. Minim Invasive Ther Allied Technol 2019; 28(3): 178-85.
[http://dx.doi.org/10.1080/13645706.2018.1498357] [PMID: 30179052]

[43]   Liu C, Liu K, Chu L, Chen L, Deng Z. Posterior percutaneous endoscopic cervical discectomy through lamina-hole approach for cervical intervertebral disc herniation. Int J Neurosci 2019; 129(7): 627-34.
[http://dx.doi.org/10.1080/00207454.2018.1503176] [PMID: 30238849]

[44]   Kong W, Xin Z, Du Q, Cao G, Liao W. Anterior percutaneous full-endoscopic transcorporeal decompression of the spinal cord for single-segment cervical spondylotic myelopathy: The technical interpretation and 2 years of clinical follow-up. J Orthop Surg Res 2019; 14(1): 461.
[http://dx.doi.org/10.1186/s13018-019-1474-5] [PMID: 31870395]

[45]   Deng ZL, Chu L, Chen L, Yang JS. Anterior transcorporeal approach of percutaneous endoscopic cervical discectomy for disc herniation at the C4-C5 levels: a technical note. Spine J 2016; 16(5): 659-66.
[http://dx.doi.org/10.1016/j.spinee.2016.01.187] [PMID: 26850173]

[46]   Yang JS, Chu L, Chen L, Chen F, Ke ZY, Deng ZL. Anterior or posterior approach of full-endoscopic cervical discectomy for cervical intervertebral disc herniation? A comparative cohort study. Spine 2014; 39(21): 1743-50.
[http://dx.doi.org/10.1097/BRS.0000000000000508] [PMID: 25010095]

[47]   Zhang C, Li D, Wang C, Yan X. Cervical endoscopic laminoplasty for cervical myelopathy. Spine 2016; 41 (Suppl. 19): B44-51.
[http://dx.doi.org/10.1097/BRS.0000000000001816] [PMID: 27656783]

[48]   Skovrlj B, Qureshi SA. Minimally invasive cervical spine surgery. J Neurosurg Sci 2017; 61(3): 325-34.
[http://dx.doi.org/10.23736/S0390-5616.16.03906-0] [PMID: 27787486]

[49]   Wilson JR, Vaccaro A, Harrop JS, *et al.* The impact of facet dislocation on clinical outcomes after cervical spinal cord injury: results of a multicenter North American prospective cohort study. Spine 2013; 38(2): 97-103.
[http://dx.doi.org/10.1097/BRS.0b013e31826e2b91] [PMID: 22895481]

[50]    Lin GX, Kotheeranurak V, Mahatthanatrakul A, *et al.* Worldwide research productivity in the field of full-endoscopic spine surgery: a bibliometric study. Eur Spine J 2020; 29(1): 153-60.
[http://dx.doi.org/10.1007/s00586-019-06171-2] [PMID: 31642995]

[51]    Odom GL, Finney W, Woodhall B. Cervical disk lesions. J Am Med Assoc 1958; 166(1): 23-8.
[http://dx.doi.org/10.1001/jama.1958.02990010025006] [PMID: 13491305]

[52]    Davis CH, Odom GL, Woodhall B. Survey of ruptured intervertebral disks in the cervical region. N C Med J 1953; 14(2): 61-6.
[PMID: 13025978]

[53]    Odom GL, Kristoff FV. Unilateral rupture of cervical disc. N C Med J 1948; 9(3): 117-22.
[PMID: 18858901]

[54]    Broekema AEH, Molenberg R, Kuijlen JMA, Groen RJM, Reneman MF, Soer R. The Odom Criteria: Validated at Last: A Clinimetric Evaluation in Cervical Spine Surgery. J Bone Joint Surg Am 2019; 101(14): 1301-8.
[http://dx.doi.org/10.2106/JBJS.18.00370] [PMID: 31318810]

[55]    Kim S, Lee JW, Chai JW, *et al.* A new mri grading system for cervical foraminal stenosis based on axial T2-weighted images. Korean J Radiol 2015; 16(6): 1294-302.
[http://dx.doi.org/10.3348/kjr.2015.16.6.1294] [PMID: 26576119]

[56]    Liu Y, Ban DX, Kan SL, Cao TW, Feng SQ. The Impact of Diabetes Mellitus on Patients Undergoing Cervical Spondylotic Myelopathy: A Meta-Analysis. Eur Neurol 2017; 77(1-2): 105-12.
[http://dx.doi.org/10.1159/000453547] [PMID: 27997913]

[57]    An HS, Silveri CP, Simpson JM, *et al.* Comparison of smoking habits between patients with surgically confirmed herniated lumbar and cervical disc disease and controls. J Spinal Disord 1994; 7(5): 369-73.
[http://dx.doi.org/10.1097/00002517-199410000-00001] [PMID: 7819635]

[58]    Park HJ, Kim SS, Lee SY, *et al.* A practical MRI grading system for cervical foraminal stenosis based on oblique sagittal images. Br J Radiol 2013; 86(1025): 20120515.
[http://dx.doi.org/10.1259/bjr.20120515] [PMID: 23410800]

[59]    Siller S, Kasem R, Witt TN, Tonn JC, Zausinger S. Painless motor radiculopathy of the cervical spine: clinical and radiological characteristics and long-term outcomes after operative decompression. J Neurosurg Spine 2018; 28(6): 621-9.
[http://dx.doi.org/10.3171/2017.10.SPINE17821] [PMID: 29570047]

[60]    Sharma SB, Lin GX, Jabri H, Siddappa ND, Kim JS. Biportal endoscopic excision of facetal cyst in the far lateral region of l5s1: 2-dimensional operative video. Oper Neurosurg (Hagerstown) 2020; 18(6): E233.
[http://dx.doi.org/10.1093/ons/opz255] [PMID: 31504842]

[61]    Lin Y, Rao S, Li Y, Zhao S, Chen B. Posterior percutaneous full-endoscopic cervical laminectomy and decompression for cervical stenosis with myelopathy: a technical note. World Neurosurg 2019; 8750(19): 30051-8.
[http://dx.doi.org/10.1016/j.wneu.2018.12.180] [PMID: 30648610]

[62]    Dahdaleh NS, Wong AP, Smith ZA, Wong RH, Lam SK, Fessler RG. Microendoscopic decompression for cervical spondylotic myelopathy. Neurosurg Focus 2013; 35(1): E8.
[http://dx.doi.org/10.3171/2013.3.FOCUS135] [PMID: 23815253]

[63]    Fessler RG, Khoo LT. Minimally invasive cervical microendoscopic foraminotomy: an initial clinical experience. Neurosurgery 2002; 51(5) (Suppl.): S37-45.
[http://dx.doi.org/10.1097/00006123-200211002-00006] [PMID: 12234428]

[64]    Abiola R, Rubery P, Mesfin A. Ossification of the posterior longitudinal ligament: etiology, diagnosis, and outcomes of nonoperative and operative management. Global Spine J 2016; 6(2): 195-204.
[http://dx.doi.org/10.1055/s-0035-1556580] [PMID: 26933622]

[65] Burkhardt BW, Wilmes M, Sharif S, Oertel JM. The visualization of the surgical field in tubular assisted spine surgery: is there a difference between HD-endoscopy and microscopy? Clin Neurol Neurosurg 2017; 158: 5-11.
[http://dx.doi.org/10.1016/j.clineuro.2017.04.010] [PMID: 28414959]

[66] Zhao T, Shen J, Zheng B, *et al.* The 100 most-cited publications in endoscopic spine surgery research. Global Spine J 2021; 11(4): 587-96.
[PMID: 32677522]

[67] Ren J, Li R, Zhu K, *et al.* Biomechanical comparison of percutaneous posterior endoscopic cervical discectomy and anterior cervical decompression and fusion on the treatment of cervical spondylotic radiculopathy. J Orthop Surg Res 2019; 14(1): 71.
[http://dx.doi.org/10.1186/s13018-019-1113-1] [PMID: 30832736]

[68] Platt A, Gerard CS, O'Toole JE. Comparison of outcomes following minimally invasive and open posterior cervical foraminotomy: description of minimally invasive technique and review of literature. J Spine Surg 2020; 6(1): 243-51.
[http://dx.doi.org/10.21037/jss.2020.01.08] [PMID: 32309662]

[69] Shen J, Telfeian AE, Shaaya E, Oyelese A, Fridley J, Gokaslan ZL. Full endoscopic cervical spine surgery. J Spine Surg 2020; 6(2): 383-90.
[http://dx.doi.org/10.21037/jss.2019.10.15] [PMID: 32656375]

[70] Kristoff FV, Odom GL. Ruptured intervertebral disk in the cervical region; a report of 20 cases. Arch Surg 1947; 54(3): 287-304.
[http://dx.doi.org/10.1001/archsurg.1947.01230070293004] [PMID: 20295734]

[71] Kang Y, Lee JW, Koh YH, *et al.* New MRI grading system for the cervical canal stenosis. AJR Am J Roentgenol 2011; 197(1): W134-40.
[http://dx.doi.org/10.2214/AJR.10.5560] [PMID: 21700974]

[72] Jho HD. Spinal cord decompression *via* microsurgical anterior foraminotomy for spondylotic cervical myelopathy. Minim Invasive Neurosurg 1997; 40(4): 124-9.
[http://dx.doi.org/10.1055/s-2008-1053432] [PMID: 9477400]

[73] Kato S, Oshima Y, Oka H, *et al.* Comparison of the japanese orthopaedic association (JOA) score and modified JOA (mJOA) score for the assessment of cervical myelopathy: a multicenter observational study. PLoS One 2015; 10(4): e0123022.
[http://dx.doi.org/10.1371/journal.pone.0123022] [PMID: 25837285]

[74] Law MD Jr, Bernhardt M, White AA III. Cervical spondylotic myelopathy: a review of surgical indications and decision making. Yale J Biol Med 1993; 66(3): 165-77.
[PMID: 8209553]

[75] Li X, An B, Gao H, *et al.* Surgical results and prognostic factors following percutaneous full endoscopic posterior decompression for thoracic myelopathy caused by ossification of the ligamentum flavum. Sci Rep 2020; 10(1): 1305.
[http://dx.doi.org/10.1038/s41598-020-58198-x] [PMID: 31992790]

[76] Roth CJ, Angevine PD, Aulino JM, *et al.* ACR appropriateness criteria myelopathy. J Am Coll Radiol 2016; 13(1): 38-44.
[http://dx.doi.org/10.1016/j.jacr.2015.10.004] [PMID: 26653797]

[77] Young WF. Cervical spondylotic myelopathy: a common cause of spinal cord dysfunction in older persons. Am Fam Physician 2000; 62(5): 1064-70-73.

[78] Choi G, Arbatti NJ, Modi HN, *et al.* Transcorporeal tunnel approach for unilateral cervical radiculopathy: a 2-year follow-up review and results. Minim Invasive Neurosurg 2010; 53(3): 127-31.
[http://dx.doi.org/10.1055/s-0030-1249681] [PMID: 20809454]

[79] Choi G, Lee SH, Bhanot A, Chae YS, Jung B, Lee S. Modified transcorporeal anterior cervical microforaminotomy for cervical radiculopathy: a technical note and early results. Eur Spine J 2007;

16(9): 1387-93.
[http://dx.doi.org/10.1007/s00586-006-0286-6] [PMID: 17203272]

[80]   Choi KC, Ahn Y, Lee CD, Lee SH. Combined anterior approach with transcorporeal herniotomy for a huge migrated cervical disc herniation. Korean J Spine 2011; 8(4): 292-4.
[http://dx.doi.org/10.14245/kjs.2011.8.4.292] [PMID: 26064148]

[81]   George B, Zerah M, Lot G, Hurth M. Oblique transcorporeal approach to anteriorly located lesions in the cervical spinal canal. Acta Neurochir (Wien) 1993; 121(3-4): 187-90.
[http://dx.doi.org/10.1007/BF01809273] [PMID: 8512017]

[82]   Kim JS, Eun SS, Prada N, Choi G, Lee SH. Modified transcorporeal anterior cervical microforaminotomy assisted by O-arm-based navigation: a technical case report. Eur Spine J 2011; 20 (Suppl. 2): S147-52.
[http://dx.doi.org/10.1007/s00586-010-1454-2] [PMID: 20490870]

[83]   Chu L, Yang JS, Yu KX, Chen CM, Hao DJ, Deng ZL. Usage of bone wax to facilitate percutaneous endoscopic cervical discectomy *via* anterior transcorporeal approach for cervical intervertebral disc herniation. World Neurosurg 2018; 118: 102-8.
[http://dx.doi.org/10.1016/j.wneu.2018.07.070] [PMID: 30026139]

CHAPTER 4

# Contemporary Clinical Decision Making in Full Endoscopic Cervical Spine Surgery

**Álvaro Dowling**[1,2], **Kai-Uwe Lewandrowski**[3,4,5,*] and **Helton Delfino**[6]

[1] *Endoscopic Spine Clinic, Santiago, Chile*

[2] *Department of Orthopaedic Surgery, USP, Ribeirão Preto, Brazil*

[3] *Center for Advanced Spine Care of Southern Arizona and Surgical Institute of Tucson, Tucson, AZ, USA*

[4] *Department of Orthopaedic Surgery, UNIRIO, Rio de Janeiro, Brazil*

[5] *Department of Orthoapedic Surgery, Fundación Universitaria Sanitas, Bogotá, D.C., Colombia, USA*

[6] *Department of Orthopaedic and Anesthesiology, Ribeirão Preto Medical School, University of São Paulo, São Paulo, Brazil*

**Abstract:** Full endoscopic surgery of the cervical spine is done in select centers where the clinical and surgical expertise is high. The procedure can be potentially dangerous in less well-trained hands, with the prospect of damage to vital vascular structures, and injury to the trachea, esophagus, cervical nerve roots, and the spinal cord. Also, cervical endoscopy is competing with traditional spinal surgeries, such as anterior cervical discectomy and fusion, or posterior cervical foraminotomy, whose clinical outcomes are reliably favorable. Therefore, most surgeons have a hard time replacing their well-performing anterior- or posterior cervical surgeries that they may very well be carrying out through open or mini-open incision or other forms of minimally invasive spinal surgery techniques. Patient satisfaction with these procedures is generally very high, and the complication rate is relatively low, and their management is well-understood. Again, is there a need for change? It is apparent that to the innovators, the answer to this question is obviously "yes" because they are looking for practical, yet less burdensome, lower cost, and more simplified outpatient cervical spine surgeries. The general push by payors and patients to transition spine care from in- to outpatient setting requires spine surgeons to rethink their approach to treating common degenerative conditions of the cervical spine. New algorithms based on updated classification systems and clinical outcome analysis of contemporary surgical techniques are required to make this transition feasible. In this chapter, the authors illustrate the application of full-endoscopic cervical spine surgery techniques, revie-

---

* **Corresponding author Kai-Uwe Lewandrowski:** Center for Advanced Spine Care of Southern Arizona and Surgical Institute of Tucson, Tucson, AZ, USA, Department of Orthopaedic Surgery, UNIRIO, Rio de Janeiro, Brazil and Department of Orthoapedic Surgery, Fundación Universitaria Sanitas, Bogotá, D.C., Colombia, USA; Tel: +1 520 204-1495; Fax: +1 623 218-1215; E-mail: business@tucsonspine.com

wing their indications, and the clinical decision-making by discussing the rationale for the procedure of choice selection ranging from patient criteria, anatomical considerations, surgeon training-, and skill level. This chapter is intended to serve as a guide for the established spine surgeons who are yet inexperienced with endoscopy and evaluates whether full endoscopy of the cervical spine should be in their armamentarium.

**Keywords:** Cervical endoscopy, Cervical herniated disc, Cervical stenosis, Clinical decision making algorithms, Myelopathy.

## INTRODUCTION

In recent years, many spine surgeons have begun to perform decompression procedures and hernia removal by cervical endoscopy, mainly through the posterior approach. some publications show that posterior foraminotomy has similar results to open traditional anterior cervical discectomy and fusion (ACDF) with the difference of having a lower cost [1, 2] but slightly higher reoperation rate [3]. On the other hand, with endoscopic techniques, one-level myelopathies began to be treated with over-the-top techniques, mainly due to the improvement of the microendoscopic Kerrison increase working channels size, and better drillings of high speed, allowing generally faster decompression central canal [4]. Traditional cervical management includes posterior cervical foraminotomy and anterior cervical discectomy and fusion (ACDF). Those procedures are exhaustively validated. However, patients may develop recurrent symptoms in some cases due to progression of the underlying degenerative disease process with vertical collapse and loss of disc height, and increasing foraminal and central stenosis, particularly at other adjacent levels. This dynaiic is known as classic adjacent segment disease or "transition syndrome". It sometimes prompts additional surgeries in the future. Nowadays, technological advances have allowed us to achieve similar clinical outcomes with shorter, more simplified surgeries through smaller incisions and less bleeding and less postoperative pain than with traditional surgery [5].

In our centers, we have performed endoscopically assisted minimally invasive cervical spine surgery for more than 15 years employing posterior foraminotomy techniques. From 2004-2010, a retrospective study was conducted on 123 Patients undergoing posterior endoscopic cervical foraminotomy (PECF) for unilateral foraminal soft and hard disc disease with or without concomitant foraminal stenosis. All patient present radicular pain at least for 3 months with an average of 7 month and follow up at least 24 months. Our results show 90% excellent or good in the Neck Disability Index (NDI) [6]. Also Visual Analogue Scale (VAS) decrease significantly after surgery. By improving the full endoscopic technology to perform the foraminotomy faster and safer, achieving the same goal than the other endoscopic assisted technique, we gradually changed the method [7, 8]. With the advent of technology advances, patient selection criteria changed, and the indications for minimally invasive posterior cervical surgery have expanded [8]. One of the most significant advantages of minimally invasive surgery (MIS) using endoscopy is the minimal muscle dissection needed to access the spine (Fig. 1). Additional advantages of MIS include reduced both operative pain and disability, decreased blood loss and soft tissue disruption, reduced surgical time and the ability to perform these surgeries in outpatient setting often under sedation and local rather than general anesthesia. The latter is of significance to most patients who now actively seek out surgeons that offering these services.

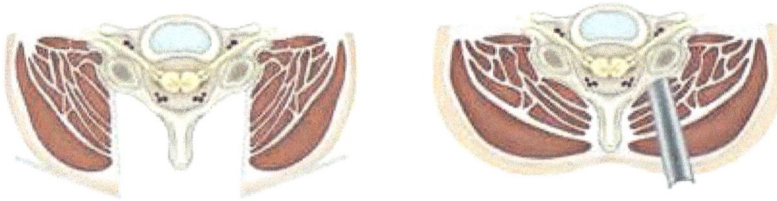

**Fig. (1).** Comparison of open cervical spine surgery to endoscopic cervical surgery. From left to right, **(a)** The amount of bone exposure and soft-tissue disruption is significantly bigger in open procedures in comparison to **(b)** endoscopic surgery, in which a working cannula reaches the surgical point without much tissue damage.

It is clear that this recent expansion of surgical indications has largely hinged on several other factors, implementation of higher definition video technology, as well as advances in the endoscopes instrumentation including working cannulas, irrigations systems, drills, Kerrisons and other rongeurs and chisels to afford more sophisticated bony decompression of neural elements with better visualization [2]. In this chapter, we will briefly review the different approaches to endoscopic surgery of the cervical spine. We will emphasize the use of clinical classification systems for stenosis and the type and localization of herniated disc and will discuss how to best approach compressive pathology in the anterior, posterior, or lateral spinal canal or the cervical foramina and how it relates to the best application of full endoscopic spinal surgery techniques including anterior endoscopic cervical discectomy (AECD), anterior endoscopic cervical foraminotomy (AECF), posterior endoscopic cervical discectomy (PECD) and other endoscopically assisted techniques which may appear more appropriate for cases with more severe stenosis of the cervical spinal canal or the foramina.

## CLINICAL AND RADIOGRAPHIC EVALUATION

It is important that all patients are evaluated clinically and radiologically. Clinical evaluation includes history and physical examination, neurological function, and neck pain, along with any other relevant symptoms. Neurological function is usually evaluated with the modified Japanese Orthopedic Association Myelopathy (mJOA) score [9], Frankel grading [10], and the Nurick scale [11]. The mJOA score provides a more comprehensive measurement of myelopathy than the Frankel score. Therefore, most authors now often use the mJOA score to quantify motor, sensory and urinary function. The Nurick scale is often used to quantify ambulatory function (Table **1**). The status of patients after surgery is graded as excellent, good, fair or poor based on the Odom criteria [12], or classified as worse, unchanged, improved or resolved. The present pain intensity score is used to assess neck pain. The neck disability index (NDI) and visual analog scale (VAS) are used to assess clinical outcomes for neck and arm pain.

Table 1. – Nurick grades for myelopathy [11].

| Grade | Signs and Symptoms |
|---|---|
| 0 | Sigs or symptoms of root involvement but without evidence of spinal cord disease |
| 1 | Signs of spinal cord disease but no difficulty in walking |
| 2 | Slight difficulty in walking which did not prevent full-time employment |
| 3 | Difficulty in walking which prevented full-time employment or the ability to do all housework, but which was not so severe as to require someone else's help to walk |
| 4 | Able to walk only with someone else's help or with the aid of a frame |
| 5 | Chair bound or bedridden |

The natural course of patients with cervical stenosis and signs of myelopathy is quite variable. In patients with no symptoms, but significant stenosis, the risk of developing myelopathy with cervical stenosis is approximately 3% per year. Myelopathic signs are useful for the clinical diagnosis of CSM. However, they are not highly sensitive and may be absent in approximately one-fifth of patients with myelopathy. Signal changes on the magnetic resonance imaging (MRI) scan and some electrophysiological tests are valuable adjuncts to diagnosis. Natural course of the CSM is still not fully understood. Although some long-term clinical outcome studies comparing non-operative to surgical treatment suggest that decompression renders more favorable outcomes in the long-run than letting the natural history play out [13]. The combination neck pain and cervical radiculopathy are common symptoms in patients with cervical myelopathy. The disease has silent periods with intermittent periods of rapid decline of neurological function. For example, minimal trauma such as trivial falls can precipitate disease progression by one or more Nurick grade. There is a consensus that patient with severe progressive symptoms need a surgical treatment. However, the role of treatment for patients with very subtle signs of myelopathy or no symptoms is not well understood.

## MAGNETIC RESONANCE IMAGING

In a retrospective study, Oshima *et al.* found that among patients with clinically mild CSM with signal change on MRI, only 44% had neurologic deterioration or underwent surgery over ten years. They suggest that the presence of such signal change in otherwise mild CSM may not necessarily warrant an operative intervention [14 - 18]. In a metanalysis investigating high signal changes in T2-weighted MRI scans and outcomes, multi-segmental and sharp increases in T2 signal changes have been found to end with poorer outcomes (Class II evidence). If the T2-weighted signal changes are regressing after surgery, better postoperative results should be expected [18]. A higher preoperative signal change ratio correlates with worse clinical outcome [19]. T2-weighted signal hyperintensity is not specific and can reflect reversible or irreversible structural changes. We know that patients may have both weak and robust T2-weighted signal hyperintensity parts (Table **2**) [20 - 23].

Table 2. Correlation between MRI signal changes and their correlations with histopathology [22].

| Imaging Type | MRI Characteristics | Pathological Correlation | Structural Change |
|---|---|---|---|
| **T2-weighted** | Weak sognal hyperintensity (without clear border) | Edema, Wallerian degeneration; demyelination; ischemia; gliosis | Reversible |
| | Strong signal hyperintensity (with sharp, clear border) | Potential cavitation; neural tissue loss; myeelomalacia; necrosis; grey matter changes | Largely irreversible |
| **T1-weighted** | Remarkable presence of signal hypointensity; appearing dark, focal, faint | Cavitation; neural tissue loww, myelomalacia; necrosis; spongiform changes in graymatter | Largely irreversible |

## ANATOMIC CONSIDERATION

### Anterior Approach

Various complications due to inadvertent injury to the structures located in the anterior part of the neck, including the esophagus recurrent laryngeal nerve, vertebral, vessels, jugulars venous injury, a carotid artery has been reported to occur during anterior cervical discectomy knowing the anatomical relationship between these structures an also their variations are significant to prevent these complications [24 - 29].

## Prevertebral Structures

The esophagus lies slightly to the left side of the C7 segment in most patients; an anterior approach from the right side is recommended. Commonly the esophagus is directly related to the anterior surface of the vertebra body and disc. Gulsen *et al.* define the closest distance of the esophagus to the cervical spine as being located in the midline of the vertebral body or disc space, with a mean of 1.1 millimeters. In terms of laterality, significantly more space is adjacent to the right longus colli [24].

The prevertebral content is very mobile due to the neck's compartmentalization and can easily displace it; the spine surgeon must separate the carotid artery an esophagus with two-finger techniques. In the case of a very wide neck, we recommend a 2 cm mini-open that allows the little finger to be inserted to ensure the disc's separation and palpation, avoiding any inadvertent damage to vital structures (Fig. **2**).

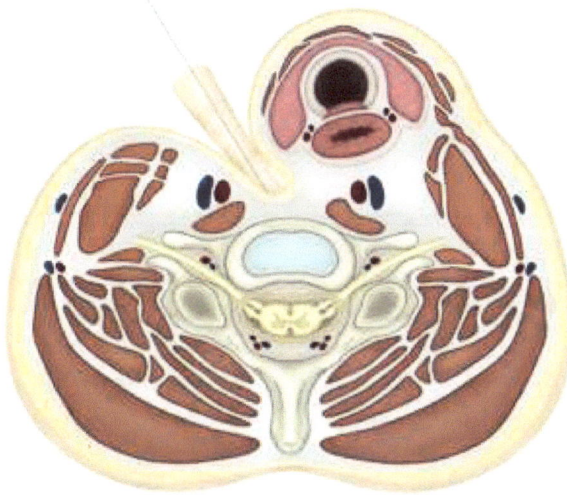

**Fig. (2).** Endoscopic anterior cervical discectomy approach with initial digital dissection aiming medially into the tracheoesophageal groove leaving the carotid sheath laterally.

## Carotid Artery Bifurcation

Most commonly located between the C 3 - C4 and C4- C5 levels but may still be at any level [24]. Various studies have demonstrated that beef bifurcation may occur as high as C1 or as low as T2, and also asymmetrical levels between right and left side. However, this anatomical variation's critical aspect is that a low bifurcation may cause complications if the surgeon is not cautious or aware of them [24].

## Posterior Approach

Anatomic relations among nerve roots, intervertebral discs, and foramina, associated with the amount of bonny resection, are useful landmarks to review posterior foraminotomy complications. However, only a few studies have reported the cervical nerve roots' location relative to the posterior aspect of the cervical spine [30, 31].

## Length of the Exposed Nerve Root

As anatomic is structures vary from one individual to another, no exact measurement has been established [32]. The mean vertical distance between the facet's medial point and the axilla of the C3 and C7 nerve root is 3.7 to 4.7 millimeters, respectively (Fig. **3**).

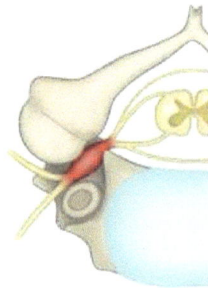

**Fig. (3).** Bone tissue surface debridement. Illustration of the burr drill polishing the lamina.

The C7 root has the most significant angle of about 68 degrees compared to C5, which usually has the smallest angle between the nerve root and the lateral margin of the dura 60 degrees approximately. However, some studies confirmed an essential difference between male and female measurements (Table **3**) [33 - 35].

**Table 3. Mean of the axilla degree and distances relative to the nerve root and intervertebral disc after half-medial facetectomy [32].**

| Measured Variable | C3 | C4 | C5 | C6 | C7 |
|---|---|---|---|---|---|
| C5 Axilla | 63 | 61 | 59 | 63 | 68 |
| Horizontal distance from point B to point C [mm] | 6.5 | 8.0 | 7.0 | 6.5 | 6.0 |
| Vertical distance from point B to point C [mm] | 3.0 | 2.0 | 1.0 | 1.0 | 2.5 |

**Point B**: medial point of the facet of the lateral mass after half-medial facetectomy. **Point C**: cross-point between medial margin of the root and inferior margin of the disc.

## Bone Resection

Surgeons have established four crucial anatomical landmarks for posterior foraminotomy, as shown in Table **4**. Although there is no exact amount of resection, Figueredo *et al.* proposed a mean percentage removal of 21,8%, 7.5%, 11.3%, and 11.5% for the superior and inferior lamina and facets, respectively [31]. Several biomechanical studies allude that the medial third of the lateral mass dissection should not exceed more than half of the lateral mass; otherwise, cervical instability might occur [1, 7]. C8 nerve root must be mainly considered where bone resection is performed because it has a longer and more lateral direction below the C7 pedicle.

**Table 4. - Posterior cervical foraminotomy landmarks.**

| Limits | Structure |
|---|---|
| **Superior** | Superior border of the superior facet |
| **Inferior** | Inferior border of the superior facet |
| **Lateral** | Vertical line linking the junction of the lamina-facet to the lateral and of the superior limit |
| **Medial** | Lateral aspect of the dural sac |

## Relation Between Nerve Root & Disc

The location of the nerve root in relation to the cervical disc changes from level to level in the cervical spine. Based on a study published by Tanaka *et al.* in 2000 the following anatomical relationship between cervical discs and nerve roots have been described [32]. Commonly, the C4-C5 discs are anterior to the C5 nerve root (shoulder type). Usually, the C6 nerve roots relates to the C5/6 disc space by forming an axillary type, followed by the anterior type in the foraminal space. The C8 root has some different because he only contacts with the disc at the exit (Table **3**). Hwang *et al.* also described the distance between the facet's medial point and the medial end of the root crossing the intervertebral disc's inferior margin [33]. After medial half facetectomy from C3 to C7, these authors established that this horizontal distance increased in the lower segments (Figs. **4** and **5**). He also measured the vertical distance among the medial margin of the root and the vertebral disc's inferior margins, as was estimated at 1mm to 3 mm for C3 to C7 nerve roots (Table **5**).

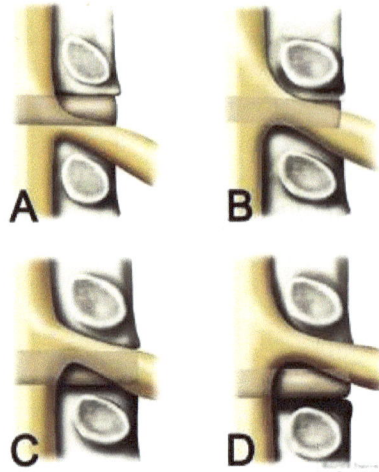

**Fig. (4).** Anatomic relations between the nerve roots and the discs in the foraminal space. **(A)** Shoulder type: when the disc is proximal to the nerve root. **(B)** Anterior type: the disc is located just anteriorly to the nerve root. **(C)** Axillary type: the disc is distal to the nerve root. **(D)** The disc does not have contact with the nerve root. (Illustration courtesy of Mauricio Sepúlveda; with permission from Hwang *et al.* [33]).

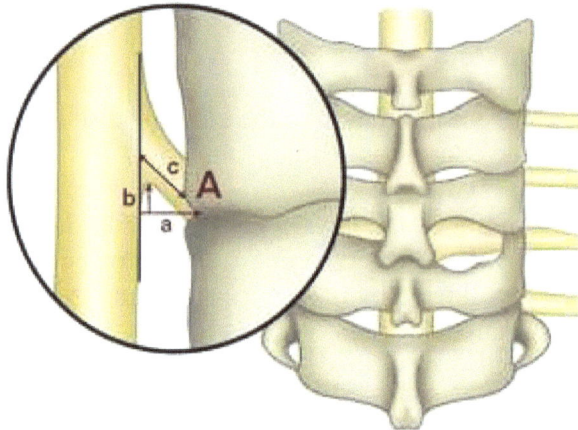

**Fig. (5).** Anatomic relations of the dura, nerve root, and the lateral mass after total laminectomy. A medial point of the lateral mass's facet after the procedure; **(a)** horizontal distance from point A to the lateral surface of the dura; **(b)**, the vertical distance from point A to the axilla; **(c)**, length of the exposed nerve root. (Illustration courtesy of Mauricio Sepúlveda; with permission from Hwang *et al.* [33]).

**Table 5. Location of the discs relative to the nerve roots at the foraminal space.**

| Nerve Root | No contact (%) | Shoulder (%) | Anterior (%) | Axillary (%) |
|:----------:|:--------------:|:------------:|:------------:|:------------:|
| C5 | - | 30 | 70 | - |
| C6 | - | 10 | 20 | 70 |

| Nerve Root | No contact (%) | Shoulder (%) | Anterior (%) | Axillary (%) |
|:---:|:---:|:---:|:---:|:---:|
| C7 | - | - | 10 | 90 |
| C8 | 80 | - | - | 20 |

## CLASSIFICATION SYSTEMS FOR SURGICAL DECISION MAKING

This chapter's first author (AD) has performed endoscopic cervical spine surgeries for over 20 years. He has developed an algorithm based on the results of the different approaches considering the location of the pathology, the number of levels compromised, and patient anatomy. It is essential to have classifications for taking clinical and surgical decisions. Based on them, you may define the anterior or posterior approach to resolve the pathology. We used four classifications to describe the pathology:

1. Park classification for foraminal stenosis,
2. Kang classification for central canal stenosis based on MRI grading,
3. Odom classification for cervical disc herniation based on soft or hard compression,
4. Crandal classification for cervical myelopathy.

### Classification of Cervical Foraminal Stenosis

In patients graded 0, Park *et al.* found 17–18% to have positive neurologic manifestations, with the remaining 82– 83% having negative neurologic manifestations [36]. In patients graded 2 or 3, we found 93–100% to have positive neurologic manifestations and 0–7% had negative neurologic findings. Therefore, we conclude that patients with MRI findings that indicate grades 2 and 3 will most likely have positive neurologic symptoms, allowing clinicians to use a grade 2 or 3 MRI finding to predict patients' clinical presentation (Fig. **6**). Therefore, using grade 0 MRI findings as a predictor of clinical findings is unreliable.

### Classification of Cervical Canal Stenosis

Kang *et al.* published an updated new grading system [37] for diagnosing and grading cervical canal stenosis that is based on the preexisting grading system [38]. The Kang classification is summarized in Fig. (**7**).

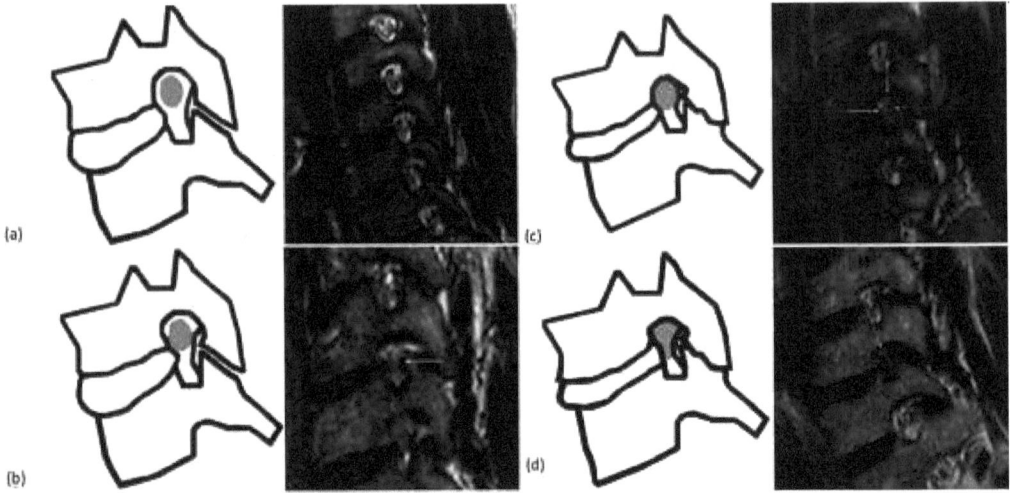

**Fig. (6).** Schematic illustrations of grading systems for cervical foraminal stenosis and MRI association. According to Park *et al.* [36] in Grade 0 **(a)**, the cervical neural foramen's oblique sagittal plane shows no significant stenosis and no perineural fat obliteration. In Grade 1 **(b)**, there is mild (below 50% of nerve root circumference) perineural fat obliteration. No morphological change of the nerve root is seen. In Grade 2 **(c)**, there is moderate (above 50% of nerve root circumference) compression, as shown by perineural fat obliteration. No morphological change of the nerve root is seen. In Grade 3 **(d)**, the nerve root is collapsed and morphologically changed. Moreover, there is severe perineural fat obliteration.

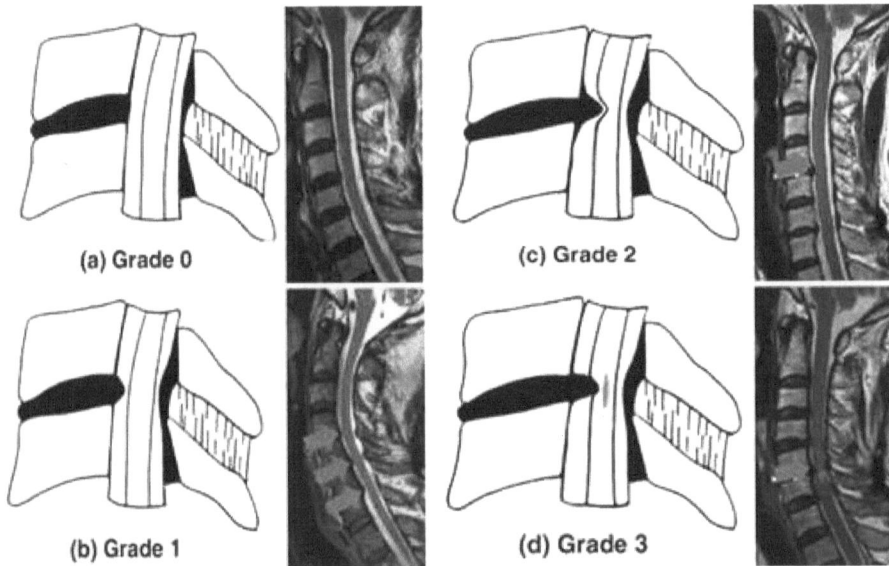

(a) Grade 0     (c) Grade 2     (b) Grade 1     (d) Grade 3

**Fig. (7).** Schematic diagrams of the grading system of cervical canal stenosis in MRI sagittal of cervical spines. Kang *et al.* **Grade 0** is normal. **Grade 1** denotes obliteration of more than 50% of subarachnoid space without any sign of cord deformity. **Grade 2** represents central canal stenosis with spinal cord deformity; the spinal cord is deformed, but no signal change is noted in the spinal cord. **Grade 3** indicates the spinal cord's increased signal intensity near the compressed level on T2- weighted images.

## Classification of Cervical Disc Herniations

According to Odom *et al.* [39], cervical disc herniation can generally be classified into four types:

1. Unilateral soft disk protrusion with nerve root compression
2. Foraminal spur, or hard disk, with nerve root compression
3. Medial smooth disk protrusion with spinal cord compression
4. Transverse ridge or cervical spondylosis with spinal cord compression

## Cervical Myelopathy Classification

Crandall *et al.* classified the pathology of cervical myelopathy into five types and his classification system has been widely accepted worldwide [40, 41]. Later, Hattori *et al.* reported that myelopathy advanced from type 1, in which damage was limited to the central part of the spinal cord, to type 2 which involves they pyramidal tract and finally to type 3 in which the damage spreads transversally in the spinal cord (Table **6**) [42 - 44]. However, many patients do not fit any of the types described in Crandall's classification or exhibit symptom changes that cannot be explained with Hattori's theory. In general, the patients with anterior or central lesion syndrome, in which the damage was limited to the grey matter, exhibited greater neurological improvements after surgical treatment. However, once the pathological changes extended into the white matter, which includes the ascending and descending tracts, surgical decompression did not result in marked recovery of neural function [45]. An additional comparison of biomechanical response to surgical procedures used for cervical radiculopathy has been classified by Chen *et al.* to aid in the decision making for posterior keyhole foraminotomy *versus* anterior foraminotomy and discectomy *versus* anterior discectomy with fusion (Fig. **8**) [46].

**Table 6. Novel classification of cervical myelopathy with prevalence of each type [42].**

| Type | Spinal Cord Involvement | Deteriorated Extremity | Number | Prevalence |
|------|-------------------------|------------------------|--------|------------|
| I | Anterior | Unilateral | 41 | 13.1% |
| II | Central | Bilateral U/E | 27 | 8.6% |
| III | Posterior | Bilateral L/E | 17 | 5.4% |
| IV | Hemilateral | Unilateral U/E & L/E | 38 | 12.1% |
| V | Transverse | All extremities | 190 | 60.7% |
| U/E: Upper extremity, L/E: Lower extremity | | | | |

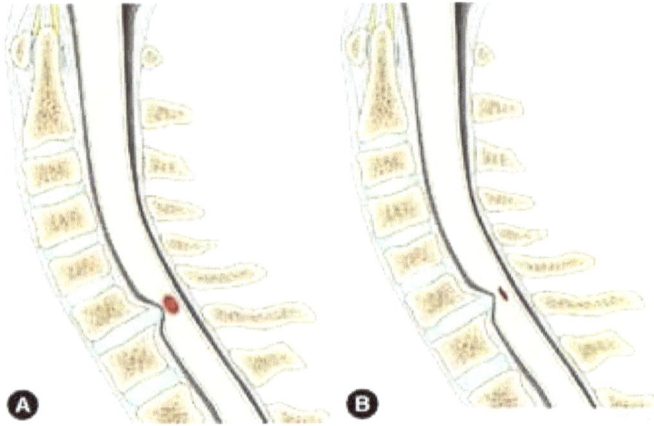

**Fig. (8).** High signal in T2-weighted magnetic resonance images has been graded by Chen *et al.* [46]: Grade 0 is no signal increase. **(A)** Grade 1 is faint, fuzzy bordered intensity increase. **(B)** Grade 2 is an intense, well-defined bordered intensity increase.

## CLINICAL DECISION MAKING

### For Herniated Disc

To treat cervical disc herniations, one must consider two fundamental factors: the problem's location and how many levels are involved. The authors found the Odom classification most useful in describing the site of the disc herniation [12, 39, 47]. Most endoscopic spine surgeons consider the anterior approach is the most appropriate approach for central disc herniations. Paramedian disc herniations, on the other hand, may be treated both from the anterior or the posterior approach. Surgeon's experience and skill level, as well as preference, may be the deciding factor. Also, in patients with multi-level involvement performing surgery simultaneously at more than one cervical intervertebral disc space through the same surgical access corridor may prove advantageous.

### For Stenosis

Patients should be stratified whether the painful condition can be attributed to a central or foraminal stenotic process. In general, both anterior and posterior approaches are feasible for foraminal stenosis, which is preferentially treated with PECD by most surgeons. In contrast, central stenosis is often attacked with AECD. However, the presence of spinal instability, loss of cervical lordosis, or even the process of focal or multilevel kyphosis, or advanced degenerative changes with loss of intervertebral disc height of less than 4 mm typically calls for concomitant fusion (ACDF).

## THE SURGEON FACTOR & HOW TO ARRIVE AT THE PREFERRED PROCEDURE

The listed recommendations for common painful degenerative conditions of the cervical spine may be treated differently based on the surgeon's training, experience, and the available equipment to support his endoscopic spine surgery program. Therefore, the authors ask the reader of this chapter not to dogmatically adhere to their recommendations for anterior (AECD) or posterior (PECD) surgery and take the patient-related factors and their situation into account when making decisions. Additional factors in deciding for the preferred endoscopic surgery approach to common cervical spine conditions may arise from the established local standards of care, reimbursement, peer-pressure, and acceptance of the procedures with patients, payors, and other involved stakeholders in the health care delivery equation locally where the prospective endoscopic spine surgeon works [48]. Surgeons' ability to execute these highly advanced minimally invasive spine procedures may not be equal across the board, and the recommendations for AECD or PECD made herein for are intended for the highly skilled surgeon who understands the anatomy, the technical issues involved and employs the clinical protocols recommended by the authors of this chapter judiciously. The first author prefers AECD while the second author favors PECD with foraminotomy for radicular arm pain due to cervical disc herniation or foraminal stenosis. For the purpose of illustrating the forgoing discussion on classification painful degenerative conditions of the cervical spine, we will showcase the first author's preferred endoscopic cervical technique – the anterior endoscopic cervical discectomy – the AECD, and the second author's posterior endoscopic cervical discectomy – PECD.

Other chapters in this textbook illustrate these various endoscopic surgery techniques and others in more detail. To keep within this chapter's scope on clinical decision-making, we will review the two methods employed by the authors for soft disc herniations in an illustrative manner in other chapters. More importantly, we emphasize that more than patient- and technique related factors may enter into the decision-making equation and that surgeons will ultimately perform procedures at their comfort- and skill level while aiming for good clinical outcomes supportive of their recognized status in their respective communities. The surgeon factor is the ultimate wild card that must be taken into account. It is often forgotten when discussing the indications and patient selection criteria for employing endoscopy in cervical spine surgery.

## DISCUSSION

Further improvement in microscopy, laser technology, endoscopy, video, and image guidance systems designed for minimally invasive procedures will inevitably lead to further applications in MIS surgery and will allow surgeons to perform complex procedures through small portals, thus reducing the morbidity for the patient. Nowadays, surgeons are trained in minimally invasive approaches, providing adequate exposure for the desired anatomic structures while minimizing the disadvantages of excessive soft-tissue stripping, dissection, and prolonged retraction from cervical spine procedures. Although anterior cervical procedures are popular among surgeons [48, 49], posterior cervical foraminotomy still provides symptomatic relief, in about 90% of patients with radiculopathy from foraminal stenosis, at a lower cost than the anterior procedure [7, 8, 50]. Posterior approach advantages compared with anterior approaches are: lower probability of damaging vital structures located in the anterior area of the cervical spine (trachea, esophagus, internal carotid artery, vertebral artery, and recurrent laryngeal nerve); less damage to structural and biomechanical properties of the vertebral disc by preserving it; no segment motion loss; and reduced occurrence of complications associated with bone graft as well as degenerative changes of the adjacent joint [48, 51 - 59]. On the other hand, the anterior approach is more suitable in central soft hernia or bilateral symptomatic foraminal stenosis and myelopathy in more than one level. The experience of the spine team is crucial to achieving a good and excellent result. There is a learning curve with the need for continuous training with the use of the cadaver lab. In the authors' opinion, the first 20 to 30 surgeries should be supervised.

## CONCLUSIONS

Clinical decision making for appropriate application of endoscopic techniques in the surgical treatment of common painful degenerative conditions of the cervical spine is complex. It cannot be reduced to a rigid, dogmatic algorithm to decide between anterior and posterior procedures. Many confounding factors impact the choice of procedure. In this chapter, the authors attempted to illustrate the pros and cons of the various techniques for common clinical entities. We recommend that surgeons engage in a shared decision on the most appropriate care based on the characteristics of the relevant pathology, surgeon skill- and comfort level, available equipment, and support protocols as they play out in their clinical setting. The authors predict that future technology advances will likely impact the clinical decision making by moving the needle to more reliable and simplified procedures that meet patients' expectations per performing them in an outpatient surgery center setting.

## CONSENT FOR PUBLICATION

Not applicable.

## CONFLICT OF INTEREST

The author declares no conflict of interest, financial or otherwise.

## ACKNOWLEDGEMENTS

Declared none.

## REFERENCES

[1]    Winder MJ, Thomas KC. Minimally invasive *versus* open approach for cervical laminoforaminotomy. Can J Neurol Sci 2011; 38(2): 262-7.
       [http://dx.doi.org/10.1017/S0317167100011446] [PMID: 21320831]

[2]    Clark JG, Abdullah KG, Steinmetz MP, Benzel EC, Mroz TE. Minimally Invasive *versus* Open Cervical Foraminotomy: A Systematic Review. Global Spine J 2011; 1(1): 9-14.
       [http://dx.doi.org/10.1055/s-0031-1296050] [PMID: 24353931]

[3]    Hussain I, Schmidt FA, Kirnaz S, Wipplinger C, Schwartz TH, Härtl R. MIS approaches in the cervical spine. J Spine Surg 2019; 5 (Suppl. 1): S74-83.
       [http://dx.doi.org/10.21037/jss.2019.04.21] [PMID: 31380495]

[4]    Ruetten S, Komp M, Merk H, Godolias G. Full-endoscopic cervical posterior foraminotomy for the operation of lateral disc herniations using 5.9-mm endoscopes: a prospective, randomized, controlled study. Spine 2008; 33(9): 940-8.
       [http://dx.doi.org/10.1097/BRS.0b013e31816c8b67] [PMID: 18427313]

[5]    Hasan S, Härtl R, Hofstetter CP. The benefit zone of full-endoscopic spine surgery. J Spine Surg 2019; 5 (Suppl. 1): S41-56.
       [http://dx.doi.org/10.21037/jss.2019.04.19] [PMID: 31380492]

[6]    Dowling A. Endoscopic anterior cervical discectomy. London: JP Brothers 2013.

[7]    Adamson TE. Microendoscopic posterior cervical laminoforaminotomy for unilateral radiculopathy: results of a new technique in 100 cases. J Neurosurg 2001; 95(1) (Suppl.): 51-7.
       [PMID: 11453432]

[8]    Zeidman SM, Ducker TB. Posterior cervical laminoforaminotomy for radiculopathy: review of 172 cases. Neurosurgery 1993; 33(3): 356-62.
       [http://dx.doi.org/10.1227/00006123-199309000-00002] [PMID: 8413864]

[9]    Kato S, Oshima Y, Oka H, *et al.* Comparison of the Japanese Orthopaedic Association (JOA) score and modified JOA (mJOA) score for the assessment of cervical myelopathy: a multicenter observational study. PLoS One 2015; 10(4): e0123022.
       [http://dx.doi.org/10.1371/journal.pone.0123022] [PMID: 25837285]

[10]   Frankel HL, Hancock DO, Hyslop G, *et al.* The value of postural reduction in the initial management of closed injuries of the spine with paraplegia and tetraplegia. I. Paraplegia 1969; 7(3): 179-92.
       [PMID: 5360915]

[11]   Nurick S. The pathogenesis of the spinal cord disorder associated with cervical spondylosis. Brain 1972; 95(1): 87-100.
       [http://dx.doi.org/10.1093/brain/95.1.87] [PMID: 5023093]

[12]   Odom GL, Finney W, Woodhall B. Cervical disk lesions. J Am Med Assoc 1958; 166(1): 23-8.

[http://dx.doi.org/10.1001/jama.1958.02990010025006] [PMID: 13491305]

[13]    Laiginhas AR, Silva PA, Pereira P, Vaz R. Long-term clinical and radiological follow-up after laminectomy for cervical spondylotic myelopathy. Surg Neurol Int 2015; 6: 162.
[http://dx.doi.org/10.4103/2152-7806.167211] [PMID: 26543671]

[14]    Oshima Y, Seichi A, Takeshita K, *et al.* Natural course and prognostic factors in patients with mild cervical spondylotic myelopathy with increased signal intensity on T2-weighted magnetic resonance imaging. Spine 2012; 37(22): 1909-13.
[http://dx.doi.org/10.1097/BRS.0b013e318259a65b] [PMID: 22511231]

[15]    Oshima Y, Takeshita K, Inanami H, *et al.* Cervical microendoscopic interlaminar decompression through a midline approach in patients with cervical myelopathy: a technical note. J Neurol Surg A Cent Eur Neurosurg 2014; 75(6): 474-8.
[http://dx.doi.org/10.1055/s-0034-1373663] [PMID: 24819630]

[16]    Oshima Y, Takeshita K, Taniguchi Y, *et al.* Effect of preoperative sagittal balance on cervical laminoplasty outcomes. Spine 2016; 41(21): E1265-70.
[http://dx.doi.org/10.1097/BRS.0000000000001615] [PMID: 27054450]

[17]    Oshina M, Oshima Y, Tanaka S, Riew KD. Radiological fusion criteria of postoperative anterior cervical discectomy and fusion: a systematic review. Global Spine J 2018; 8(7): 739-50.
[http://dx.doi.org/10.1177/2192568218755141] [PMID: 30443486]

[18]    Oshina M, Tanaka M, Oshima Y, Tanaka S, Riew KD. Correlation and differences in cervical sagittal alignment parameters between cervical radiographs and magnetic resonance images. Eur Spine J 2018; 27(6): 1408-15.
[http://dx.doi.org/10.1007/s00586-018-5550-z] [PMID: 29572735]

[19]    Wang LF, Zhang YZ, Shen Y, *et al.* Using the T2-weighted magnetic resonance imaging signal intensity ratio and clinical manifestations to assess the prognosis of patients with cervical ossification of the posterior longitudinal ligament. J Neurosurg Spine 2010; 13(3): 319-23.
[http://dx.doi.org/10.3171/2010.3.SPINE09887] [PMID: 20809723]

[20]    Nouri A, Cheng JS, Davies B, Kotter M, Schaller K, Tessitore E. Degenerative cervical myelopathy: a brief review of past perspectives, present developments, and future directions. J Clin Med 2020; 9(2): E535.
[http://dx.doi.org/10.3390/jcm9020535] [PMID: 32079075]

[21]    Nouri A, Gondar R, Cheng JS, Kotter MRN, Tessitore E. Degenerative cervical myelopathy and the aging spine: introduction to the special issue. J Clin Med 2020; 9(8): E2535.
[http://dx.doi.org/10.3390/jcm9082535] [PMID: 32781513]

[22]    Nouri A, Tetreault L, Côté P, Zamorano JJ, Dalzell K, Fehlings MG. Does magnetic resonance imaging improve the predictive performance of a validated clinical prediction rule developed to evaluate surgical outcome in patients with degenerative cervical myelopathy? Spine 2015; 40(14): 1092-100.
[http://dx.doi.org/10.1097/BRS.0000000000000919] [PMID: 25893357]

[23]    Nouri A, Tetreault L, Singh A, Karadimas SK, Fehlings MG. Degenerative cervical myelopathy: epidemiology, genetics, and pathogenesis. Spine 2015; 40(12): E675-93.
[http://dx.doi.org/10.1097/BRS.0000000000000913] [PMID: 25839387]

[24]    Gulsen S, Caner H, Altinors N. An anatomical variant : low-lying bifurcation of the common carotid artery, and its surgical implications in anterior cervical discectomy. J Korean Neurosurg Soc 2009; 45(1): 32-4.
[http://dx.doi.org/10.3340/jkns.2009.45.1.32] [PMID: 19242568]

[25]    Fraser JF, Härtl R. Anterior approaches to fusion of the cervical spine: a metaanalysis of fusion rates. J Neurosurg Spine 2007; 6(4): 298-303.
[http://dx.doi.org/10.3171/spi.2007.6.4.2] [PMID: 17436916]

[26]   Mayfield FH. Cervical spondylosis: a comparison of the anterior and posterior approaches. Clin Neurosurg 1965; 13: 181-8.
[PMID: 5870806]

[27]   Ito H, Mataga I, Kageyama I, Kobayashi K. Clinical anatomy in the neck region--the position of external and internal carotid arteries may be reversed. Okajimas Folia Anat Jpn 2006; 82(4): 157-67.
[http://dx.doi.org/10.2535/ofaj.82.157] [PMID: 16526574]

[28]   Yao N, Wang C, Wang W, Wang L. Full-endoscopic technique for anterior cervical discectomy and interbody fusion: 5-year follow-up results of 67 cases. Eur Spine J 2011; 20(6): 899-904.
[http://dx.doi.org/10.1007/s00586-010-1642-0] [PMID: 21153596]

[29]   Du Q, Lei LQ, Cao GR, *et al.* Percutaneous full-endoscopic anterior transcorporeal cervical discectomy and channel repair: a technique note report. BMC Musculoskelet Disord 2019; 20(1): 280.
[http://dx.doi.org/10.1186/s12891-019-2659-0] [PMID: 31182078]

[30]   Zdeblick TA, Zou D, Warden KE, McCabe R, Kunz D, Vanderby R. Cervical stability after foraminotomy. A biomechanical *in vitro* analysis. J Bone Joint Surg Am 1992; 74(1): 22-7.
[http://dx.doi.org/10.2106/00004623-199274010-00004] [PMID: 1734010]

[31]   Figueiredo EG, Castillo De la Cruz M, Theodore N, Deshmukh P, Preul MC. Modified cervical laminoforaminotomy based on anatomic landmarks reduces need for bony removal. Minim Invasive Neurosurg 2006; 49(1): 37-42.
[http://dx.doi.org/10.1055/s-2006-932146] [PMID: 16547881]

[32]   Tanaka N, Fujimoto Y, An HS, Ikuta Y, Yasuda M. The anatomic relation among the nerve roots, intervertebral foramina, and intervertebral discs of the cervical spine. Spine 2000; 25(3): 286-91.
[http://dx.doi.org/10.1097/00007632-200002010-00005] [PMID: 10703098]

[33]   Hwang JC, Bae HG, Cho SW, Cho SJ, Park HK, Chang JC. Morphometric study of the nerve roots around the lateral mass for posterior foraminotomy. J Korean Neurosurg Soc 2010; 47(5): 358-64.
[http://dx.doi.org/10.3340/jkns.2010.47.5.358] [PMID: 20539795]

[34]   Xu R, Ebraheim NA, Nadaud MC, Yeasting RA, Stanescu S. The location of the cervical nerve roots on the posterior aspect of the cervical spine. Spine 1995; 20(21): 2267-71.
[http://dx.doi.org/10.1097/00007632-199511000-00001] [PMID: 8553111]

[35]   Barakat M, Hussein Y. Anatomical study of the cervical nerve roots for posterior foraminotomy: cadaveric study. Eur Spine J 2012; 21(7): 1383-8.
[http://dx.doi.org/10.1007/s00586-012-2158-6] [PMID: 22270247]

[36]   Park HJ, Kim SS, Lee SY, *et al.* A practical MRI grading system for cervical foraminal stenosis based on oblique sagittal images. Br J Radiol 2013; 86(1025): 20120515.
[http://dx.doi.org/10.1259/bjr.20120515] [PMID: 23410800]

[37]   Kang Y, Lee JW, Koh YH, *et al.* New MRI grading system for the cervical canal stenosis. AJR Am J Roentgenol 2011; 197(1): W134-40.
[http://dx.doi.org/10.2214/AJR.10.5560] [PMID: 21700974]

[38]   Muhle C, Weinert D, Falliner A, *et al.* Dynamic changes of the spinal canal in patients with cervical spondylosis at flexion and extension using magnetic resonance imaging. Invest Radiol 1998; 33(8): 444-9.
[http://dx.doi.org/10.1097/00004424-199808000-00004] [PMID: 9704283]

[39]   Odom GL, Kristoff FV. Unilateral rupture of cervical disc. N C Med J 1948; 9(3): 117-22.
[PMID: 18858901]

[40]   Crandall PH, Hanafee WN. Cervical spondylotic myelopathy studies by air myelography. Am J Roentgenol Radium Ther Nucl Med 1964; 92: 1261-9.
[PMID: 14237481]

[41]   Crandall PH, Batzdorf U. Cervical spondylotic myelopathy. J Neurosurg 1966; 25(1): 57-66.

[http://dx.doi.org/10.3171/jns.1966.25.1.0057] [PMID: 5947048]

[42]    Hattori S, Kawai K, Mabuchi Y, Shibayama M. The relationship between magnetic resonance imaging and quantitative electromyography findings in patients with compressive cervical myelopathy. Spine 2010; 35(8): E290-4.
        [http://dx.doi.org/10.1097/BRS.0b013e3181c84700] [PMID: 20354473]

[43]    Hattori T, Sakakibara R, Yasuda K, Murayama N, Hirayama K. Micturitional disturbance in cervical spondylotic myelopathy. J Spinal Disord 1990; 3(1): 16-8.
        [http://dx.doi.org/10.1097/00002517-199003000-00003] [PMID: 2134406]

[44]    Hattori S, Saiki K, Kawai S. Diagnosis of the level and severity of cord lesion in cervical spondylotic myelopathy. Spinal evoked potentials. Spine 1979; 4(6): 478-85.
        [http://dx.doi.org/10.1097/00007632-197911000-00005] [PMID: 515838]

[45]    Fang W, Huang L, Feng F, *et al.* Anterior cervical discectomy and fusion *versus* posterior cervical foraminotomy for the treatment of single-level unilateral cervical radiculopathy: a meta-analysis. J Orthop Surg Res 2020; 15(1): 202.
        [http://dx.doi.org/10.1186/s13018-020-01723-5] [PMID: 32487109]

[46]    Chen BH, Natarajan RN, An HS, Andersson GB. Comparison of biomechanical response to surgical procedures used for cervical radiculopathy: posterior keyhole foraminotomy *versus* anterior foraminotomy and discectomy *versus* anterior discectomy with fusion. J Spinal Disord 2001; 14(1): 17-20.
        [http://dx.doi.org/10.1097/00002517-200102000-00004] [PMID: 11242270]

[47]    Davis CH, Odom GL, Woodhall B. Survey of ruptured intervertebral disks in the cervical region. N C Med J 1953; 14(2): 61-6.
        [PMID: 13025978]

[48]    Epstein NE. A review of complication rates for Anterior Cervical Diskectomy and Fusion (ACDF). Surg Neurol Int 2019; 10: 100.
        [http://dx.doi.org/10.25259/SNI-191-2019] [PMID: 31528438]

[49]    Lee HC, Chen CH, Wu CY, Guo JH, Chen YS. Comparison of radiological outcomes and complications between single-level and multilevel anterior cervical discectomy and fusion (ACDF) by using a polyetheretherketone (PEEK) cage-plate fusion system. Medicine (Baltimore) 2019; 98(5): e14277.
        [http://dx.doi.org/10.1097/MD.0000000000014277] [PMID: 30702590]

[50]    Li C, Tang X, Chen S, Meng Y, Zhang W. Clinical application of large channel endoscopic decompression in posterior cervical spine disorders. BMC Musculoskelet Disord 2019; 20(1): 548.
        [http://dx.doi.org/10.1186/s12891-019-2920-6] [PMID: 31739780]

[51]    Ranson WA, Neifert SN, Cheung ZB, Mikhail CM, Caridi JM, Cho SK. Predicting in-hospital complications after anterior cervical discectomy and fusion: a comparison of the elixhauser and charlson comorbidity indices. World Neurosurg 2020; 134: e487-96.
        [http://dx.doi.org/10.1016/j.wneu.2019.10.102] [PMID: 31669536]

[52]    Ramírez León JF, Rugeles Ortíz JG, Martínez CR, Alonso Cuéllar GO, Lewandrowski KU. Surgical treatment of cervical radiculopathy using an anterior cervical endoscopic decompression. J Spine Surg 2020; 6 (Suppl. 1): S179-85.
        [http://dx.doi.org/10.21037/jss.2019.09.24] [PMID: 32195426]

[53]    Narain AS, Hijji FY, Haws BE, *et al.* Risk factors for medical and surgical complications after 1--level anterior cervical discectomy and fusion procedures. Int J Spine Surg 2020; 14(3): 286-93.
        [http://dx.doi.org/10.14444/7038] [PMID: 32699749]

[54]    Ebot J, Domingo R, Nottmeier E. Post-operative dysphagia in patients undergoing a four level anterior cervical discectomy and fusion (ACDF). J Clin Neurosci 2020; 72: 211-3.
        [http://dx.doi.org/10.1016/j.jocn.2019.12.002] [PMID: 31839384]

[55]   Al Eissa S, Konbaz F, Aldeghaither S, *et al.* Anterior cervical discectomy and fusion complications and thirty-day mortality and morbidity. Cureus 2020; 12(4): e7643.
[PMID: 32411545]

[56]   Yew AY, Nguyen MT, Hsu WK, Patel AA. Quantitative risk factor analysis of postoperative dysphagia after anterior cervical discectomy and fusion (ACDF) using the eating assessment tool-10 (EAT-10). Spine 2019; 44(2): E82-8.
[http://dx.doi.org/10.1097/BRS.0000000000002770] [PMID: 29965886]

[57]   Kashkoush A, Mehta A, Agarwal N, *et al.* Perioperative neurological complications following anterior cervical discectomy and fusion: clinical impact on 317,789 patients from the national inpatient sample. World Neurosurg 2019; 128: e107-15.
[http://dx.doi.org/10.1016/j.wneu.2019.04.037] [PMID: 30980979]

[58]   Khanna R, Kim RB, Lam SK, Cybulski GR, Smith ZA, Dahdaleh NS. Comparing short-term complications of inpatient *versus* outpatient single-level anterior cervical discectomy and fusion: an analysis of 6940 patients using the ACS-NSQIP database. Clin Spine Surg 2018; 31(1): 43-7.
[http://dx.doi.org/10.1097/BSD.0000000000000499] [PMID: 28079682]

[59]   Kelly MP, Eliasberg CD, Riley MS, Ajiboye RM, SooHoo NF. Reoperation and complications after anterior cervical discectomy and fusion and cervical disc arthroplasty: a study of 52,395 cases. Eur Spine J 2018; 27(6): 1432-9.
[http://dx.doi.org/10.1007/s00586-018-5570-8] [PMID: 29605899]

# CHAPTER 5

# Indications and Outcomes with Endoscopic Posterior Cervical Rhizotomy

**Kai-Uwe Lewandrowski**[1,2,3]**, Ralf Rothoerl**[4]**, Stefan Hellinger**[5] **and Hyeun Sung Kim**[6,7,8,9,10,*]

[1] *Center for Advanced Spine Care of Southern Arizona and Surgical Institute of Tucson, Tucson, AZ, USA*

[2] *Department of Orthopaedic Surgery, UNIRIO, Rio de Janeiro, Brazil*

[3] *Department of Orthoapedic Surgery, Fundación Universitaria Sanitas, Bogotá, D.C., Colombia, USA*

[4] *Department of Neurosurgery, Isar Clinic, Munich, Germany*

[5] *Department of Orthopedic and Spine Surgery, Arabellaklinik, Munich, Germany*

[6] *Department of Neurosurgery, Nanoori Gangnam Hospital, Seoul, Republic of Korea*

[7] *A President of the Korean Research Society of the Endoscopic Spine Surgery (KOSESS), South Korea*

[8] *A Faculty of the KOrean Minimally Invasive Spine Surgery Society (KOMISS), South Korea*

[9] *A Chairman of the Nanoori Hospital Group Scientific Team, South Korea*

[10] *An Adjunct Professor of the Medical College of the Chosun University, Gwangju, South Korea*

**Abstract:** Axial neck pain without much radicular shoulder arm pain is a somewhat tricky situation for spine care providers. Patients often have the early-stage degenerative disease of the cervical intervertebral disc and facet joints, with minimal spinal alignment changes and without instability. Yet such patients may have legitimate symptoms and may have failed multiple rounds of physical therapy, spinal injections, activity modifications, non-steroidal anti-inflammatories, and other medical and supportive care measures. These patients may not fit traditional image-based spinal care protocols and are mostly left untreated. This chapter presents the authors' indications, and clinical outcomes with an endoscopically visualized combined mechanical and radiofrequency facet ablation with a minimal laminotomy at the symptomatic levels. They offer their rationale behind their strategies to attend to these patients with minimal cervical spine disease on advanced images but with unmanageable complaints who ordinarily have been falling into this watershed area of

* **Corresponding author Hyeun Sung Kim:** Department of Neurosurgery, Nanoori Gangnam Hospital, Seoul, Republic of Korea, A President of the Korean Research Society of the Endoscopic Spine Surgery (KOSESS), South Korea, A Faculty of the KOrean Minimally Invasive Spine Surgery Society (KOMISS), South Korea and A Chairman of the Nanoori Hospital Group Scientific Team, South Korea;
E-mail: neurospinekim@gmail.com

traditional spine care and reviewing possible pain relief mechanisms. The latter may be achieved not only by the combined mechanical and radiofrequency ablation of the cervical facet joint complex but also rely on modulation of the activity of the dorsal root ganglion of the cervical nerve root at the affected level. Outcomes are favorable in most patients, suggesting the authors' approach to treating these patients has merits; thus, warranting further clinical validation.

**Keywords:** Axial neck pain, Cervical spine, Decompression, Degeneration, Disc herniation, Endoscopic, Impingement, Minimally invasive, Open, Radiofrequency, Rhizotomy, Stenosis.

## INTRODUCTION

Chambers *et al.* has described the cervical rhizotomy for axial neck pain. As a treatment modality as early as in 1954. Others have reported on their clinical outcomes in the 1960ies. Early on, the treatment was used to treat torticollis due to spasticity or dyskinetic syndromes of the neck [1, 2]. Initial treatments were directed at the cervical nerve roots to modulate their activity. In 1977, Fraioli *et al.* reported their results with the bilateral cervical posterior rhizotomy, which they performed in 16 dystonia and athetosis infantile cerebral palsy (CP) patients [3]. As a result of their rhizotomy procedures ranging from C1 to C6, their patients experienced a significant decrease in muscle spasms and athetoid movements, and improved posture and voluntary mobility. However, the authors also reported complications in 5 patients who suffered from uneven and irregular breathing associated with lethargy immediately postoperatively due to reduced diaphragmatic activity in 4 of these five patients. The latter four patients developed pneumonia, of which only one patient recovered. The other three of their pneumonia patients eventually died. Urinary retention for up to 3 months was also observed in 4 of the five patients. The authors concluded that the lesion of ascending reticular fibers in the posterior cervical roots could have been responsible for the observations. This early report by Fraioli *et al.* indicates that there are potentially severe side effects from cervical rhizotomy procedure when used to treat CP-related problems [3].

Later, the procedure was used to manage intractable pain in the face and cervical region caused by malignant tumors. Mracek *et al.* reported a transverse separation of the tract of the cerebral nerves V, IX, X, and VII [4]. They performed the procedure with stimulation at several levels under local anesthesia. Besides, the authors severed sensitive cervical roots 1 to 3. The authors explained that the extent of the separation should depend on the extent of the painful area and the effect of the individual separations. The authors reported reasonable pain control in 13 patients, of which 4 had laryngeal carcinomas, 2 parotid carcinomas, 2 tongue carcinomas, one carcinoma of the pharynx, 1 of the maxilla, 1 of the lip, 1 of the tonsil, and 1 of the Os occipitale, in most cases with submandibular metastases [4]. Another application of rhizotomy in treating intractable shoulder pain was demonstrated by Grunert *et al.* in 1985 [5]. Their publication entitled "Results of cervical chordotomy with and without rhizotomy in therapy-resistant pain in the shoulder and arm," the authors reported 39 patients of theirs who they treated with the upper cervical cordotomy at the C1/C2 level. The majority of them (30 patients) were cancer patients with intractable pain of the shoulder and arm region. The remaining 9 had a benign lesion. The authors performed a simultaneous cordotomy and rhizotomy in 9 of their tumor patients and 2 patients with benign lesions. They concluded that the upper cervical cordotomy effectively reduced the pain of cancer patients whose pain cannot be controlled adequately in any other way. However, they found that the addition of the rhizotomy did not provide a further advantage [5]. Kapoor *et al.* reported on CT-guided nerve block before dorsal cervical rhizotomy they performed on 17 occipital neuralgia patients who underwent 32 C2 or C2 and C3 nerve root blocks achieving temporary pain relief [6]. The authors performed unilateral (n = 16) or bilateral (n = 1) intradural C1 (n = 9), C2 (n = 17), C3 (n = 17), or C4 (n = 7) dorsal rhizotomies. At an average final follow-up of 20 months, 11 patients (64.7%) reported complete relief, two (11.8%) had partial relief, and four (23.5%) had no relief. The authors concluded that the proper selection of patients for intradural cervical dorsal rhizotomy might produce good pain relief [6]. Gande *et al.* corroborated these findings in a long-term 14-year follow-up study of 70 patients who underwent intradural cervical dorsal root rhizotomy for refractory occipital neuralgia [7].

Less aggressive pain management applications were reported in the early 1990s. Babur *et al.* reported facet rhizotomy for cervical radiculitis in the Mount Sinai Medical Journal in 1994 [8]. They had performed 166 successful cervical facet denervations or cervical facet rhizotomies on 133 patients suffering from intractable cervical facet pain. Li *et al.* reported on endoscopic dorsal ramus rhizotomy in facetogenic chronic low back pain patients [9]. Duff *et al.* demonstrated percutaneous radiofrequency rhizotomy for cervical zygapophyseal joint mediated neck pain *via* radiofrequency (RF) rhizotomy of the medial branches of the dorsal rami from the spinal nerves [10]. These authors set out to determine the duration of complete pain relief, analgesic consumption, and any procedure-related problems. The authors found that at 12 months, 63.64% of their patients were still pain-free. The one-year follow-up time point was also the median duration of complete pain relief. Typically, these patients with pain relief stopped using prescription analgesics by six weeks after the rhizotomy procedures. The authors did not report any repeat cervical RF rhizotomies, infections, or unplanned admissions to a hospital. They concluded that percutaneous cervical RF rhizotomy is an effective treatment for cervical zygapophyseal joint mediated neck pain [10]. Radiofrequency ablation of the cervical facet pillars has since become mainstream as shown by Palea *et al.* in his 2018 report [11]. These authors commented that the percutaneous radiofrequency probe is traditionally positioned at the anterior lateral capsule of the cervical facet joint using an oblique access approach to position the electrode as closed as possible at the proximal location of the recurrent branch after its take-off from the exiting nerve root as it loops back to the cervical facet joints. The authors explained that with the oblique technique, testing of both motor and sensory function is needed to position the electrode in such a way that the more anterior nerve roots or the vertebral artery are not damaged. In contrast, the recommended direct posterior approach, which they discussed, allowed the radiofrequency electrodes to be positioned over the entire facet joint while minimizing the risk to the nerve root or vertebral artery injury. In their four-year study, the authors demonstrated that radiofrequency lesioning along the larger posterior area of the facet capsule is as effective as the traditional target point closer to the nerve root but technically more straightforward and less risky [11].

In this chapter, the authors present their endoscopic version of this technique validated by Palea *et al.* [11] who reviewed the anatomy and innervation of the cervical facet joint and capsule in detail by showing that there is a more diffuse and extensive nerve supply extending into the capsule of the cervical facet joint than just those provided by the recurrent medial sensory branches that have been the focus of traditional radiofrequency lesioning. The authors of this chapter stipulated that the spinal endoscope's direct visualization adds to the safety of the procedure by allowing the surgeon to observe the ablation process on the video screen. Moreover, the additional use of endoscopic abrasion tools, including burrs or drills, may benefit in providing more durable pain relief due to the more thorough mechanical denervation effect.

## SURGICAL TECHNIQUE

The endoscopic rhizotomy is performed under local anesthesia with sedation with the patient in a prone position in a cervical foam cushion. Some patients may undergo the proedure with a laryngeal airway mask (LMA) and others may be intubated at the dicretion of the anesthesiologist to maintain adequate ventilation. The patients are prepped and draped in standard surgical fashion. A sterile draped fluoroscopy unit is brought into the field and used in the posterior-anterior (PA) and lateral (LAT) projection to identify and confirm the planes' surgical level. A spinal needle is placed in the mid-portion of the surgical cervical facet pillars in a direct posterior approach. A guidewire is introduced through the spinal needle after applying a 0.5 to 1 cc of 1% bupivacaine. The second author does not use local anesthesia since his patients are under general anesthesia. A small 6 to 11 mm skin incision is then made around the guidewire. Serial dilators are then introduced and pushed onto the cervical facet joint to directly place the endoscopic working cannula at the junction with the cervical lamina and the facet joint. The cervical endoscope is then introduced for direct visualization of the cervical facet joint capsule and the junction with the lamina medially (Figs. **1** and **2**). Care is taken not to advance anteriorly and laterally. Slipping of the cervical facet joint pillar should be avoided. The authors then introduce a high-speed surgical drill to carefully debride any adventitial tissue of the posterior facet joint capsule without destroying it. The authors' preference also is to combine this mechanical denervation procedure with a small laminotomy with the same drill and at times with a Kerrison rongeur (Fig. **3**) to address the diffuse and extensive nerve supply extending into the capsule of the cervical facet joint described by Palea [11] and the ventral innervation reported by Yin *et al.* [12]. If the diagnostic workup suggested multilevel involvement in the pain syndrome, adjacent levels are included in this denervation procedure to address any cross-innervation from adjacent cervical painful levels [12 - 18]. After the mechanical denervation with the drill with exposure of the facet joint pillars' bony surface is completed, a pulsed radiofrequency probe is inserted to shrink and ablate the capsular fibers that are debrided of the cervical facet joint complex. The same radiofrequency may also be used for hemostasis. The small skin incision is closed with a 3-0 absorbable monofilament suture after removing the endoscopic working cannula.

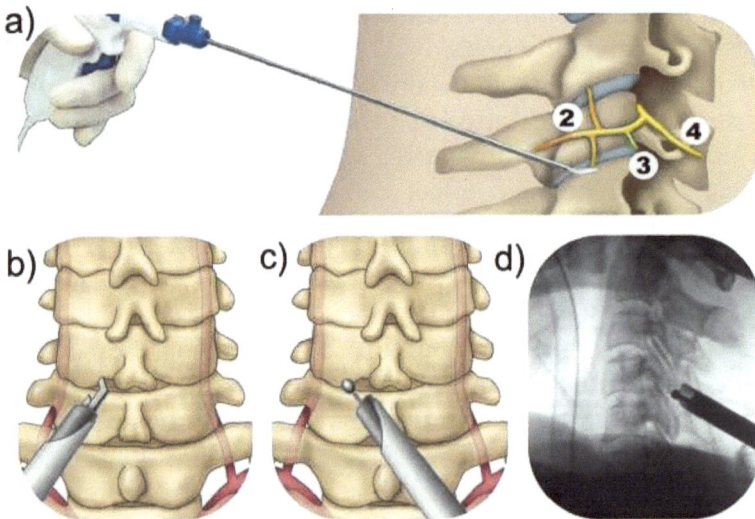

**Fig. (1).** Schematic of the radiofrequency ablation of the soft tissue of the posterior aspect of the cervical facet joint complex is shown **(a)** followed by mechanical debridement of the facet capsule Kerrison rongeur **(b)** and a high-speed drill for a limited laminotomy **(c, d)**. In panel (a), #2 indicates the innervation of the cervical facet joint complex by fibers arising from the medial branch. #3 shows the ventral sinuvertebral branch, #4 marks the anteriorly exiting cervical nerve root.

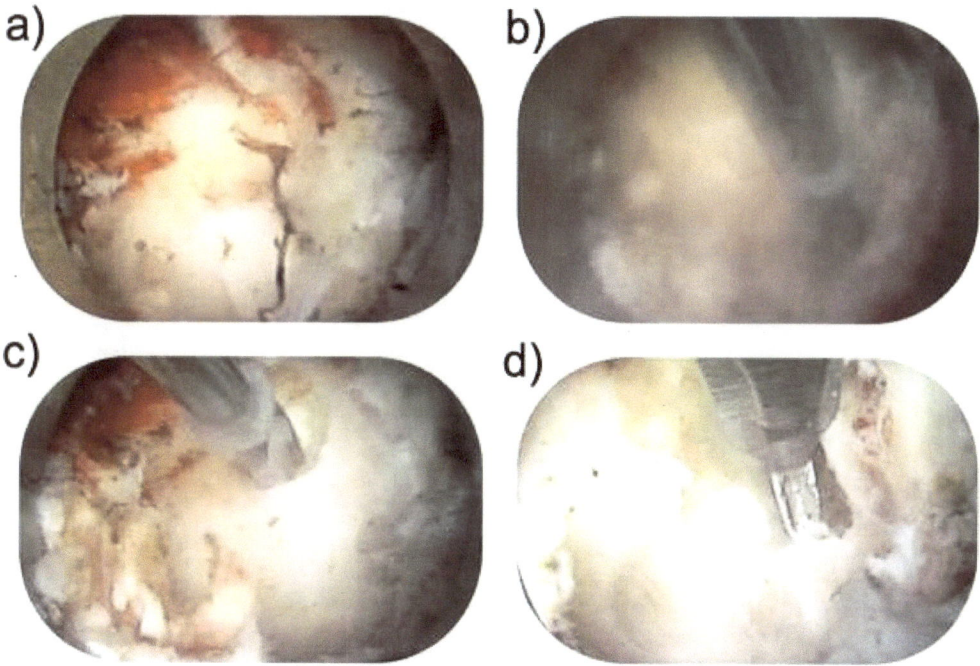

**Fig. (2).**   View through the endoscopic working cannular after the initial docking **(a)** followed by debridement of the facet capsule and hemostasis with the pulsed radiofrequency probe **(b)**. A high-speed drill was used to mechanically debride the facet joint complex down to bare bone without destroying the facet capsule **(c)**. After exposure of the ligamentum flavum a limited laminotomy was begun **(d)**.

## CLINICAL SERIES

The Inclusion criteria for inclusion for endoscopic cervical rhizotomy were axial neck pain for more than three months; (1) failed six weeks of conservative treatment with physical therapy and non-steroidal anti-inflammatories (NSAIDs); (2) absence of overt neurological deficit; (3) advanced imaging studies demonstrating early-stage degenerative changes in the cervical spine (4) and more than 50% pain relief after diagnostic cervical medial branch block with 0.5 ml 1%. Patients were excluded from inclusion in this case series if they had (1) an infectious process, (2) fracture or any other traumatic injury, (3) a severe stenotic process in the spinal canal or foramen, (4) medical comorbidities including hematological diseases, diabetes, and gastrointestinal ulcers, (5) age less than 18 years, and (6) pregnant women.

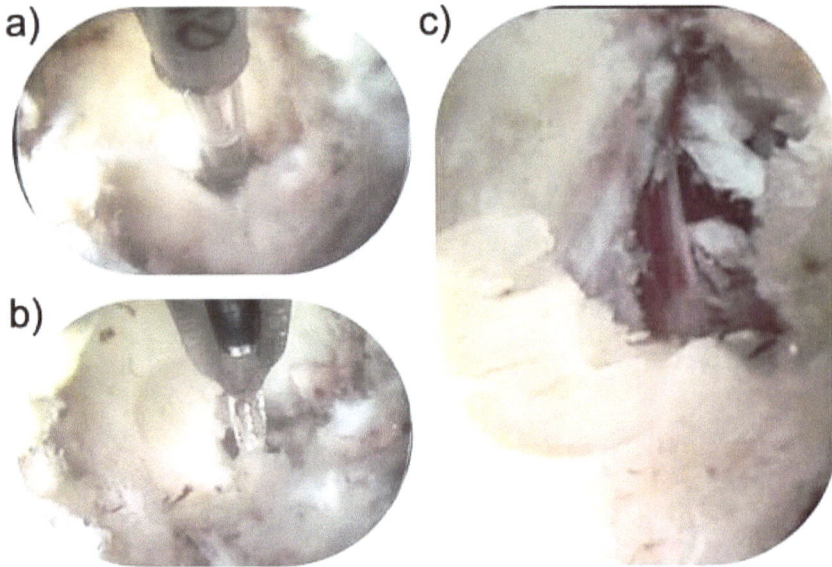

**Fig. (3).** The pulsed radiofrequency is used for hemostasis of the venous complex in the lateral cervical spinal canal **(a)**. A Kerrison rongeur is used to expand the laminotomy to just expose the lateral cervical spinal cord **(b)** and the exiting nerve root **(c)**.

From 2015 to 2019, the authors were able to enroll 371 patients, of which 187 (50.4%) were female, and the remaining 184 (49.6%) were male. The average age was 46.2 years ranging from 33 to 62 years of age. The average follow-up period was 27.9 months, ranging from 24 to 53 months. Patient outcomes were assessed with the neck disability index (NDI) and the VAS for axial neck pain and VAS for arm pain. The authors established clinical protocol that essentially selected patients for the combination mechanical rhizotomy with the drill followed by the pulsed radiofrequency ablation of at least one but more often two-level denervation procedure who were deemed not "bad enough" based on traditional image-based clinical treatment guidelines for anterior cervical discectomy and fusion (ACDF), or posterior cervical foraminotomy decompression with or without fusion. These patients were typically at a loss with no definitive treatment being offered since they were deemed candidates for physical therapy, NSAIDs, and chronic pain management. The authors observed that many patients were frustrated with the lack of more definitive treatment. Therefore, patients were offered the denervation procedure described herein if they had a diagnostic medial branch block with at least 50% pain relief. The authors' patient selection was most likely suffering from hindsight [19, 20] and selection bias [21 - 23]. They attempted to offer some treatment compassionately, particularly in those patients with significant disability, chronic pain, and unable to work and needed narcotics to control their pain. While patients were selected according to the inclusion/exclusion criteria, the authors did not attempt to distinguish between actual facetogenic axial neck pain with radiation into the shoulders and possibly the arm *versus* radicular pain from an inflamed or compromised cervical nerve root whose extension was limited to the neck without much radiation into the arms. In reality, it was impractical to make that distinction [24]. It was also irrelevant as a diagnostic injection with adequate pain relief was expected to be of high accuracy and positive predictive value, as observed and reported in other areas of the spine.

There were no injuries to the cervical nerve roots or the vertebral artery, wound complications, or excessive postoperative pain. All patients were discharged from the recovery room at the ambulatory surgery center typically within 30 to 60 minutes after surgery. Analysis of the primary outcome measures, which significantly reduced the NDI from an average preoperative value of 49.4% ± 11.9 (moderate disability) to 14.1% ± 6.3% (mild disability). The majority (75.5%; 139) of the 184 patients had a moderate disability as their NDI score was between 15 and 24 points (30% – 48%). Fifteen patients (8.15%) had severe disability from the neck (between 25 – 34 points; 50% - 64%). The remaining 30 patients had mild neck disability (5 – 14 points; 10% – 28%). All patients improved at least by one disability grade, and of the 184 patients, 122 (66.3%) patients had no pain at the final follow-up of 27.9 months. More importantly, none of the 184 patients had any repeat cervical rhizotomy with the follow-up period studies. Notably, the patient with the longest follow-up of 53 three months was still pain-free at that time. Similar improvements of the VAS-Neck and the VAS-Arm scores were observed from preoperative values of 7.9±1.8 and 3.6±1.1 postoperative values of 2.4±0.9 and 1.9±0.4, respectively.

## DISCUSSION

Chronic neck pain with or without radiation into the shoulders or arms can be disabling and incredibly frustrating to aging patients [25] who are told that there is no structural correlate on advanced imaging studies to explain their symptoms [24]. In those cases, the authors' endoscopic combination mechanical and radiofrequency denervation procedure is an attractive alternative to repetitive rounds of physical therapy, NSAIDs, and interventional and medical pain management. Real facetogenic neck pain can be quite severe and may radiate into the shoulders and the upper arm and muscular compartments and myofascial planes [26]. Our endoscopic denervation protocol following a diagnostic injection with at least 50% reduction in the patient's symptoms was successfully employed in all of the 184 patients with a significant decrease in symptoms and with complete pain relief in 66.3% (122) of the patients and minimal disability in the remaining patients without any repeat procedures at final follow-up available for each patient.

The most significant limitation of this case series study is that the authors had no way of determining whether their patients suffered from axial facetogenic neck pain or suffered from radicular pain or both [26]. It was entirely impractical to make that distinction and, in the authors' opinion, not essential in providing sufficient proof of the feasibility of using the endoscopic platform for the cervical denervation procedure. It has been demonstrated by others in the lumbar [9, 27]. The durability of the treatment benefit speaks for itself with no additional denervation or decompression fusion procedures performed in any of our study patients. This leaves the remainder of the discussion to focus on potential mechanisms of providing our patients with such compelling and durable pain relief. The most likely reason is the thorough disruption of the innervation of the facet capsule. The use of an endoscopic power drill to debride and ablate down to the bone of the cervical facet joint pillar from medial to lateral and the inclusion of a small laminotomy to kill any cross-innervation from any adjacent levels or innervation that could be provided by other nerve fibers arising from the exiting cervical nerve root as it takes off from the spinal cord and exits the cervical spine underneath the facet joint complex. Other mechanisms described in the interventional pain management literature could apply to the modulation of the dorsal root ganglion activity of the symptomatic cervical nerve root [28 - 31], particularly with the application of the pulsed radiofrequency during the directly visualized endoscopic cervical denervation procedure described by the authors [32 - 36].

Besides durable and effective pain relief, the endoscopic combined mechanical and radiofrequency denervation procedure using the authors' direct posterior approach in their 5-year consecutive case series study was extremely safe with no injuries to the cervical nerve roots or the vertebral artery. While the exact mechanism of pain relief is not entirely known to the authors it is conceivable that a combination of radicular and facetogenic symptoms contributed to the symptoms in all patients. The authors' theory is supportive of the additional pain relief they observed early on in the study with the addition of the laminotomy procedure. Therefore, the authors continued its use regardless of whether they did or did not fully understand how exactly that additional step in the denervation procedure provided additional benefit.

## CONCLUSION

The surgical protocol the authors presented in this book chapter is time-proven in their hands. A formal clinical validation in more extensive clinical trials across multiple ambulatory surgical centers is indicated to mainstream the endoscopic combined mechanical and rhizotomy denervation of the cervical facet joint complex.

## CONSENT FOR PUBLICATION

Not applicable.

## CONFLICT OF INTEREST

The author declares no conflict of interest, financial or otherwise.

## ACKNOWLEDGEMENTS

Declared none.

## REFERENCES

[1]     Benedetti A, Carbonin C, Colombo F. Extended posterior cervical rhizotomy for severe spastic syndromes with dyskinesias. Appl Neurophysiol 1977-1978; 40(1): 41-7.
[PMID: 666311]

[2]     Heimburger RF, Slominski A, Griswold P. Cervical posterior rhizotomy for reducing spasticity in cerebral palsy. J Neurosurg 1973; 39(1): 30-4.
[http://dx.doi.org/10.3171/jns.1973.39.1.0030] [PMID: 4717140]

[3]     Fraioli B, Nucci F, Baldassarre L. Bilateral cervical posterior rhizotomy: effects on dystonia and athetosis, on respiration and other autonomic functions. Appl Neurophysiol 1977-1978; 40(1): 26-40.
[PMID: 666310]

[4]     Mracek Z. Cervical tractotomy V, IX, X and VII and accompanying rhizotomy in incurable pain due to malignant tumors of the facial-cervical reagion. Zentralbl Neurochir 1978; 39(3): 311-6.
[PMID: 86250]

[5]     Grunert P, Sunder-Plassmann M. Results of cervical chordotomy with and without rhizotomy in therapy-resistant pain in the shoulder and arm. Zentralbl Neurochir 1985; 46(3): 267-71.
[PMID: 4090809]

[6]     Kapoor V, Rothfus WE, Grahovac SZ, Amin Kassam SZ, Horowitz MB. Refractory occipital neuralgia: preoperative assessment with CT-guided nerve block prior to dorsal cervical rhizotomy. AJNR Am J Neuroradiol 2003; 24(10): 2105-10.
[PMID: 14625243]

[7]     Gande AV, Chivukula S, Moossy JJ, *et al.* Long-term outcomes of intradural cervical dorsal root rhizotomy for refractory occipital neuralgia. J Neurosurg 2016; 125(1): 102-10.
[http://dx.doi.org/10.3171/2015.6.JNS142772] [PMID: 26684782]

[8]     Babur H. Facet rhizotomy for cervical radiculitis. Mt Sinai J Med 1994; 61(3): 265-71.
[PMID: 8072511]

[9]     Li ZZ, Hou SX, Shang WL, Song KR, Wu WW. Evaluation of endoscopic dorsal ramus rhizotomy in managing facetogenic chronic low back pain. Clin Neurol Neurosurg 2014; 126: 11-7.
[http://dx.doi.org/10.1016/j.clineuro.2014.08.014] [PMID: 25194305]

[10]    Duff P, Das B, McCrory C. Percutaneous radiofrequency rhizotomy for cervical zygapophyseal joint mediated neck pain: a retrospective review of outcomes in forty-four cases. J Back Musculoskeletal Rehabil 2016; 29(1): 1-5.

[http://dx.doi.org/10.3233/BMR-150597] [PMID: 26406215]

[11]   Palea O, Andar HM, Lugo R, Granville M, Jacobson RE. Direct posterior bipolar cervical facet radiofrequency rhizotomy: a simpler and safer approach to denervate the facet capsule. Cureus 2018; 10(3): e2322.
[http://dx.doi.org/10.7759/cureus.2322] [PMID: 29765790]

[12]   Yin W, Willard F, Dixon T, Bogduk N. Ventral innervation of the lateral C1-C2 joint: an anatomical study. Pain Med 2008; 9(8): 1022-9.
[http://dx.doi.org/10.1111/j.1526-4637.2008.00493.x] [PMID: 18721172]

[13]   Kallakuri S, Li Y, Chen C, Cavanaugh JM. Innervation of cervical ventral facet joint capsule: histological evidence. World J Orthop 2012; 3(2): 10-4.
[http://dx.doi.org/10.5312/wjo.v3.i2.10] [PMID: 22470845]

[14]   Zhou HY, Chen AM, Guo FJ, Liao GJ, Xiao WD. Sensory and sympathetic innervation of cervical facet joint in rats. Chin J Traumatol 2006; 9(6): 377-80.
[PMID: 17096935]

[15]   Casatti CA, Frigo L, Bauer JA. Origin of sensory and autonomic innervation of the rat temporomandibular joint: a retrograde axonal tracing study with the fluorescent dye fast blue. J Dent Res 1999; 78(3): 776-83.
[http://dx.doi.org/10.1177/00220345990780031001] [PMID: 10096453]

[16]   Yoshida N, Nishiyama K, Tonosaki Y, Kikuchi S, Sugiura Y. Sympathetic and sensory innervation of the rat shoulder joint: a WGA-HRP tracing and CGRP immunohistochemical study. Anat Embryol (Berl) 1995; 191(5): 465-9.
[http://dx.doi.org/10.1007/BF00304431] [PMID: 7625615]

[17]   Wiberg M, Widenfalk B. An anatomical study of the origin of sympathetic and sensory innervation of the elbow and knee joint in the monkey. Neurosci Lett 1991; 127(2): 185-8.
[http://dx.doi.org/10.1016/0304-3940(91)90790-Z] [PMID: 1881630]

[18]   Widenfalk B, Wiberg M. Origin of sympathetic and sensory innervation of the temporo-mandibular joint. A retrograde axonal tracing study in the rat. Neurosci Lett 1990; 109(1-2): 30-5.
[http://dx.doi.org/10.1016/0304-3940(90)90533-F] [PMID: 1690367]

[19]   Zwaan L, Monteiro S, Sherbino J, Ilgen J, Howey B, Norman G. Is bias in the eye of the beholder? A vignette study to assess recognition of cognitive biases in clinical case workups. BMJ Qual Saf 2017; 26(2): 104-10.
[http://dx.doi.org/10.1136/bmjqs-2015-005014] [PMID: 26825476]

[20]   Henriksen K, Kaplan H. Hindsight bias, outcome knowledge and adaptive learning. Qual Saf Health Care 2003; 12 (Suppl. 2): ii46-50.
[http://dx.doi.org/10.1136/qhc.12.suppl_2.ii46] [PMID: 14645895]

[21]   Noseworthy PA, Attia ZI, Brewer LC, et al. Assessing and mitigating bias in medical artificial intelligence: the effects of race and ethnicity on a deep learning model for ECG analysis. Circ Arrhythm Electrophysiol 2020; 13(3): e007988.
[http://dx.doi.org/10.1161/CIRCEP.119.007988] [PMID: 32064914]

[22]   Sibbald M, Sherbino J, Ilgen JS, et al. Correction to: Debiasing *versus* knowledge retrieval checklists to reduce diagnostic error in ECG interpretation. Adv Health Sci Educ Theory Pract 2019; 24(3): 441-2.
[http://dx.doi.org/10.1007/s10459-019-09884-7] [PMID: 30915640]

[23]   Sibbald M, Cavalcanti RB. The biasing effect of clinical history on physical examination diagnostic accuracy. Med Educ 2011; 45(8): 827-34.
[http://dx.doi.org/10.1111/j.1365-2923.2011.03997.x] [PMID: 21752079]

[24]   Jensen RK, Jensen TS, Grøn S, et al. Prevalence of MRI findings in the cervical spine in patients with persistent neck pain based on quantification of narrative MRI reports. Chiropr Man Therap 2019; 27:

13.
[http://dx.doi.org/10.1186/s12998-019-0233-3] [PMID: 30873276]

[25]   Moskovich R. Neck pain in the elderly: common causes and management. Geriatrics 1988; 43(4): 65-70.

[26]   LaGrew J, Balduyeu P, Vasilopoulos T, Kumar S. Incidence of cervicogenic headache following lower cervical radiofrequency neurotomy. Pain Physician 2019; 22(2): E127-32.
[PMID: 30921990]

[27]   Haufe SM, Mork AR. Endoscopic facet debridement for the treatment of facet arthritic pain--a novel new technique. Int J Med Sci 2010; 7(3): 120-3.
[http://dx.doi.org/10.7150/ijms.7.120] [PMID: 20567612]

[28]   Hampton DW, Steeves JD, Fawcett JW, Ramer MS. Spinally upregulated noggin suppresses axonal and dendritic plasticity following dorsal rhizotomy. Exp Neurol 2007; 204(1): 366-79.
[http://dx.doi.org/10.1016/j.expneurol.2006.11.017] [PMID: 17258709]

[29]   Song XJ, Cao JL, Li HC, Zheng JH, Song XS, Xiong LZ. Upregulation and redistribution of ephrinB and EphB receptor in dorsal root ganglion and spinal dorsal horn neurons after peripheral nerve injury and dorsal rhizotomy. Eur J Pain 2008; 12(8): 1031-9.
[http://dx.doi.org/10.1016/j.ejpain.2008.01.011] [PMID: 18321739]

[30]   Wang TH, Wang XY, Li XL, Chen HM, Wu LF. Effect of electroacupuncture on neurotrophin expression in cat spinal cord after partial dorsal rhizotomy. Neurochem Res 2007; 32(8): 1415-22.
[http://dx.doi.org/10.1007/s11064-007-9326-9] [PMID: 17406982]

[31]   Zhou X, Yang JW, Zhang W, *et al.* Role of NGF in spared DRG following partial dorsal rhizotomy in cats. Neuropeptides 2009; 43(5): 363-9.
[http://dx.doi.org/10.1016/j.npep.2009.07.001] [PMID: 19664821]

[32]   Kwak SG, Lee DG, Chang MC. Effectiveness of pulsed radiofrequency treatment on cervical radicular pain: A meta-analysis. Medicine (Baltimore) 2018; 97(31): e11761.
[http://dx.doi.org/10.1097/MD.0000000000011761] [PMID: 30075599]

[33]   O'Gara A, Leahy A, McCrory C, Das B. Dorsal root ganglion pulsed radiofrequency treatment for chronic cervical radicular pain: a retrospective review of outcomes in fifty-nine cases. Ir J Med Sci 2020; 189(1): 299-303.
[http://dx.doi.org/10.1007/s11845-019-02087-4] [PMID: 31441007]

[34]   Park J, Lee YJ, Kim ED. Clinical effects of pulsed radiofrequency to the thoracic sympathetic ganglion *versus* the cervical sympathetic chain in patients with upper-extremity complex regional pain syndrome: a retrospective analysis. Medicine (Baltimore) 2019; 98(5): e14282.
[http://dx.doi.org/10.1097/MD.0000000000014282] [PMID: 30702594]

[35]   Wang F, Zhou Q, Xiao L, *et al.* A randomized comparative study of pulsed radiofrequency treatment with or without selective nerve root block for chronic cervical radicular pain. Pain Pract 2017; 17(5): 589-95.
[http://dx.doi.org/10.1111/papr.12493] [PMID: 27739217]

[36]   Yang S, Chang MC. Effect of bipolar pulsed radiofrequency on chronic cervical radicular pain refractory to monopolar pulsed radiofrequency. Ann Palliat Med 2020; 9(2): 169-74.
[http://dx.doi.org/10.21037/apm.2020.02.19] [PMID: 32156143]

# CHAPTER 6

# Anterior Endoscopic Cervical Discectomy

**Malcolm Pestonji[1], Álvaro Dowling[2,3], Helton Delfino[4] and Kai-Uwe Lewandrowski[5,6,7]**

[1] *Mahatma Gandhi Memorial University of Health Sciences, Navi Mumbai, Kamothe Maharashtra, India*

[2] *Endoscopic Spine Clinic, Santiago, Chile*

[3] *Department of Orthopaedic Surgery, USP, Ribeirão Preto, Brazil*

[4] *Department of Orthopaedic and Anesthesiology, Ribeirão Preto Medical School, University of São Paulo, São Paulo, Brazil*

[5] *Center for Advanced Spine Care of Southern Arizona and Surgical Institute of Tucson, Tucson, AZ, USA*

[6] *Department of Orthopaedic Surgery, UNIRIO, Rio de Janeiro, Brazil*

[7] *Department of Orthoapedic Surgery, Fundación Universitaria Sanitas, Bogotá, D.C., Colombia, USA*

**Abstract:** Anterior endoscopic cervical discectomy (AECD) is a surgical procedure born in the era of minimally invasive spine surgery. A cervical discectomy through a 4 mm incision, in skilled hands, can be an ambulatory outpatient procedure where the patient may be discharged the same day from the surgical facility. Recent advances in video-endoscopic equipment and decompression tools have facilitated endoscopic spinal surgery techniques to common soft disc herniations in the cervical spine. The authors review the procedural steps of the procedure and position it as a motion preservation surgery that may alleviate radicular symptoms in the upper extremities that have not responded to non-operative care. Unrelenting arm pain in the younger patient with early degeneration of the cervical spine motion segments may be the most appropriate indication for the AECD. Procedural details and outcomes from a clinical series are reviewed to illustrate technical pearls and postoperative problems common to the procedure – with segmental kyphosis and vertical collapse of the disc space being the most relevant – if not carried out with attention to detail.

**Keywords:** Anatomy cervical spine, Anterior endoscopy, Cervical disc herniation.

* **Corresponding author Kai-Uwe Lewandrowski:** Center for Advanced Spine Care of Southern Arizona and Surgical Institute of Tucson, Tucson, AZ, USA, Department of Orthopaedic Surgery, UNIRIO, Rio de Janeiro, Brazil and Department of Orthoapedic Surgery, Fundación Universitaria Sanitas, Bogotá, D.C., Colombia, USA; Tel: +1 520 204-1495; Fax: +1 623 218-1215; E-mail: business@tucsonspine.com

## INTRODUCTION

Anterior endoscopic cervical discectomy is probably the most demanding surgery amongst all the endoscopic surgeries in the cervical spine. Knowledge of the applied surgical anatomy of the anterior cervical spine is critical to avoid injury to the vital structures which are at risk when the endoscopic working cannula is traversing the anterior neck in a path to the anterior cervical spine. Once the cervical disc spaces are approached *via* percutaneous dissection with serial dilation, the placement of the work cannula into the disc space may be difficult due to reduced disc height in segments with advanced degeneration. Anterior osteophytes or calcifications of the anterior longitudinal ligament may increase the level of difficulty with the procedure. When done in younger patients it carries the advantage of a motion preservation procedure. In this chapter, the authors review the indications, the surgical steps, the inclusion- and exclusion criteria, and postoperative care.

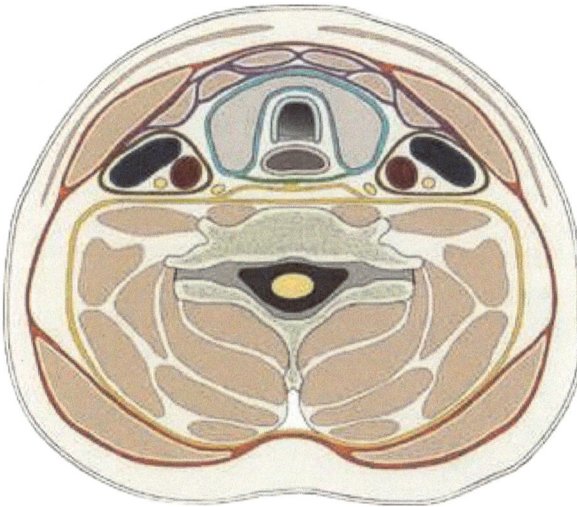

**Fig. (1).** Schematic drawing of the cross-section through the neck showing the cervical spinal motion segment at the C5/6 level. The turquoise line indicates the content of the tracheoesophageal groove. The purple outlines the anterior strap muscles, and the red line traces the superficial cervical muscles, *i.e.*, the platysma in the anterior cervical spine (top). The carotic sheet content is outlined on both sides by the brown line.

## ANATOMICAL CONSIDERATIONS

The superficial cervical fascia is very thin and covers the platysma. The four layers of the deep cervical fascia invest the neck muscles. This fascial system is composed of fibroareolar tissue filling up the empty spaces among muscles, vessels, and the neck's viscera. This fibroareolar tissue is variable, forming thin fascial layers or loosely arranged connective tissue matrix. It can easily be dissected. The superficial layer surrounds the sternocleidomastoid muscles uniting in the midline. The middle layer covers the strap muscles and forms a visceral fascia for the trachea, the esophagus, and the recurrent laryngeal nerve. The alar fascia is attached on both sides to this visceral fascia medially and the carotid sheaths laterally. The deep layer is the prevertebral fascia, covering the spine's anterior surface, longus colli, and scalene muscles (Figs. **5** and **2**).

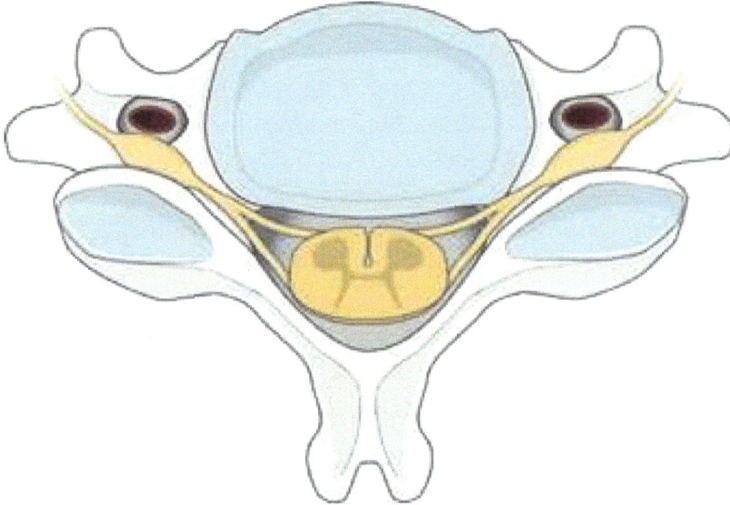

**Fig. (2).** Schematic drawing of the cross-section through the C5/6 level showing the spinal cord and nerve roots which in the cervical spine exit anteriorly but posteriorly to the vertebral artery.

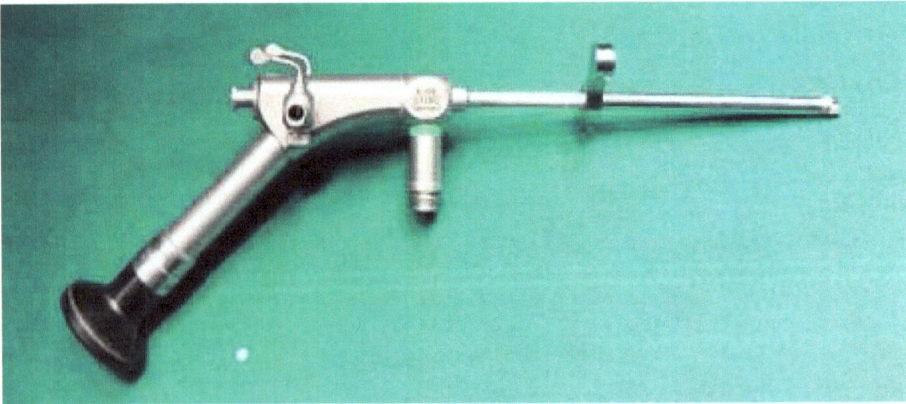

**Fig. (3).** Photo of a 4-mm Storz cervical endoscope with an inner central working channel measuring 2.7 mm accommodating 2.5 mm instruments. The endoscope has an ocular attachment for commonly available CCD video cameras. The light is attached to the bottom quick connect. The endoscope has two stop-cocks for irrigation fluid and suction channel attachments. The working sleeve has a beveled tip and a vane to help manipulate the working cannular during surgery.

## ENDOSCOPIC INSTRUMENTATION

The authors employ a variety of endoscopes. Since this team of authors is from Chile, Brazil, USA, and India, several vendors are available in their respective countries. The surgeon authors of this chapter have developed a preference for different types of cervical spinal endoscopes. An example is shown in Fig. (3). Typically, the cervical endoscope consists of a 4 mm rigid scope with a rod lens system. The smaller construction with less light-carrying fibers which may impact image resolution and distortion.

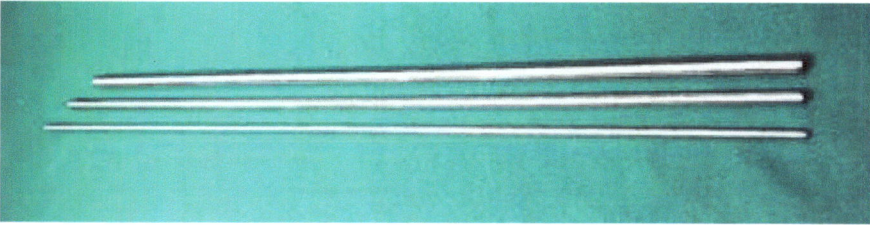

**Fig. (4).** Photo of the serial dilators used for placement of the working sleeve and the 4-mm Storz cervical endoscope.

Each cervical endoscope comes with standard set of serial dilators, working cannula, and operative instruments (Fig. **4**). These include graspers, tubular Kerrison, hooks and dissector. Some power burrs and drills have also recently become available.

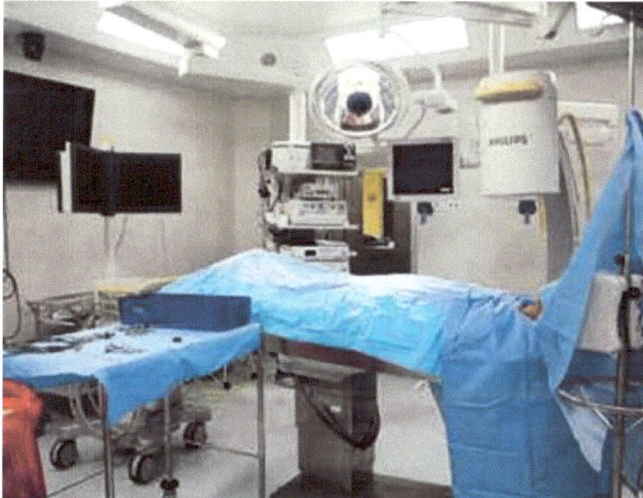

**Fig. (5).** Operation room equipment distribution. The anterior surface of the patient's neck is exposed in supine position. Fluoroscope C-arm is placed on the opposite side of the surgical approach and the surgeon.

## POSITIONING & SETUP

For the AECD procedure, the patient must be in a supine position with the neck mildly extended. A 7-cm-thick, short, rolled drape is put under the neck. For strict patient immobilization, both knees are fixed to the surgical table, and the two arms lie along the patient's trunk. Fluoroscopic C-arm goes on the opposite side of the cervical procedure. The surgeon's position may vary depending on how comfortable he or she is performing the surgery but is usually localized on the same side of the surgical approach with monitors in front (Fig. **5**).

Lines are drawn on anteroposterior (AP) and in a lateral fluoroscopic views are marked considering the location of the sternocleidomastoid muscle's inner edge, the median axis of the neck, and the upper edge of the sternum. The patient's draped with a sterile drape, leaving the anesthesiologist's access to the patient's head to observe and speak to the patient during surgery if needed. Local anesthesia is applied in the skin and in the surgical field. The details of these anesthesia nuances and how they apply to cervical endoscopic spine surgery are discussed in a separate chapter within this text.

## PEARLS OF SETUP & ACCESS

- Position the patient in the reverse Trendelenburg position. The patient must be distally supported with foot supports to avoid the patient sliding downwards. This position reduces blood pressure and bleeding at the surgical site.
- The spine must not be subjected to excessive traction or extension to ensure that the anterior structures (trachea and esophagus) remain mobile.
- Keep a pad between two shoulder blades to allow for the extension of the cervical spine with a pillow under the head.
- The shoulders must always be pulled in a downward position using adhesive/stretch tape from the shoulder downwards to visualize the lower segments, as the shoulders may obstruct the lateral C-arm view.
- Avoid using wrist traction and cause subsequent stretching of the neural structures resulting from excessive traction along the nerve at rest under anesthesia.
- The surgeon can benefit from the use of an endotracheal tube. It acts as a guide to safe lateralization of the trachea and esophagus away from the midline during access.
- Also, since neck movement is not desirable during endoscopy, it is essential to tape the head to the table, keeping the head center.

## TWO FINGER MOBILIZATION & NEEDLE PLACEMENT

First, the surgeon must mobilize the content of the tracheoesophageal complex medially and the content of the carotid sheath laterally. The access side may be chosen based on the location of the herniated disc. Typically, a posterolateral disc herniation is access from the opposite side. As the longus colli muscles are on the lateral aspects of the cervical vertebra, rolling the surgeon's two fingers over these muscles may facilitate the mobilization and palpation of the front of the cervical spine. The investing fascial layers and loose alveolar tissue between the anterior neck layers allow this freehand medial to lateral mobilization and stretching of the tracheoesophageal groove for placement of the access needle. Fluoroscopic views in both planes may also aid in assessing the tissue mobilization and whether it is adequate. In the authors' opinion, practicing the surgical access corridor's mobilization and initial needle placement is the key to unlocking endoscopic access to the anterior cervical spine. Once the access needle and guidewire are placed into the surgical cervical disc space, the remainder of the access procedure is straightforward with the serial dilators' placement and the endoscopic working cannula (Fig. **6**).

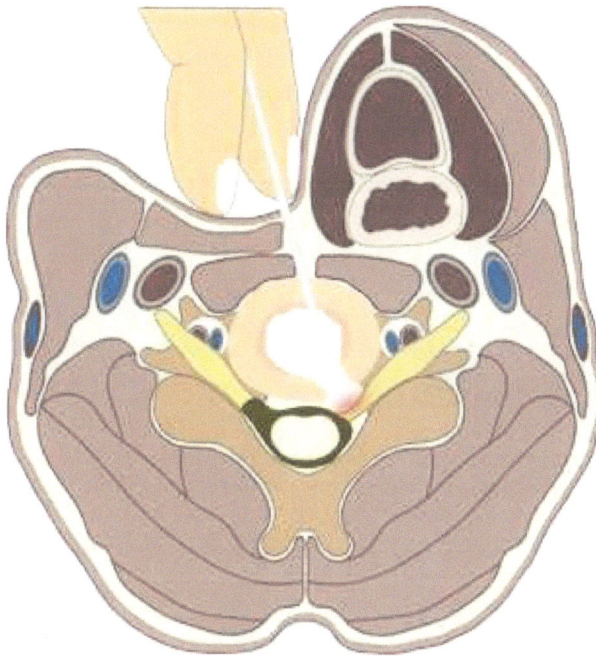

**Fig. (6).** A schematic drawing is shown showing the two-finger mobilization of the prevertebral tissues in the tracheoesophageal groove. The fingers are to maintain contact with the anterior cervical spine palpation of the bilateral longus colli muscle. The access needle is introduced under biplanar fluoroscopic views.

With AP and lateral fluoroscopic images, the surgical cervical level is defined. The entry point may be ipsilateral or contralateral to the hernia, depending on the surgeon's preference. Digital pressure toward the anterior vertebral surface is applied between the sternocleidomastoid muscle and the trachea. The larynx and trachea are displaced medially, and the carotid artery laterally. An access needle – for example an 18 gauge trocar – is inserted at the edge of the index finger, oriented at about 25° into the disc space, and confirmed through fluoroscopy. A provocation pain test may be performed if the patient is sedated and not under general anesthesia. A 5-mm skin incision is made, and a guidewire is placed. Once the trocar is removed, 2.5- to 3.5-mm diameter (depending on the height of the disc) dilation tubes are sequentially introduced over the wire and into the disc space. The final working cannula is inserted, and discectomy may be started. Sometimes anterior bone spurs impede instrument insertion, so it must be tabbed. From this point, the surgeon visualizes every step through a high-definition video. Disc annular fibers are first opened with radiofrequency, and, once inside the discal substance, extraction of hernia slices is made with the endoscopic forceps (Fig. **7**).

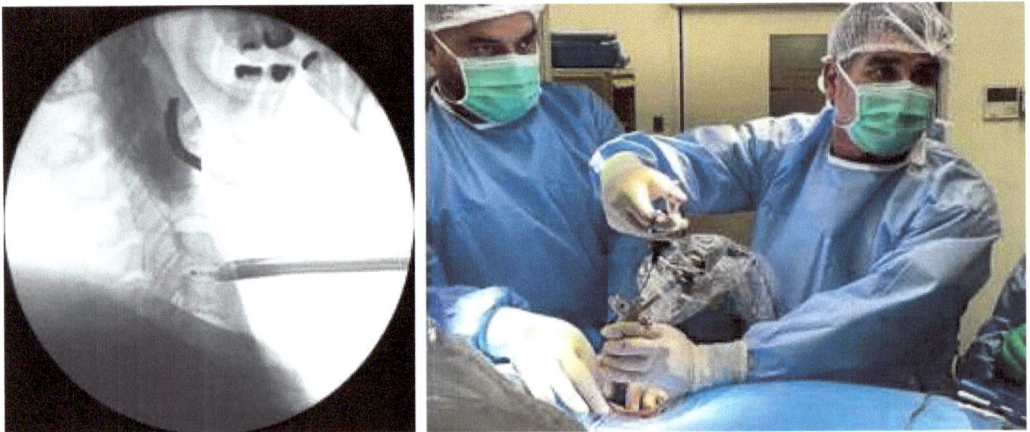

**Fig. (7).** From left to right, **(a)** Lateral fluoroscopic images are used to verify the correct positioning into the disc mass of the endoscopic forceps once the trocar has been removed. Dilation tubes are sequentially inserted, and a final working cannula is left. **(b)** While the surgeon visualizes every step of the discectomy through a high-definition video, an endoscopic forceps is inserted through surgery is done under direct visualization using the videoendoscopic system and high-definition video equipment.

There are some technical pearls worth mentioning. The authors use a 2 mm cannulated dilator as the first dilator. The first dilator should be gradually rolled over the guidewire with a gentle forward pushing movement, thereby advancing it deeper towards the cervical spine while pushing away the tracheoesophageal complex with fingers of one hand. Once the annulus is reached, the first dilator should be pushed into the surgical disc level no more than 50% of its depth on the lateral fluoroscopic projection. The other serial dilator of 3 mm and 4 mm in diameter is introduced over the 2 mm dilator, again advancing no further than approximately 50% of the lateral depth. Limiting the advancement to 50% or less is an essential step since the cumulative increase in the serial dilators' diameter may push deranged discal tissue into the neuroforamen or, worse, into the spinal canal. Similar care should be taken when the endoscopic working cannula is inserted, and the dilators are removed. At this stage, the working cannula may be carefully advanced further with a mallet (Fig. **8**).

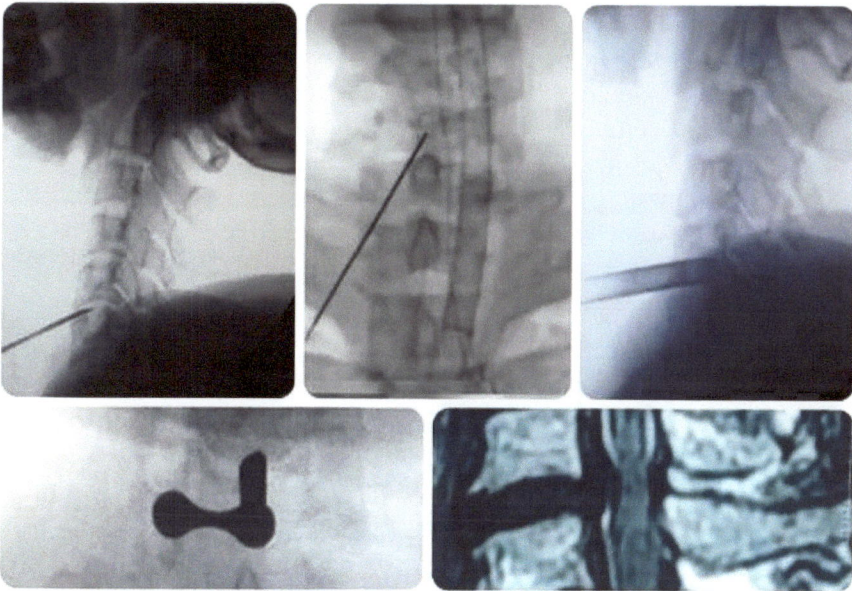

**Fig. (8).** Lateral and AP fluoroscopic images of the access needle placement and the endoscopic working cannula positioned into the C5/6 surgical level, where the sagittal MRI scan showed a herniated disc.

## ENDOSCOPIC SURGERY PEARLS

Frequently, there are two scenarios that could present some degree of difficulty to the endoscopic spine surgeon. How to pull in a fragment which has herniated through a small annular rent only visable by a small tail, and how to remove a sequestrated fragment with no tail or continuity with the main disc? The authors recommend the following procedural pearls to mobilize and gain better access to the herniated disc:

• Carefully push the cannula deeper into the disc and gently tap it in between the posterior ring apophysis to further contribute to the disc space's vertical dilation. The working cannula may be pushed 1 mm past the cervical vertebral body's posterior edge on the lateral fluoroscopic projection.

- A nerve hook may now be introduced since the posterior longitudinal ligament (PLL) is stretched, thus, facilitating access to the herniated disc.
- The herniated disc may be gradually teased out of the foramen or central cervical canal by rotating the nerve hook carefully away from the spinal cord.
- The PLL may be sharply dissected by pulling the nerve hook sharply into the disc space, thus tearing its fibers, making the rent in the PLL larger.
- The herniated disc fragment may then be pulled into the surgical view and, once liberated, may be removed with a small grasper.
- At this juncture, the posterior vertebral ring apophysis, which is typically hypertrophied, may be removed to increase the decompression further using a 1mm tubular Kerrison. These maneuvers may increase the space for the endoscope, allowing maneuvering it carefully within the disc space by directing it towards additional sequestered fragments by gentle hooking, grasping, and even pulling (Fig. **9**).
- Additional advancement of the working cannula and resection of the PLL complex may allow direct visualization of the dura. Side-firing lasers, such as a Holmium: YAG and neodymium lasers, may come in useful when trying to increase the size of the rent in the PLL.
- Additional use of flexible curettes or hooks may facilitate the removal of hard-to-reach sequestered disc fragments.

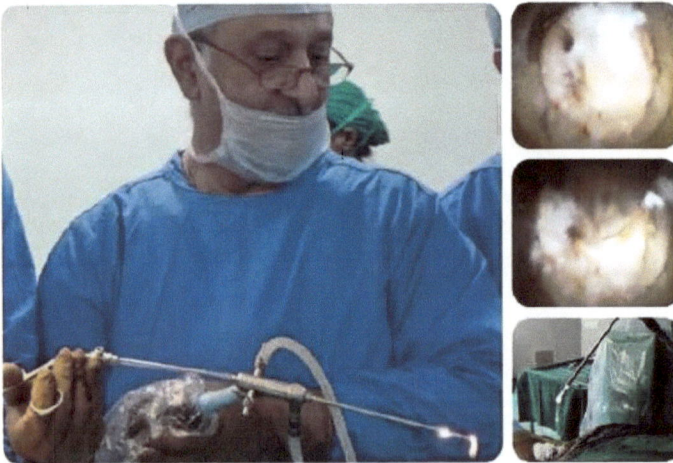

**Fig. (9).** Removal of a cervical herniated disc *via* AECD. The intraoperative images show the rent in the posterior annulus and posterior longitudinal ligament, and the removal of the sequestered disc with a grasper.

## POSTOPERATIVE MANAGEMENT

Upon withdrawal of the endoscope and working cannula, the surgeon should put gentle pressure for a couple of minutes and apply a small surgical dressing. The authors of this chapter do not use surgical drains. Patients are rapidly mobilized after recovery from anesthesia. The anesthesia recovery protocols may vary depending on whether the patient underwent AECD under general anesthesia or monitored anesthesia care (MAC). A soft cervical collar is applied, and the patient is instructed to wear it when up and about until his first postoperative visit with in one or two weeks postoperatively. Patients are advised to commence a regular diet beginning with soft mechanical foods. Typically, patients are discharged home with a cervical collar on the same day with non-narcotic pain medication. Physical therapy is order during the first postoperative visit at the discretion of the surgeon. Postoperative rehabilitation is often uncomplicated since most patients have little pain and regain function quickly in the absence of radicular pain.

## CLINICAL SERIES

From January 2015 to September 2019, the second author's group evaluated 23 patients who underwent anterior cervical discectomy performed through endoscopic technique under conscious sedation. All patients presented with neck and arm pain and no response to conservative treatment for at least 4 months. Patients with central cervical stenosis due to marked spondylosis and with myelopathy were excluded. The mean follow-up was 29 months, with a minimum of 6 and a maximum of 48 months. Clinical outcomes were determined using the neck disability index (NDI) and visual analog scale (VAS) for neck and arm pain. The mean surgical time was 40 min (range: 30–70 min), and the average hospital stay was five hours post-surgery. The NDI mean scores improved from 49% to 16%. The VAS scores for neck and arm pain also significantly decreased from pre- to post-surgery mean of 6 ($p < 0.05$). There were no intraoperative complications, dysphasia, or esophageal injury in this study group. Two patients developed post-surgery related complications: both we performed fusion after progressive radicular arm pain, in Odom's criteria excellent result 52% good 40%, poor 8%. No vascular or esophagus complications were found.

## DISCUSSION

AECD is a minimally invasive endoscopic decompression surgery of the cervical spine which is suitable for younger patients in whom motion preservation is of higher relevance than in older patients with advanced degenerative changes of the cervical spine including loss or lordosis, vertical disc collapse, and extensive osteophytosis contributing to the compromise of neural elements. However, isolated soft cervical disc herniations may still be a reasonable indication for surgery. The criteria for establishing the surgical indications for AECD and the algorithms for selecting appropriate patients for the procedure have been described in detail in two separate chapters in this text authored by the second author of this chapter.

What is evident from the detailed technical and procedural description of the AECD that the clinical success with this ultra-minimally invasive surgery is highly dependent on the surgeon's skill level and understanding of the applied surgical anatomy. The proximity of vital vascular structures, the trachea, and the esophagus to the surgical corridor put these structures at risk and has the potential for devastating complications that could arise from unfamiliarity with the procedure or the anatomy. Therefore, the authors recommend that the prospective novice endoscopic spine surgeon engages in formal postgraduate training programs wherever available in their respective countries and study side-by-side next to experienced veteran endoscopic spine surgeons who have done AECD routinely shorten the learning curve to mitigate and reduce the risk for the patient. The most dangerous aspect of AECD is placing the endoscopic working access cannula into the surgical cervical intervertebral disc. Once this access has been successfully established, injury to vital structures in the front of the cervical spine is less likely as long as the surgeon and their assistant maintain control of the working cannula within the disc space. Executing the endoscopic cervical discectomy with endoscopic rongeurs, graspers, and pituitary- or Kerrison rongeurs under videoendoscopic visualization on a large video screen may be more familiar to the endoscopic spine surgeon, who has a great deal of experience with endoscopy in other areas of the spine. Surgeons without any experience with spinal endoscopy should not begin to perform cervical endoscopy. Instead, the surgeon authors of this chapter recommend that the novice prospective spine surgeon completely agnostic to spinal endoscopy begin with straightforward lumbar discectomy cases to familiarize him- or herself with the technology and its videoendoscopic visualization on the screen. The latter aspect may seem trivial, but surgeons without any endoscopic surgery experience, whether knee- or shoulder arthroscopy for orthopedic surgeons, or endoscopic surgery of cranial cavities for neurosurgeons [1], may not easily be able to identify familiar neural structures on the video screen that they are used to seeing and identifying with loupes or the operating microscope.

As part of the expanding endoscopic surgery portfolio of the cervical spine [1 - 14], AECD has shown reliable clinical outcome improvements in skilled hands [7, 9 - 13]. In 2011, Tzaan *et al.* reported on a series of 107 consecutive patients who underwent AECD [11]. Complete one-year follow-up data was available in 86 patients (80%) which ranged from 12 to 60 months and a mean follow-up period of 22.4 months for the entire patient group. The authors of that study reported significant visual analog scale (VAS) and Neck Disability Index (NDI) improvements (p<0.001). They also assessed postoperative AECD outcomes using the modified MacNab criteria. Excellent and good results were achieved in 29 (34%) and 49 (57%) patients. Only two patients (2 of 107, 2%) had a surgical complication. One patient sustained an injury to the carotid artery, which was successfully was treated with an angiographically placed stent. The second patient developed postoperative headaches but recovered without treatment. Tzaan *et al.* cautioned that AECD, while providing comparable outcomes to open cervical discectomy, carries the risk of major complications and recommended attention to detail concerning patient selection and meticulous surgical techniques [11]. These findings were corroborated by Yang *et al.*, which enrolled 84 patients from March 2010 to July 2012 [12]. They applied AECD 42 patients comparing outcomes to posterior approach endoscopy in another 42 patients. In the AECD group, the surgery time was slightly shorter (63.5 min *vs.* 78.5 min) than in the PECD group. Moreover, the mean volume of disc removal (0.6 g *vs.* 0.3 g) was higher in the AECD *versus* PECD group. However, the postoperative loss in disc height was higher in AECD than in PECD (1.0 mm *vs.* 0.5 mm). The hospital stay was also more extended (4.9 d *vs.* 4.5 days) in AECD than PECD. Macnab outcomes were improved in both groups without any statistically significant difference (P = 0.211 and P = 0.257). Yang *et al.* reported four surgery-related complications (2 in the AECD and 2 in the PECD group) with an overall complication rate of 4.8% [12]. Application of these endoscopic techniques to anterior cervical discectomy and fusion (ACDF) has been demonstrated by others. While discussing these herein was beyond the scope of this chapter, endoscopic ACDF has been described in another chapter of this text.

## CONCLUSIONS

AECD is technically feasible, and patients may regain function quickly after surgery, which often can be done in an outpatient surgery center. The minimal pain inflicted by the procedure and effective pain relief allows mobilizing patients expeditiously and discharging them from the recovery room typically within one hour with minimal immobilization of the cervical spine. Nonetheless, AECD carries significant surgical risks and, in untrained hands, may put the patient at risk from injury to the content of the carotid sheath, the trachea, or esophagus. Vascular injury can be devastating if not diagnosed and treated rapidly. The management of these complications has been discussed in a separate chapter in this text. Surgeons interested in becoming proficient at AECD should engage in formal postgraduate training wherever possible and train with master surgeons to acquire the skills necessary to maximize patients' clinical improvements and minimize the risks associated with AECD.

## CONSENT FOR PUBLICATION

Not applicable.

## CONFLICT OF INTEREST

The author declares no conflict of interest, financial or otherwise.

## ACKNOWLEDGEMENTS

Declared none.

## REFERENCES

[1]    Srinivasan VM, Kan P, Germanwala AV, *et al.* Key perspectives on Woven EndoBridge device for wide-necked bifurcation aneurysms, endoscopic endonasal clipping of intracranial aneurysms, retrosigmoid *versus* translabyrinthine approaches for acoustic neuromas, and impact of local intraoperative steroid administration on postoperative dysphagia following anterior cervical discectomy and fusion. Surg Neurol Int 2016; 7 (Suppl. 27): S720-4.
[http://dx.doi.org/10.4103/2152-7806.192511] [PMID: 27857863]

[2]    Ahn Y, Keum HJ, Shin SH. Percutaneous endoscopic cervical discectomy *Versus* anterior cervical discectomy and fusion: a comparative cohort study with a five-year follow-up. J Clin Med 2020; 9(2): E371.
[http://dx.doi.org/10.3390/jcm9020371] [PMID: 32013206]

[3]    Chu L, Yang JS, Yu KX, Chen CM, Hao DJ, Deng ZL. Usage of bone wax to facilitate percutaneous endoscopic cervical discectomy *via* anterior transcorporeal approach for cervical intervertebral disc herniation. World Neurosurg 2018; 118: 102-8.
[http://dx.doi.org/10.1016/j.wneu.2018.07.070] [PMID: 30026139]

[4]    Deng ZL, Chu L, Chen L, Yang JS. Anterior transcorporeal approach of percutaneous endoscopic cervical discectomy for disc herniation at the C4-C5 levels: a technical note. Spine J 2016; 16(5): 659-66.
[http://dx.doi.org/10.1016/j.spinee.2016.01.187] [PMID: 26850173]

[5]    Du Q, Lei LQ, Cao GR, *et al.* Percutaneous full-endoscopic anterior transcorporeal cervical discectomy and channel repair: a technique note report. BMC Musculoskelet Disord 2019; 20(1): 280.
[http://dx.doi.org/10.1186/s12891-019-2659-0] [PMID: 31182078]

[6]    Erwood MS, Walters BC, Connolly TM, *et al.* Assessment of the reliability of the fiberoptic endoscopic evaluation of swallowing as an outcome measure in patients undergoing revision anterior cervical discectomy and fusion. World Neurosurg 2019; 130: e199-205.
[http://dx.doi.org/10.1016/j.wneu.2019.06.028] [PMID: 31203083]

[7]    Liu KX, Massoud B. Endoscopic anterior cervical discectomy under epidurogram guidance. Surg Technol Int 2010; 20: 373-8.
[PMID: 21082589]

[8]    Ren J, Li R, Zhu K, *et al.* Biomechanical comparison of percutaneous posterior endoscopic cervical discectomy and anterior cervical decompression and fusion on the treatment of cervical spondylotic radiculopathy. J Orthop Surg Res 2019; 14(1): 71.
[http://dx.doi.org/10.1186/s13018-019-1113-1] [PMID: 30832736]

[9]    Tacconi L, Giordan E. A novel hybrid endoscopic approach for anterior cervical discectomy and fusion and a meta-analysis of the literature. World Neurosurg 2019; 131: e237-46.
[http://dx.doi.org/10.1016/j.wneu.2019.07.122] [PMID: 31349080]

[10]   Tan J, Zheng Y, Gong L, Liu X, Li J, Du W. Anterior cervical discectomy and interbody fusion by endoscopic approach: a preliminary report. J Neurosurg Spine 2008; 8(1): 17-21.
[http://dx.doi.org/10.3171/SPI-08/01/017] [PMID: 18173342]

[11]   Tzaan WC. Anterior percutaneous endoscopic cervical discectomy for cervical intervertebral disc

herniation: outcome, complications, and technique. J Spinal Disord Tech 2011; 24(7): 421-31.
[http://dx.doi.org/10.1097/BSD.0b013e31820ef328] [PMID: 21430567]

[12]     Yang JS, Chu L, Chen L, Chen F, Ke ZY, Deng ZL. Anterior or posterior approach of full-endoscopic cervical discectomy for cervical intervertebral disc herniation? A comparative cohort study. Spine 2014; 39(21): 1743-50.
[http://dx.doi.org/10.1097/BRS.0000000000000508] [PMID: 25010095]

[13]     Yao N, Wang C, Wang W, Wang L. Full-endoscopic technique for anterior cervical discectomy and interbody fusion: 5-year follow-up results of 67 cases. Eur Spine J 2011; 20(6): 899-904.
[http://dx.doi.org/10.1007/s00586-010-1642-0] [PMID: 21153596]

[14]     Yuchi CX, Sun G, Chen C, *et al.* Comparison of the biomechanical changes after percutaneous full-endoscopic anterior cervical discectomy *versus* posterior cervical foraminotomy at C5-C6: A finite element-based study. World Neurosurg 2019; 128: e905-11.
[http://dx.doi.org/10.1016/j.wneu.2019.05.025] [PMID: 31096026]

# CHAPTER 7

# Anterior Transcorporeal Approach of Percutaneous Endoscopic Cervical Discectomy

**Zhong-Liang Deng[1],\*, Lei Chu[1], Liang Chen[1] and Jun-Song Yang[2]**

*[1] Department of Orthopaedics, the Second Affiliated Hospital, Chongqing Medical University, Chongqing 400010, China*

*[2] Department of Spinal Surgery, Hong-Hui Hospital, Medical College of Xi'an Jiaotong University, Xi'an 710054, China*

**Abstract:** Percutaneous endoscopic cervical discectomy (PECD) was designed to bridge the gap between failed medical- and interventional care for cervical radiculopathy due to small herniated discs and traditional open anterior cervical discectomy surgery many of which employ fusion and far fewer motion preservation strategies. PECD can be divided into the anterior transdiscal- and the posterior interlaminar approach. Anterior PECD has been criticized for the potential propagation of cervical disc collapse due to the more aggressive disruption of the anterior annulus. Additional limitations of the anterior transdiscal PECD may become relevant when upward or downward disc fragments are entrapped behind the vertebral body. Even during ACDF, a corpectomy may be required to remove these far-migrated disc fragments. Therefore, the authors advocated for the anterior transcorporeal approach through a small bony channel through a cervical vertebral body. The surgical trajectory can be freely aimed at the compressed pathology giving the surgeon more flexibility to remove the herniated disc while preserving the motion of the surgical- and possibly adjacent segments by limiting the bony resection required to gain access to the disc herniation. The authors present case examples to illustrate the involved surgical steps, required equipment, discuss pitfalls, and technical details to achieve reliable clinical improvements without complications. This simplified anterior cervical decompression procedure improved their patients without surgery-related complications, such as dysphagia, Horner's syndrome, recurrent laryngeal nerve palsy, vagal nerve injury, tracheoesophageal injury, or anterior cervical hematoma. The authors concluded that the transcorporeal PECD is suitable for the outpatient setting in an ambulatory surgery center, provides excellent direct visualization of the herniated disc with little iatrogenic injury to the cervical spine. Thus, it minimizes the risk of secondary decline of intervertebral height due to access-induced advanced cervical disc degeneration commonly seen with anterior transdiscal approaches.

---

\* **Corresponding author Zhong-Liang Deng:** Department of Orthopaedics, the Second Affiliated Hospital, Chongqing Medical University, Chongqing 400010, China; Tel: 86-13608367586; E-mail: zhongliang.deng@yahoo.com

**Keywords:** Cervical spine, Discectomy, Endoscopy, Herniated disc, Minimally invasive surgery, Transcorporeal approach.

## INTRODUCTION

While most spine surgeons accept anterior cervical discectomy and fusion (ACDF) as the gold standard operation for the treatment of symptomatic cervical disc herniations refractory to conservative care [1 - 8], well-recognized problems with the procedure including adjacent segment disease, failure and subsidence of the implants, pseudoarthrosis, and loss of intervertebral height have motivated the development of minimally invasive and simplified alternatives. Some have advocated the percutaneous endoscopic cervical discectomy (PECD) as such an alternative intended to provide treatment to those patients who have failed non-operative medical-, and interventional care. However, who by conventional medical necessity criteria are still not eligible candidates for the ACDF [9 - 12]. PECD permits to approach the cervical spine both from the anterior transdiscal and the posterior interlaminar approach. The anterior approach also carries the risk of injury to the anterior annulus and nucleus pulposus of the cervical intervertebral disc, which has been linked to advanced degeneration of the surgical disc level with the propagation of progressive vertical collapse and in some cases with recurrence of symptoms [13 - 17].

In an attempt to prevent these problems, the anterior endoscopic transcorporeal approach was advocated by George [17, 18]. A myriad of publications employing this transcorporeal approach have been published describing successful clinical outcomes with this anterior cervical decompression and its modified versions, including thee microforaminotomy, and the transuncal technique [19 - 28]. Preservation of the cervical disc structure and maintaining the medial wall of the cervical transverse process containing the transverse foramen is the common element to all of these transcorporeal procedures – may of which were with traditional open surgery, or microsurgical technique rather than under direct endoscopic visualization.

In this chapter, the authors present their percutaneous endoscopic version of the anterior transcorporeal approach to a symptomatic cervical disc herniation with illustrative case examples highlighting the clinical advantages of the procedure. The authors will demonstrate how the PECD lends itself to be carried out in an ambulatory surgery center because of shorter operative time and lower surgical risks for intraoperative iatrogenic injury because of the direct magnified endoscopic visualization the painful pathology – the cervical herniated disc.

## SURGICAL TECHNIQUE

First, the authors attempted the percutaneous endoscopic anterior cervical discectomy (PECD) in a cadaver study to adopt the endoscopic application technique. The surgery is performed in a supine position with the patient on a radiolucent table and the cervical spine in slight extension and under general anesthesia and continuous electroneurophysiological neuromonitoring. The patient is set up such that intraoperative fluoroscopy images can quickly be taken in the anterior and lateral projection without impeding the surgeon's ability to operate without obstruction by surgical equipment (Fig. **1**). The assistant should be on the side of the surgeon. The authors' preferred endoscopic equipment is the cervical set from SPINENDOS GmbH. The surgical level is marked after it has been located on biplanar fluoroscopy views—an 8-mm transverse skin incision, just the sternocleidomastoid muscle, and slightly below the surgical level. The content of the tracheoesophageal groove is pushed medial and the carotid sheath lateral employing the two-finger technique. This technique allows the creation of a small safe window to advance a spinal needle to target the surgical cervical vertebral body in a trajectory best suited for accessing the surgical pathology. A right-handed surgeon should push the entire tracheoesophageal content is pushed to the opposite side with the left-hand index- and middle finger.

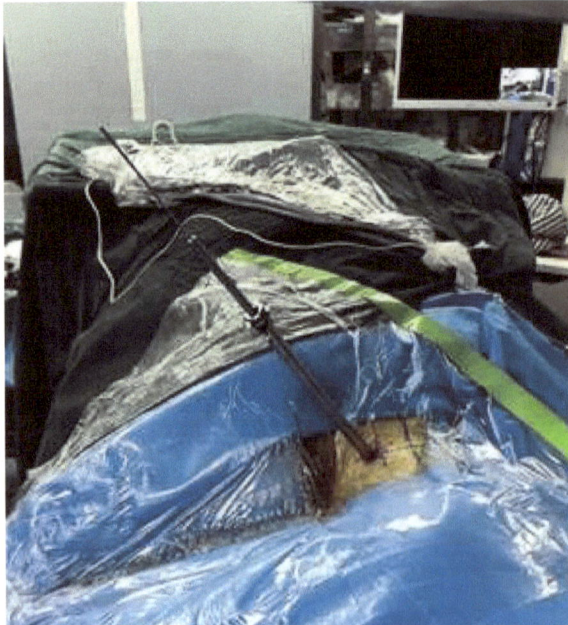

**Fig. (1).** Along with the guidewire, the dilator sheath and the outer working sheath were inserted sequentially *via* the created intracorporeal hole into the targeted vertebral body.

Through the skin incision, a puncture-needle-obturator assembly, incorporating a non-beveled sheath of a thoracolumbar vertebroplasty needle is advanced over a blunt K-wire to the anterior aspect of the cervical vertebral body (Fig. 2). Once on the anterior cervical spine, this large access needle is then carefully migrated cranially and medially under fluoroscopic control to be positioned strategically over the vertebral body adjacent and inferior to the surgical disc level as to aim towards the painful compressive pathology in the lateral cervical canal (Fig. 3). When the desired position of the vertebroplasty sheath is confirmed with intraoperative fluoroscopy, the blunt inner K-wire removed, and the sharp stylet of the vertebroplasty needle is then tapped into the target cervical vertebral body to anchor on the anterior surface. The outer sheath of the vertebroplasty needle is advanced through the vertebral body of C5 until the tip of the sharp stylet has reached the proximity of the posterosuperior edge of C5 on biplanar fluoroscopic imaging. Then, the obturator is removed vertebroplasty needle. A blunt guidewire is introduced to probe the posterior wall of the cervical vertebral body to check under fluoroscopy on whether or not the sharp vertebroplasty puncture needle penetrated the posterior wall of C5 (Figs. 3 and 4). Ideally, the blunt guidewire is contained within the surgical vertebral body. Serial dilators and the working cannula of the cervical endoscope are then introduced and place to the desired final position over this blunt guidewire (Fig. 4). Once the endoscopic working sheath is satisfactorily positioned, both the dilator sheath and the inner guidewire are removed. The cervical endoscope is introduced to facilitate direct and continuous visualization of the decompression site intended to gain access to the painful compressive bony pathology or herniated disc. This is done under continuous irrigation with 0.9% saline solution.

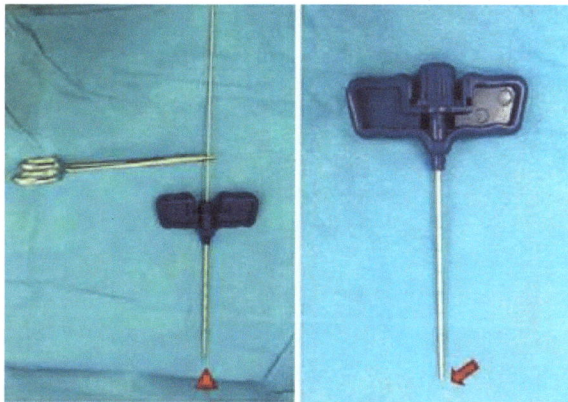

**Fig. (2).** A self-designed puncture needle complex incorporates a nonbeveled sheath of a vertebroplasty needle on the outside and a blunted K-wire on the inside (left). The red arrowhead shows the blunted tip, which was replaced with a sharp stylet (middle, red arrow).

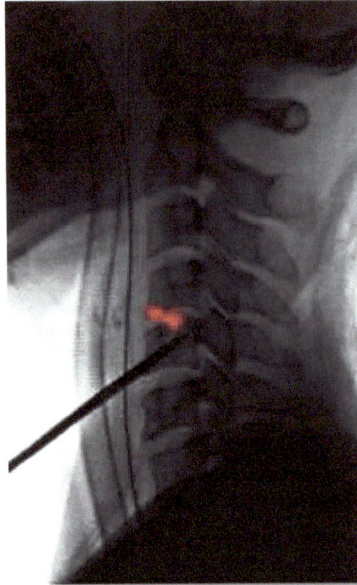

**Fig. (3).** Lateral intraoperative fluoroscopic view showing the puncture needle complex incorporating a nonbeveled sheath of a vertebroplasty needle on the outside and a blunted K-wire on the inside. The red arrowhead shows the when the puncture needle complex was placed near the posterosuperior edge of the targeted vertebral body (right, red arrow). Note the endotracheal tube and the gastric tube are visualized and should be used as landmark during the initial puncture.

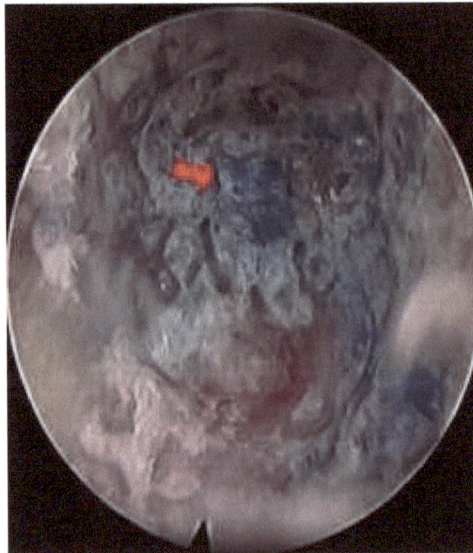

**Fig. (4).** Because of the blue color, bone wax containing indigo carmine (red arrow) was easily visible under endoscopy, which could guide the drilling process along the designed trajectory.

At this juncture, enlarging the hole within the surgical cervical vertebral body may have to be expanded. The authors accomplished with a diamond high-speed following the same surgical corridor previously established to establish access to the compressive pathology. Under continuous fluoroscopic control, the cervical vertebral body's posterosuperior wall is penetrated (Fig. **5**). At this juncture, a blunt hook could be employed to verify whether the posterior wall of the cervical vertebral body was opened. If further decompression is needed, an endoscopic Kerrison rongeur can be employed to enlarge the orifice. Bleeding may be controlled with a low-energy pulsed bipolar radiofrequency probe (Elliquence, LLC Long Island NY) to maintain a clear visual field. Sometimes incising the posterior longitudinal ligament may be necessary to mobilize and extirpate extruded disc herniations after the herniated nucleus pulposus is removed with a pituitary rongeur (Fig. **6**). The spinal cord's decompression by dural sac expansion and the exiting nerve root is visually inspected and palpated with a blunt nerve hook. Before removing the endoscopic instruments, meticulous hemostasis should be achieved. This can be achieved by placing bone wax into the tunnel (Fig. **7**). A JP-type tubing-suction system is placed into the transosseous access channel to avoid a postoperative surgical site hematoma. Typically, this transcorporeal endoscopic decompression can be completed in approximately 75 minutes. The wound is then closed with an intracuticular suture and covered with a water-impermeable dressing. The drainage tube is removed 24 hours postoperatively.

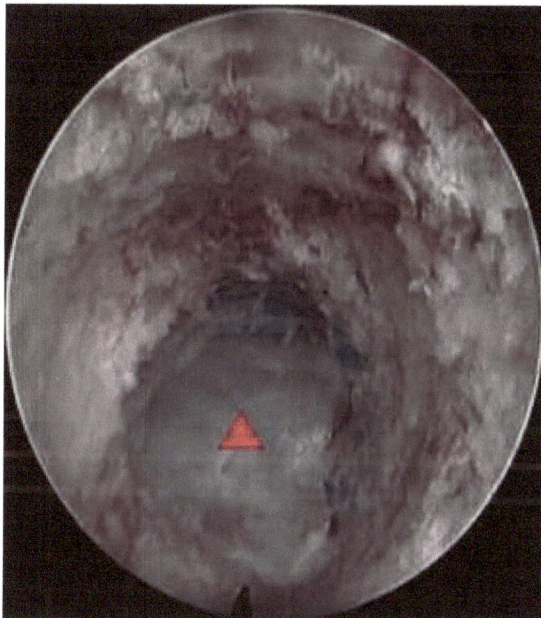

**Fig. (5).** View through the orifice of the posterosuperior wall of the vertebral body (red arrowhead) exposing the herniated disc.

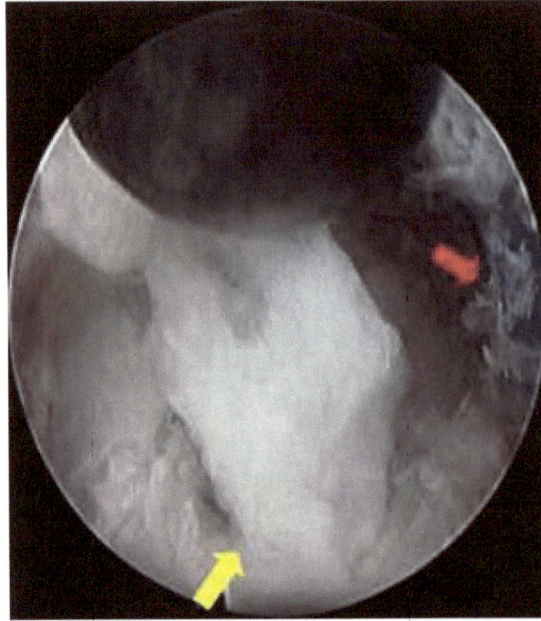

**Fig. (6).** Intraoperative endoscopic view through the orifice of the posterosuperior wall of the vertebral body showing the herniated disc (yellow arrow) being removed with a pituitary rongeur. Notably, the surrounding bone wax containing indigo carmine was visible (red arrow).

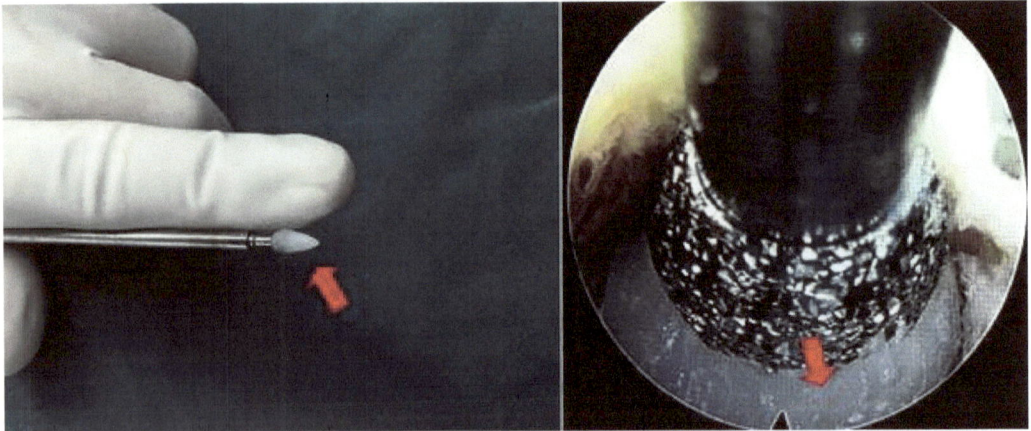

**Fig. (7).** Bone wax smeared on the endoscopic burr (left) (red arrow) could facilitate hemostasis during the drilling process (right).

## CLINICAL SERIES

The authors investigated initial clinical outcomes with the PECD procedure in a small case series of 5 consecutive patients who had surgery by the participating surgeons from October 2014 to March 2015 [29]. The ethics committee approved the study of the Second Affiliated Hospital of Chongqing Medical University and

Honghui Hospital of Xi'an Jiaotong University. There were three female and two male patients with cervical disc herniations who underwent PECD *via* the anterior transcorporeal tunnel approach (Table 1). The patients' mean patient age was 42.8 ± 5.0 years, ranging from 37 to 50 years. The mean follow-up was 10.4 ± 3.9 months, ranging from 6 to 16 months. Three patients were suffering from radiculopathy refractory to conservative care, and two patients were suffering from cervical myelopathy as a result of severe spinal cord compression. Therefore, the neurologic status of patients was carefully evaluated an recorded by employing the American Spinal Injury Association scoring system. Patients were asked to indicate the severity of their neck- and arm pain on the visual analog scale (VAS) ranging from 0 (no pain) to 10 (extreme severe pain). Postoperatively, patients were evaluated clinically at 1, 3, 6, and 12 months postoperatively at which time plain radiograph, computed tomography (CT), and magnetic resonance imaging (MRI) examinations were recommended. The inclusion criteria were failed conservative therapy for at least six weeks or sudden deterioration of neurologic function with unbearable pain, symptoms consistent with preoperative MRI scan, a single-level central or paramedian disc herniation. The exclusion criteria were challenging to reach disc herniations, downward migrated disc herniations at the C6-7 level, presence of associated foraminal stenosis, lateral disc herniations, severe obesity, a short neck where it would be difficult to push the tracheoesophageal visceral sheath to the opposite side, and calcified disc herniations.

**Table 1. Demographic Characteristics of Patients Before and After Percutaneous Endoscopic Cervical Discectomy.**

| Age (Years) | Sex | Indications for Surgery | Surgical Level | Preoperative VAS Neck & Arm | Preoperative JOA Score | VAS 6 Months Postoperatively | JOA Score 6 Months Postoperatively |
|---|---|---|---|---|---|---|---|
| 37 | F | Myelopathy | C4-5 | 7 | 10 | 2 | 14 |
| 40 | M | Radiculopathy | C5-6 | 8 | 14 | 1 | 15 |
| 45 | F | Radiculopathy | C4-5 | 7 | 13 | 2 | 15 |
| 42 | F | Radiculopathy | C5-6 | 8 | 14 | 1 | 16 |
| 50 | M | Myelopathy | C5-6 | 6 | 11 | 2 | 15 |

VAS, visual analog scale; JOA, Japanese Orthopaedic Association; F, female; M, male.

The PECD was successfully complete in all of the five patients. The mean preoperative VAS score was 7.2 ± 0.8, and JOA score was 12.4 ± 1.8, respectively. At six months postoperatively, the mean VAS for neck- and arm pain was 1.6 ± 1.1 and the mean JOA score 15.0 ± 0.7, respectively. The authors did not encounter any surgery-related complications. In the absence of dysphagia, Horner syndrome, recurrent laryngeal nerve palsy, vagus nerve injury, tracheoesophageal- and vascular injury, cervical hematoma, intervertebral disc infection, or postoperative headaches the authors deemed to PECD procedure as safe and effective. At postoperative 3-month follow-up, there was also no discernable radiographic evidence of disc space narrowing nor instability at the surgical level. Postoperative CT scans showed partial healing of thee bony tunnel created to accommodate the endoscopic working cannula. Generally, it appeared healed at 6 months postoperatively (Fig. **8**).

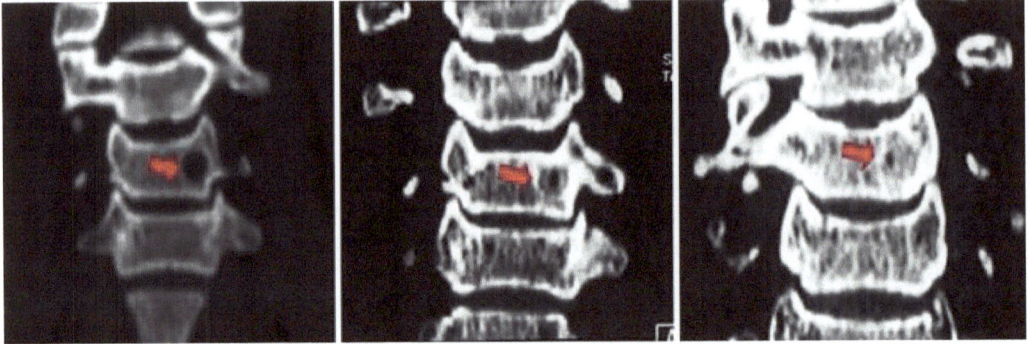

**Fig. (8).** Computed tomography coronal reconstruction views of 1 (left), 3 (middle), and 6 (right) months postoperatively showed the process of bone healing dynamically. Notably, the intracorporeal hole almost disappeared at 6 months postoperatively. The red arrow showed the drilling tunnel is gradually shrank and healed.

The exemplary case is referenced earlier in this chapter, illustrates the treatment of a cervical disc herniation with the PECD procedure in a 37-year-old female patient who presented with posterior neck pain and weakness of the extremities for nine months preceding here PECD surgery [30]. The patient complained of tingling and numbness in the upper extremity with a globally decreased motor strength of 3/5. In the presence of a positive Hoffman's sign and other upper motor neuron signs, the patient was diagnosed with spinal cord dysfunction due to cervical myelopathy. The preoperative MRI scan showed a huge C4/5 disc herniation causing severe spinal cord compression. Calcifications within this disc herniations were also noted on the patient's preoperative CT scan. A brief attempt at conservative care was made by asking the patient to wear a soft cervical collar for three weeks, which did not produce noticeable clinical improvements. Then, the patient underwent successful PECD and noted immediate relief of neck and arm pain after the operation. Her VAS rating for the neck- and arm pain had reduced from a preoperative score of 7/10 to 3/10 postoperatively. Her gait and control of the extremities improved gradually and in a stepwise manner with an over reduced spasticity and diminished upper motor neuro signs on physical examination. At the final follow-up, the surgeon noted the complete recovery of neurological function and near-complete pain relief. A postoperative MRI scan confirmed the total removal of the herniated disc. The transcorporeal drill tunnel was proved to be intact on postoperative CT scanning. At postoperative 3-month follow-up, there was no radiographic evidence of disc space narrowing, or instability. The CT scan showed partial closure of the transcorporeal bone tunnel. This patient had none of the previously listed possible surgery-related complications.

## DISCUSSION

PECD has recently received significant attention as a viable alternative to ACDF [28, 31 - 35]. It has gained traction because of its potential to obviate some of the disadvantages of cervical fusion surgery – most importantly, adjacent segment disease (ASD) [36, 37]. Besides this long-term problem, there are other perioperative problems with ACDF, such as dysphagia, recurrent laryngeal nerve palsy, Horner syndrome, vagal nerve injury, tracheoesophageal- and vascular injury, postoperative hematoma, intervertebral disc infection, or postoperative headaches [38 - 46]. Traditionally, endoscopic discectomy in the cervical spine has been done from the anterior transdiscal- [28, 31] or the posterior interlaminar [47 - 49] approach. Clinical outcomes with both techniques have been reported as favorable [14, 31, 50]. Notably, decrease in vertical disc height with the anterior transdiscal approach has been reported to occur later in follow-up several months later, which is most likely attributable to the fact that more disc tissue is removed during the anterior transdiscal approach. Moreover, the transdiscal approach may create more damage to the residual healthy disc, thereby leading to further iatrogenic discal degeneration and, ultimately, to loss of intervertebral disc height. This problem has motivated the clinical application of the anterior transcorporeal approach but raised concerns for the need to repair the transosseous surgical access corridor or whether it can heal by spontaneous osteogenesis without the need for a bone graft. While all these issues are undoubtedly relevant, investigators in the prior literature employed open or microsurgical techniques [19 - 28]. In comparison, the authors' contribution is having to further miniaturized the surgical approach by the application of endoscopic procedures and in overcoming its limitations because endoscopic manipulation and removal of a herniated disc through a small transcorporeal channel through a small narrow surgical field inside a small hole in the posterior superior vertebral call may prove difficult and troublesome particularly if disc fragments are large or calcified [29, 34].

There are several advantages of using an endoscopic technology platform to execute the transcorporeal approach. First, the illumination, magnification, and clearance of the surgical field of view by continuous saline irrigation provide much better visualization of the surgical compressive pathology with the hydraulic pressure from the irrigation, reducing bleeding. The authors discourage the use of bipolar electrocautery close to the spinal cord. Instead, the application of Avitene™ [51] is recommended. Intermittent aspiration of any blood accumulated in the drill hole may also be useful in maintaining clear visualization. Occasionally, pulsed bipolar radiofrequency can be employed to control bleeding from the anterior cervical epidural venous plexus. Typically, pulsating neural tissue and epidural fat floating indicates adequate endoscopic decompression. Another desirable side effect of the irrigated endoscopy is the potentially lower risk of infection since the surgical site is constantly lavaged. The ability to adjust the viewing angle also improves the surgeon's ability to visualize, manipulate, and safely extirpate the disc herniation while reducing the risk of intraoperative iatrogenic injury.

There may also be some limitations to the transcorporeal PECD. The authors limited the application of this endoscopic technique exclusively to the treatment of central disc herniations. In comparison, an open transdiscal approach gives the surgeon more flexibility at attacking paracentral disc herniations or lateral canal stenosis, however, at the expense of destroying more intact disc tissue. Besides, the transcorporeal PECD may prove useful in cases of relative and absolute contraindications to the transdiscal approach. For example, the reduced height of the cervical interspace of less than 4 mm or large anterior cervical disc osteophytes may prove to be relative or absolute contraindications depending on the equipment requirements and surgeon's skill level. The latter may also determine whether a surgeon should approach large central- and paracentral cervical disc herniations better with the anterior transdiscal version of the open or microendoscopic PECD technique. Alternatively, the posterior interlaminar approach may be more appropriate for lateral herniation directly amenable to the foraminotomy exposure and discectomy regardless of whether the decompression is done openly, endoscopically, or with the use of other MIS techniques. However, the posterior approach's utility may be limited, particularly if a sizeable central herniation causing spinal cord compression needs to be removed. Notably, large upward- or downward migrated herniations as shown in the authors' illustrative case example seem best suited for the anterior transcorporeal PECD technique since the transosseous channel can be directly aimed at the surgical pathology without excessive bony resection and preservation of cervical motion – a step that would be virtually unavoidable during conventional ACDF surgery likely turning that surgery into a multilevel operation and, thus, increasing the risk of ASD.

There are a few technical details and risks of the surgical approach and exposure worth discussing. For example, the risk of injuring the content of the carotid sheath - more dangerously of the jugular vein, but also the vagus nerve, and the sympathetic plexus (Horner's syndrome) – is undeniably real during the initial blunt finger dissection and the percutaneous placement of the vertebroplasty trochar needle. Therefore, the authors recommend that beginners create a mini-open exposure with a more familiar blunt dissection of the tracheoesophageal groove, perhaps under microscopic visualization to expose the anterior cervical spine and facilitate the placement of the endoscopic working cannula. The authors modified the vertebroplasty puncture needle with a non-beveled tip and validated its safety during C1 vertebroplasty employing the anterior retropharyngeal approach under C-arm fluoroscopic control [32]. This modified blunt vertebroplasty trocar is to be introduced over a guidewire to minimize the risk for iatrogenic injury during this step of the surgery. Another pearl to be considered is to place a gastric tube into the esophagus and intubate the patient with an endotracheal tube. Both are easily identified on fluoroscopic images and should assist the surgeon in placing the trochar safely in front of the anterior cervical spine. Another potential pitfall of the anterior transcorporeal PECD is the possible violation of the medial wall of the transverse process, which contains the vertebral artery within the transverse foramen. Exposure of the vertebral artery when employing the transuncal technique has been recommended [52 - 57]. Instead, the authors suggest not to jeopardize the vertebral artery and modified the method with attention to this detail. The cervical body's width may range from 19 to 22 mm and is considerably smaller than thoracic or lumbar vertebral bodies for that matter. Hence, staying on course with the transcorporeal decompression is of utmost importance to assure the safety of the anterior endoscopic PECD procedure [58]. Another consideration is the transverse release of the longus colli muscle (LCM), which may be necessary at times. The need for LCM release has been reported in open transcorporeal discectomy procedures where retractors need to be placed to maintain a surgical access corridor. However, the authors caution the reader since there is the risk of sympathetic plexus injury, which could propagate Horner's syndrome since it lies mostly at the lateral border of the LCM. Again, the endoscopic, percutaneous procedure through a 7 or 8 mm incision may prevent these problems. Conceivably, the risk of recurrent laryngeal nerve palsy and dysphagia may also be lower than observed with open anterior cervical surgery.

What is clear from the author's consecutive case series is that a precise drilling trajectory is extremely important for the ease of this operation. The hole is so narrow that the removal of the herniated disc can be unnecessarily complicated. The judicious use and careful interpretation of intraoperative fluoroscopy and endoscopic images is recommended to facilitate the transcorporeal PECD. Kim *et al.* suggested using intraoperative O-arm-based navigation to increase further the accuracy of the initial placement of the drill channel to gain access to the posterior superior cervical vertebral body wall. Cadaver training is also recommended for the novice surgeon; particularly those who have no experience in spinal endoscopy [23]. The authors have no doubt that with increasing comfort level and confidence in their skills, surgeons should be able to take full advantage of the low morbidity associated with the minimal endoscopic access. Minimizing iatrogenic injury to the anterior visceral content of the neck and the anterior cervical spine is the key advantage of the endoscopic PECD technique making this treatment method ideal for applications in an outpatient ambulatory surgery center. Utilization of modern ERAS anesthesia protocols [59 - 61] may facilitate early discharge from the ASC and allow for faster overall recovery, shorter time to postoperative narcotic independence, and faster social reintegration and return to work.

This case series suffers from the limitation of consisting of only five patients. While the feasibility of this anterior transcorporeal approach under endoscopy was established, further study with a larger patient sample needs to be conducted if it is efficacious, safe, and reliable. Long-term follow-up studies need to ascertain whether there are any unforeseen risks to patients. At least theoretically, there is a risk of postoperative kyphosis or instability of the cervical vertebral body through which the transcorporeal access channel was placed. In our series with limited one-year follow-up, postoperative instability was not observed, and in only one patient was there progressive collapse of the disc space. Thus far, the clinical data generated by the authors suggests a low propensity of postoperative decrease of disc height. However, a comparative study is warranted to ascertain whether the anterior transcorporeal tunnel approach, when carried out with the utilization of endoscopic techniques, is indeed beneficial in terms of long-term symptom relief while maintaining the disc space height.

## CONCLUSIONS

The anterior transcorporeal approach is a novel access concept employed in the treatment of cervical intervertebral disc herniations. This approach's advantages are multiple, and range improved visualization of the surgical pathology to decreased perioperative burden to the patient and a lower risk of iatrogenic injury to vital structures residing in the anterior neck. Theoretically, the potential of the secondary collapse of the cervical intervertebral disc, often seen with transdiscal discectomy techniques and development of adjacent level disease common to ACDF may also be lower. Larger scale studies with longer follow-up need to validate the notions.

## CONSENT FOR PUBLICATION

Not applicable.

## CONFLICT OF INTEREST

The author declares no conflict of interest, financial or otherwise.

## ACKNOWLEDGEMENTS

This work was partially supported by a grant from the Key Project of Chongqing Municipal Healthy Bureau (No. 2011-1-053) for ZL Deng.

## REFERENCES

[1]     De la Garza-Ramos R, Xu R, Ramhmdani S, *et al*. Long-term clinical outcomes following 3- and 4-level anterior cervical discectomy and fusion. J Neurosurg Spine 2016; 24(6): 885-91.
        [http://dx.doi.org/10.3171/2015.10.SPINE15795] [PMID: 26895527]

[2]     Findlay C, Ayis S, Demetriades AK. Total disc replacement *versus* anterior cervical discectomy and fusion: a systematic review with meta-analysis of data from a total of 3160 patients across 14 randomized controlled trials with both short- and medium- to long-term outcomes. Bone Joint J 2018; 100-B(8): 991-1001.
        [http://dx.doi.org/10.1302/0301-620X.100B8.BJJ-2018-0120.R1] [PMID: 30062947]

[3]     Grasso G, Landi A. Long-term clinical and radiological outcomes following anterior cervical discectomy and fusion by zero-profile anchored cage. J Craniovertebr Junction Spine 2018; 9(2): 87-92.
        [http://dx.doi.org/10.4103/jcvjs.JCVJS_36_18] [PMID: 30008525]

[4]     Hu Y, Lv G, Ren S, Johansen D. Mid-to long-term outcomes of cervical disc arthroplasty *versus* anterior cervical discectomy and fusion for treatment of symptomatic cervical disc disease: a systematic review and meta-analysis of eight prospective randomized controlled trials. PLoS One 2016; 11(2): e0149312.
        [http://dx.doi.org/10.1371/journal.pone.0149312] [PMID: 26872258]

[5]     Lee CJ, Boody BS, Demeter J, Smucker JD, Sasso RC. Long-term radiographic and functional outcomes of patients with absence of radiographic union at 2 years after single-level anterior cervical discectomy and fusion. Global Spine J 2020; 10(6): 741-7.
        [http://dx.doi.org/10.1177/2192568219874768] [PMID: 32707013]

[6]     Bohlman HH, Emery SE, Goodfellow DB, Jones PK. Robinson anterior cervical discectomy and arthrodesis for cervical radiculopathy. Long-term follow-up of one hundred and twenty-two patients. J Bone Joint Surg Am 1993; 75(9): 1298-307.
        [http://dx.doi.org/10.2106/00004623-199309000-00005] [PMID: 8408151]

[7]     Emery SE, Fisher JR, Bohlman HH. Three-level anterior cervical discectomy and fusion: radiographic and clinical results. Spine 1997; 22(22): 2622-4.
        [http://dx.doi.org/10.1097/00007632-199711150-00008] [PMID: 9399447]

[8]     Zdeblick TA, Hughes SS, Riew KD, Bohlman HH. Failed anterior cervical discectomy and arthrodesis. Analysis and treatment of thirty-five patients. J Bone Joint Surg Am 1997; 79(4): 523-32.
        [http://dx.doi.org/10.2106/00004623-199704000-00007] [PMID: 9111396]

[9]     Epstein NE. A review of complication rates for Anterior Cervical Diskectomy and Fusion (ACDF). Surg Neurol Int 2019; 10: 100.
        [http://dx.doi.org/10.25259/SNI-191-2019] [PMID: 31528438]

[10]    Laxer EB, Brigham CD, Darden BV, *et al*. Adjacent segment degeneration following ProDisc-C total disc replacement (TDR) and anterior cervical discectomy and fusion (ACDF): does surgeon bias effect radiographic interpretation? Eur Spine J 2017; 26(4): 1199-204.
        [http://dx.doi.org/10.1007/s00586-016-4780-1] [PMID: 27650387]

[11] Yang Y, Ma L, Liu H, *et al.* Comparison of the incidence of patient-reported post-operative dysphagia between ACDF with a traditional anterior plate and artificial cervical disc replacement. Clin Neurol Neurosurg 2016; 148: 72-8.
[http://dx.doi.org/10.1016/j.clineuro.2016.07.020] [PMID: 27428486]

[12] Yew AY, Nguyen MT, Hsu WK, Patel AA. Quantitative risk factor analysis of postoperative dysphagia after Anterior Cervical Discectomy and Fusion (ACDF) using the Eating Assessment Tool-10 (EAT-10). Spine 2019; 44(2): E82-8.
[http://dx.doi.org/10.1097/BRS.0000000000002770] [PMID: 29965886]

[13] Ruetten S, Komp M, Merk H, Godolias G. Full-endoscopic anterior decompression *versus* conventional anterior decompression and fusion in cervical disc herniations. Int Orthop 2009; 33(6): 1677-82.
[http://dx.doi.org/10.1007/s00264-008-0684-y] [PMID: 19015851]

[14] Ahn Y, Lee SH, Shin SW. Percutaneous endoscopic cervical discectomy: clinical outcome and radiographic changes. Photomed Laser Surg 2005; 23(4): 362-8.
[http://dx.doi.org/10.1089/pho.2005.23.362] [PMID: 16144477]

[15] Tzaan WC. Anterior percutaneous endoscopic cervical discectomy for cervical intervertebral disc herniation: outcome, complications, and technique. J Spinal Disord Tech 2011; 24(7): 421-31.
[http://dx.doi.org/10.1097/BSD.0b013e31820ef328] [PMID: 21430567]

[16] Ahn Y, Keum HJ, Shin SH. Percutaneous endoscopic cervical discectomy *versus* anterior cervical discectomy and fusion: a comparative cohort study with a five-year follow-up. J Clin Med 2020; 9(2): E371.
[http://dx.doi.org/10.3390/jcm9020371] [PMID: 32013206]

[17] George B, Zerah M, Lot G, Hurth M. Oblique transcorporeal approach to anteriorly located lesions in the cervical spinal canal. Acta Neurochir (Wien) 1993; 121(3-4): 187-90.
[http://dx.doi.org/10.1007/BF01809273] [PMID: 8512017]

[18] George B, Lot G, Mourier KL, Reizine D. Cervical spondylosis. Resection by oblique transcorporeal approach. Neurochirurgie 1993; 39(3): 171-7.
[PMID: 8295649]

[19] Hakuba A. Trans-unco-discal approach. A combined anterior and lateral approach to cervical discs. J Neurosurg 1976; 45(3): 284-91.
[http://dx.doi.org/10.3171/jns.1976.45.3.0284] [PMID: 781189]

[20] Kishi H, Hakuba A. A combined anterior and lateral approach for cervical spondylosis; trans-unc--discal approach (TUD method). No Shinkei Geka 1992; 20(8): 843-8.
[PMID: 1508310]

[21] Jho HD, Kim WK, Kim MH. Anterior microforaminotomy for treatment of cervical radiculopathy: part 1--disc-preserving "functional cervical disc surgery". Neurosurgery 2002; 51(5) (Suppl.): S46-53.
[http://dx.doi.org/10.1097/00006123-200211002-00007] [PMID: 12234429]

[22] Choi G, Lee SH, Bhanot A, Chae YS, Jung B, Lee S. Modified transcorporeal anterior cervical microforaminotomy for cervical radiculopathy: a technical note and early results. Eur Spine J 2007; 16(9): 1387-93.
[http://dx.doi.org/10.1007/s00586-006-0286-6] [PMID: 17203272]

[23] Kim JS, Eun SS, Prada N, Choi G, Lee SH. Modified transcorporeal anterior cervical microforaminotomy assisted by O-arm-based navigation: a technical case report. Eur Spine J 2011; 20 (Suppl. 2): S147-52.
[http://dx.doi.org/10.1007/s00586-010-1454-2] [PMID: 20490870]

[24] Hong WJ, Kim WK, Park CW, *et al.* Comparison between transuncal approach and upper vertebral transcorporeal approach for unilateral cervical radiculopathy - a preliminary report. Minim Invasive Neurosurg 2006; 49(5): 296-301.

[http://dx.doi.org/10.1055/s-2006-954828] [PMID: 17163344]

[25] Choi KC, Ahn Y, Lee CD, Lee SH. Combined anterior approach with transcorporeal herniotomy for a huge migrated cervical disc herniation. Korean J Spine 2011; 8(4): 292-4.
[http://dx.doi.org/10.14245/kjs.2011.8.4.292] [PMID: 26064148]

[26] Choi G, Arbatti NJ, Modi HN, *et al.* Transcorporeal tunnel approach for unilateral cervical radiculopathy: a 2-year follow-up review and results. Minim Invasive Neurosurg 2010; 53(3): 127-31.
[http://dx.doi.org/10.1055/s-0030-1249681] [PMID: 20809454]

[27] Du Q, Lei LQ, Cao GR, *et al.* Percutaneous full-endoscopic anterior transcorporeal cervical discectomy and channel repair: a technique note report. BMC Musculoskelet Disord 2019; 20(1): 280.
[http://dx.doi.org/10.1186/s12891-019-2659-0] [PMID: 31182078]

[28] Ren Y, Yang J, Chen CM, *et al.* Outcomes of discectomy by using full-endoscopic visualization technique *via* the transcorporeal and transdiscal approaches in the treatment of cervical intervertebral disc herniation: a comparative study. BioMed Res Int 2020; 2020: 5613459.
[http://dx.doi.org/10.1155/2020/5613459] [PMID: 32596328]

[29] Chu L, Yang JS, Yu KX, Chen CM, Hao DJ, Deng ZL. Usage of bone wax to facilitate percutaneous endoscopic cervical discectomy *via* anterior transcorporeal approach for cervical intervertebral disc herniation. World Neurosurg 2018; 118: 102-8.
[http://dx.doi.org/10.1016/j.wneu.2018.07.070] [PMID: 30026139]

[30] Deng ZL, Chu L, Chen L, Yang JS. Anterior transcorporeal approach of percutaneous endoscopic cervical discectomy for disc herniation at the C4-C5 levels: a technical note. Spine J 2016; 16(5): 659-66.
[http://dx.doi.org/10.1016/j.spinee.2016.01.187] [PMID: 26850173]

[31] Yang JS, Chu L, Chen L, Chen F, Ke ZY, Deng ZL. Anterior or posterior approach of full-endoscopic cervical discectomy for cervical intervertebral disc herniation? A comparative cohort study. Spine 2014; 39(21): 1743-50.
[http://dx.doi.org/10.1097/BRS.0000000000000508] [PMID: 25010095]

[32] Yang JS, Chu L, Xiao FT, *et al.* Anterior retropharyngeal approach to C1 for percutaneous vertebroplasty under C-arm fluoroscopy. Spine J 2015; 15(3): 539-45.
[http://dx.doi.org/10.1016/j.spinee.2014.12.014] [PMID: 25523378]

[33] Yu KX, Chu L, Yang JS, *et al.* Anterior transcorporeal approach to percutaneous endoscopic cervical diskectomy for single-level cervical intervertebral disk herniation: case series with 2-Year follow-up. World Neurosurg 2019; 122: e1345-53.
[http://dx.doi.org/10.1016/j.wneu.2018.11.045] [PMID: 30448574]

[34] Yang J, Chu L, Deng Z, *et al.* Clinical study of single-level cervical disc herniation treated by full-endoscopic decompression *via* anterior transcorporeal approach. Zhongguo Xiu Fu Chong Jian Wai Ke Za Zhi 2020; 34(5): 543-9.
[PMID: 32410418]

[35] Yang JS, Chu L, Chen H, Liu P, Hao DJ. Comment on "effective range of percutaneous posterior full-endoscopic paramedian cervical disc herniation discectomy and indications for patient selection". BioMed Res Int 2020; 2020: 3548194.
[PMID: 32337243]

[36] Verma K, Gandhi SD, Maltenfort M, *et al.* Rate of adjacent segment disease in cervical disc arthroplasty *versus* single-level fusion: meta-analysis of prospective studies. Spine 2013; 38(26): 2253-7.
[http://dx.doi.org/10.1097/BRS.0000000000000052] [PMID: 24335631]

[37] Shriver MF, Lubelski D, Sharma AM, Steinmetz MP, Benzel EC, Mroz TE. Adjacent segment degeneration and disease following cervical arthroplasty: a systematic review and meta-analysis. Spine J 2016; 16(2): 168-81.
[http://dx.doi.org/10.1016/j.spinee.2015.10.032] [PMID: 26515401]

[38]  Arshi A, Wang C, Park HY, *et al.* Ambulatory anterior cervical discectomy and fusion is associated with a higher risk of revision surgery and perioperative complications: an analysis of a large nationwide database. Spine J 2018; 18(7): 1180-7.
[http://dx.doi.org/10.1016/j.spinee.2017.11.012] [PMID: 29155340]

[39]  Kelly MP, Eliasberg CD, Riley MS, Ajiboye RM, SooHoo NF. Reoperation and complications after anterior cervical discectomy and fusion and cervical disc arthroplasty: a study of 52,395 cases. Eur Spine J 2018; 27(6): 1432-9.
[http://dx.doi.org/10.1007/s00586-018-5570-8] [PMID: 29605899]

[40]  Khanna R, Kim RB, Lam SK, Cybulski GR, Smith ZA, Dahdaleh NS. Comparing short-term complications of inpatient *versus* outpatient single-level anterior cervical discectomy and fusion: an analysis of 6940 patients using the ACS-NSQIP database. Clin Spine Surg 2018; 31(1): 43-7.
[http://dx.doi.org/10.1097/BSD.0000000000000499] [PMID: 28079682]

[41]  Rumalla K, Smith KA, Arnold PM. Cervical total disc replacement and anterior cervical discectomy and fusion: reoperation rates, complications, and hospital resource utilization in 72 688 patients in the United States. Neurosurgery 2018; 82(4): 441-53.
[http://dx.doi.org/10.1093/neuros/nyx289] [PMID: 28973385]

[42]  Kashkoush A, Mehta A, Agarwal N, *et al.* Perioperative neurological complications following anterior cervical discectomy and fusion: clinical impact on 317, 789 patients from the national inpatient sample. World Neurosurg 2019; 128: e107-15.
[http://dx.doi.org/10.1016/j.wneu.2019.04.037] [PMID: 30980979]

[43]  Lee HC, Chen CH, Wu CY, Guo JH, Chen YS. Comparison of radiological outcomes and complications between single-level and multilevel anterior cervical discectomy and fusion (ACDF) by using a polyetheretherketone (PEEK) cage-plate fusion system. Medicine (Baltimore) 2019; 98(5): e14277.
[http://dx.doi.org/10.1097/MD.0000000000014277] [PMID: 30702590]

[44]  Al Eissa S, Konbaz F, Aldeghaither S, *et al.* Anterior cervical discectomy and fusion complications and thirty-day mortality and morbidity. Cureus 2020; 12(4): e7643.
[PMID: 32411545]

[45]  Narain AS, Hijji FY, Haws BE, *et al.* Risk factors for medical and surgical complications after 1--level anterior cervical discectomy and fusion procedures. Int J Spine Surg 2020; 14(3): 286-93.
[http://dx.doi.org/10.14444/7038] [PMID: 32699749]

[46]  Ranson WA, Neifert SN, Cheung ZB, Mikhail CM, Caridi JM, Cho SK. Predicting in-hospital complications after anterior cervical discectomy and fusion: a comparison of the elixhauser and charlson comorbidity indices. World Neurosurg 2020; 134: e487-96.
[http://dx.doi.org/10.1016/j.wneu.2019.10.102] [PMID: 31669536]

[47]  Liao C, Ren Q, Chu L, *et al.* Modified posterior percutaneous endoscopic cervical discectomy for lateral cervical disc herniation: the vertical anchoring technique. Eur Spine J 2018; 27(6): 1460-8.
[http://dx.doi.org/10.1007/s00586-018-5527-y] [PMID: 29478117]

[48]  Liu C, Liu K, Chu L, Chen L, Deng Z. Posterior percutaneous endoscopic cervical discectomy through lamina-hole approach for cervical intervertebral disc herniation. Int J Neurosci 2019; 129(7): 627-34.
[http://dx.doi.org/10.1080/00207454.2018.1503176] [PMID: 30238849]

[49]  Yu KX, Chu L, Chen L, Shi L, Deng ZL. A novel posterior trench approach involving percutaneous endoscopic cervical discectomy for central cervical intervertebral disc herniation. Clin Spine Surg 2019; 32(1): 10-7.
[http://dx.doi.org/10.1097/BSD.0000000000000680] [PMID: 29979215]

[50]  Ruetten S, Komp M, Merk H, Godolias G. Full-endoscopic cervical posterior foraminotomy for the operation of lateral disc herniations using 5.9-mm endoscopes: a prospective, randomized, controlled study. Spine 2008; 33(9): 940-8.
[http://dx.doi.org/10.1097/BRS.0b013e31816c8b67] [PMID: 18427313]

[51] Watanabe G, Misaki T, Kotoh K. Microfibrillar collagen (Avitene) and antibiotic-containing fibrin-glue after median sternotomy. J Card Surg 1997; 12(2): 110-1.
[http://dx.doi.org/10.1111/j.1540-8191.1997.tb00104.x] [PMID: 9271731]

[52] Jho HD. Microsurgical anterior cervical foraminotomy for radiculopathy: a new approach to cervical disc herniation. J Neurosurg 1996; 84(2): 155-60.
[http://dx.doi.org/10.3171/jns.1996.84.2.0155] [PMID: 8592215]

[53] Jho HD. Spinal cord decompression *via* microsurgical anterior foraminotomy for spondylotic cervical myelopathy. Minim Invasive Neurosurg 1997; 40(4): 124-9.
[http://dx.doi.org/10.1055/s-2008-1053432] [PMID: 9477400]

[54] Jho HD. Decompression *via* microsurgical anterior foraminotomy for cervical spondylotic myelopathy. Technical note. J Neurosurg 1997; 86(2): 297-302.
[http://dx.doi.org/10.3171/jns.1997.86.2.0297] [PMID: 9010435]

[55] Taşçioğlu AO, Attar A, Taşçioğlu B. Microsurgical anterior cervical foraminotomy (uncinatectomy) for cervical disc herniation. Report of three cases. J Neurosurg 2001; 94(1) (Suppl.): 121-5.
[PMID: 11147846]

[56] Saringer W, Nöbauer I, Reddy M, Tschabitscher M, Horaczek A. Microsurgical anterior cervical foraminotomy (uncoforaminotomy) for unilateral radiculopathy: clinical results of a new technique. Acta Neurochir (Wien) 2002; 144(7): 685-94.
[http://dx.doi.org/10.1007/s00701-002-0953-2] [PMID: 12181702]

[57] Grigorian Iu A, Stepanian MA, Onopchenko EV, Kadin LA, Khimochko EB, Lunina ES. Microsurgical anterior cervical foraminotomy in spondylogenous cervical radiculopathy. Vopr Neirokhir 2008; (2): 31-5.

[58] Sampath P, Bendebba M, Davis JD, Ducker T. Outcome in patients with cervical radiculopathy. Prospective, multicenter study with independent clinical review. Spine 1999; 24(6): 591-7.
[http://dx.doi.org/10.1097/00007632-199903150-00021] [PMID: 10101827]

[59] Huang M, Brusko GD, Borowsky PA, *et al.* The University of Miami spine surgery ERAS protocol: a review of our journey. J Spine Surg 2020; 6 (Suppl. 1): S29-34.
[http://dx.doi.org/10.21037/jss.2019.11.10] [PMID: 32195411]

[60] Wang MY, Chang HK, Grossman J. Reduced acute care costs with the ERAS® minimally invasive transforaminal lumbar interbody fusion compared with conventional minimally invasive transforaminal lumbar interbody fusion. Neurosurgery 2018; 83(4): 827-34.
[http://dx.doi.org/10.1093/neuros/nyx400] [PMID: 28945854]

[61] Wang MY, Tessitore E, Berrington N, Dailey A. Introduction. Enhanced recovery after surgery (ERAS) in spine. Neurosurg Focus 2019; 46(4): E1.
[http://dx.doi.org/10.3171/2019.1.FOCUS1957] [PMID: 30933910]

# CHAPTER 8

# Anterior Endoscopic Cervical Discectomy and Foraminoplasty for Herniated Disc and Lateral Canal Stenosis

**Jorge Felipe Ramírez León[1,2,*], José Gabriel Rugeles Ortíz[1], Carolina Ramírez Martínez[1], Nicolás Prada Ramírez[1,3], Enrique Osorio Fonseca[4] and Gabriel Oswaldo Alonso Cuéllar[1]**

[1] *Minimally Invasive Spine Center for Latinamerican Endoscopic Spine Surgeons, LESS Invasiva Academy, Bogotá, D.C., Colombia*

[2] *Fundación Universitaria Sanitas, Bogotá, D.C., Colombia*

[3] *Colombia Clínica Foscal, Bucaramanga, Colombia*

[4] *Universidad El Bosque, Bogotá, D.C., Colombia*

**Abstract:** Cervical foraminotomy is a popular procedure with surgeons to treat patients with refractory cervical radicular pain. Traditionally, it has been performed from the posterior approach. With the advent of minimally invasive spinal surgery techniques (MISST), anterior methods have also been employed to approach the compressive pathology from the axilla of the painful cervical nerve root. The authors of this chapter present their technique of transdiscal endoscopic anterior cervical discectomy foraminoplasty using an instrument system comprised of serial dilators, trephines, rongeurs, and a pulsed radiofrequency probe. They demonstrate the steps of the procedure from patient positioning, placement of surgical access, the employment of the individual surgical instruments, and their clinical outcomes. The authors briefly describe their clinical experience over a twenty-one year period. They performed a total of 232 procedures on 169 patients with single and up to 4 level surgeries herniate disc (219/232; 94.39%). An additional 13 patients (4.9%) had procedures for the treatment of lateral cervical canal stenosis. At a one-year follow-up, 90% of patients were rated to have had Excellent and Good Macnab outcomes, whereas Fair and Poor results were reported by 7%, and 3% of patients, respectively. In the absence of intraoperative or postoperative complications or reoperations associated with the procedure, the authors recommended it as a simplified outpatient alternative to anterior cervical discectomy and fusion.

---

[*] **Corresponding author Jorge Felipe Ramírez León:** Minimally Invasive Spine Center for Latinamerican Endoscopic Spine Surgeons, LESS Invasiva Academy, Bogotá, D.C., Colombia; Tel: +57 1 6002555; E-mail: academy@lessinvasiva.com

**Keywords:** Anterior approach, Cervical disc herniations, Endoscopic surgery, Foraminal stenosis, Outpatient, Pulsed radiofrequency, Radicular pain.

## INTRODUCTION

Robinson and Smith in 1955 first reported the anterior cervical discectomy and fusion (ACDF) technique [1]. ACDF has become the principal surgery for cervical herniated disc and stenosis in the anterior central and lateral canal stenosis. Although clinical outcomes with ACDF are generally good with the procedure being considered one of the better spinal surgeries with high patient satisfaction, concerns of developing adjacent segment disease (ASD) and the need for another fusion surgery remains [2 - 8]. Many strategies to avoid ASD following ACDF with open surgery have been entertained. Several minimally invasive spinal surgery technologies (MISST) have received attention due to significant technological advances in both endoscopic equipment and implants [2, 3, 6]. However, the burden of proof of the superiority of one MISST over another in treating cervical herniated disc and stenosis still rests with their advocates.

## BACKGROUND

Cervical lateral stenosis refers to the narrowing of the neuroforamen for the exiting nerve roots at each respective level. This pathology can be caused by a herniated disc, presence of osteophytes. The latter are often induced by degeneration or microfractures of adjacent bony structures, or occur in combination herniated disc. Periosteal distention due to bulging disc has also been recognized as a stimulus to the formation of osteophytic bone spurs, which can encroach on the cervical neural elements. In its early stages, cervical stenosis may be asymptomatic [9], but when radiculopathy develops, the predominant symptom is axial neck pain radiating to the arm in its corresponding dermatome. Radiating pain and its dermatomal distribution correspond to the affected level. Concomitant cervical myelopathy is uncommon but can be observed in some cases. The diagnosis is based on a detailed history and physical examination (H&P). The onset and type of pain and corresponding diagnostic information, including radiography (A-P, lateral, extension & flexion views) MRI and CT scans. Although the course of cervical radiculopathy is generally favorable, approximately 25% of patients with degenerative processes of the cervical spine may require surgery once persistent symptoms are non-responsive to conservative care such as the use of analgesics, physiotherapy, soft collar, epidural steroid injections, and selective nerve blocks [10]. Therefore, non-operative therapeutic measures should be tried first. Surgery is generally considered when non-operative measures for the patient's intense, unrelenting pain or progressive neurological deficit have failed. Typically, a minimum of 6 weeks of non-operative treatment is thought to be appropriate before considering surgery [11, 12]. The choice of surgical procedure depends on individual surgeon training and preference and the availability of necessary surgical instruments and implants.

## OBJECTIVE

Surgical options for cervical decompression can generally be divided into three groups: open, mini-open, and endoscopic procedures. The open or conventional technique was developed in 1950 and is now widely accepted as gold standard surgical treatment for cervical foraminal stenosis [13 - 15]. Open surgical treatment options include open foraminotomy or anterior cervical discectomy and fusion (ACDF) combined with decompression and/or fusion procedure. With the intent of minimizing morbidity associated with conventional open procedures, minimally invasive techniques have been recently developed for lateral stenosis. These included mini-open and endoscopic techniques. Both mini-open and endoscopic cervical decompression techniques have recently gained more popularity because of decreased approach related problems, including blood loss, postoperative pain, and muscle atrophy [16, 17]. In this chapter, the authors will discuss their results and compare them to those of endoscopic cervical foraminoplasty procedure. The authors have used endoscopic methods for the treatment of cervical radicular pain for the last 19 years.

## ANTERIOR ENDOSCOPIC CERVICAL FORAMINOPLASTY

Anterior Endoscopic Cervical Foraminoplasty (AECF) is the removal of degenerated tissue compressing nerve structures in the foraminal area under an endoscope view from an anterior percutaneous approach. The surgical principle is the same as in open decompression and aims to expand the foraminal window, remove the hypertrophic tissue and osteophytes to achieve decompression of neural structures. One of its advantages is that it can be performed on one or several levels without a fusion need.

### Indications

We have initial indications for the anterior cervical endoscopic approach: contained or extruded non migrated discal hernias or hernias with lateral fragments [18, 19] and stenosis foraminal produced by osteophytes [18, 20]. Recently some authors described the feasibility of the use of an anterior endoscopic approach for ossified posterior longitudinal ligament (OPLL) and cervical spondylotic myelopathy (CSM) using anterior full-endoscopic percutaneous trans corporeal procedure, the approach has been successfully used in a case report of OPLL and in a study with 2 years follow-up for single segment CSM [21, 22].

## Contraindications

There are diseases and morpho-physiological factors in which endoscopic technique is not recommended, including cases of cervical discogenic pain with greater than 50% loss of height, intervertebral space collapse, segmental instability, infection, uncontrollable disorders relating to coagulation disease and bleeding, anatomic alterations, severe neurological deficit, extruded and migrated hernia, progressive myelopathy, calcified discal protrusion, and ossification of the posterior longitudinal ligament [23]. Most importantly, MIS should not be performed on patients whose diagnostic workup was non-conclusive.

## Patient Positioning & Anesthesia

The patient is positioned in the prone position and prepped and draped such that the entire neck area from the chin to the upper chest is left accessible for surgical access planning. Surgical landmarks, including the lateral border of the sternocleidoid muscle in its entirety, the sternal notch, and the clavicular heads, should be visible within the surgical field. The authors recommend to draped out the entire anterior neck area from left to right to help the surgeon with orientation and assessment of the best surgical access point and trajectories to the painful surgical disc. The surgery is performed under local anesthesia and sedation under modern monitored anesthesia care (MAC) protocols without an airway. Since the patient is positioned in the prone position, an oxygen mask typically suffices to maintain proper oxygenation. Local anesthesia to the skin and the surgical tract is applied with 1% bupivacaine. The patient should be sufficiently alert to talk to the surgeon and verbalize any complaints during the procedure.

## Equipment & Instrumentation

Cervical spine endoscopic surgery requires high-tech devices for its implementation. Among the key devices we have: video-endoscopic tower, source of heat energy, and cervical endoscope with their respective instrumental set. The tower used by the authors in the cervical foraminoplasty includes equipment such as a monitor, video processor, light source and camera, shaver console and irrigation pump, devices, all of them, available in several brands. For thermal therapy, a bipolar radiofrequency console is used. This device allows coagulation, annuloplasty, and nucleoplasty with a fiber that passes through the endoscope's working channel and reaches the intradiscal space. The instrumental complementary is a set of spinal needles, dilators, cannula, trephines, burr, and punch clamps (Fig. **1**).

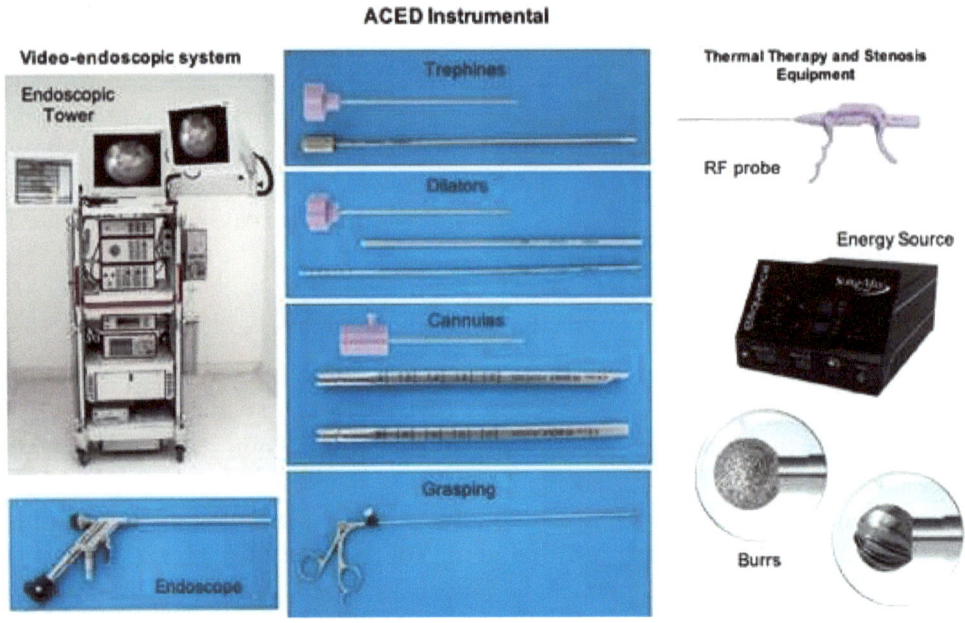

**Fig. (1).**  Set of instruments needed for AECF.

## SURGICAL TECHNIQUE

The patient is placed in a supine position in cervical extension. A pillow is placed under the shoulders to facilitate cervical lordosis. Typically, there is no need to use any type of mechanical hyperextension system. Intervertebral level and point of entry of the blunt-ended cannula is determined previously using biplanar fluoroscopy. Anatomical landmarks correspond to the intersection of the level affected and medial edge of the sternocleidomastoid muscle (Fig. **2**).

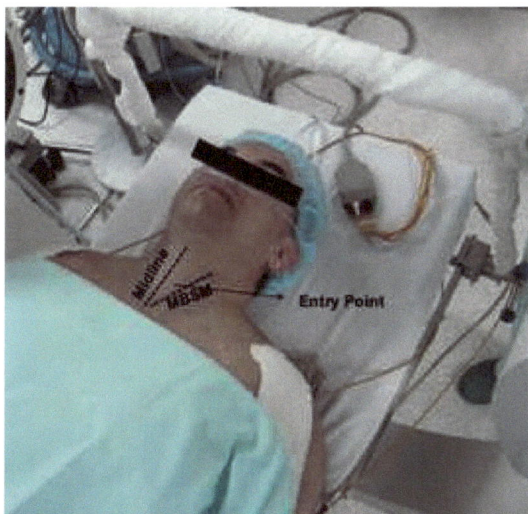

**Fig. (2).** Entry point for anterior cervical approach just lateral to the midline The latteral border of the trachea and the medial border of the sternocleidoid muscle are outlined and indicated by the dotted lines.

Once the point for the small skin incision is identified, the patient's head is slightly tilted toward the approach's contralateral side. The esophagus and trachea need to be mobilized medially and the neurovascular bundle laterally. Therefore, the surgeon's finger firmly pressed on the space between the muscle and the trachea (tracheoesophageal groove). Under an abundant local anesthetic infiltration, a 4 mm skin incision is made. Then, turning gently, a cannula together with the dilator is joined until the anterior edge of the annulus. (Fig. **3**). Cannula, dilator, and trephine are part of the MiniDiscFx™ system for cervical thermodiscoplasty.

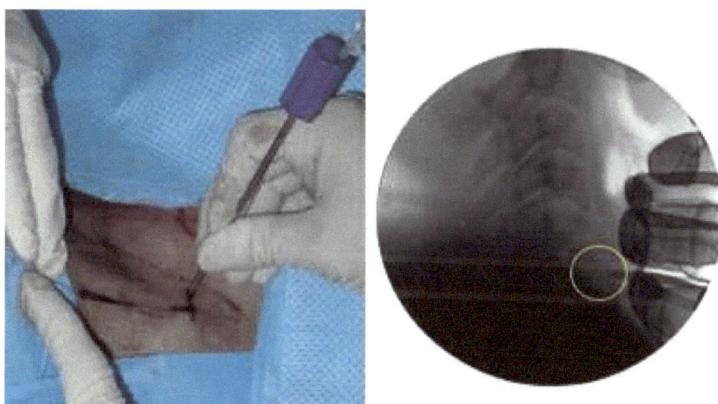

**Fig. (3).** Advance with blunt-tipped cannula within the intervertebral disc. The blunt-tipped cannula is softly advanced up to the annulus anterior edge with circular movements and fluoroscopic view aid.

With the dilator blunt tip just in front of the disc, the needle is advanced through the cannula up to the posterior third of the disc. This step is very important to reach a blunt technique to avoid an undesirable puncture of a vascular structure (Fig. **4**) [24].

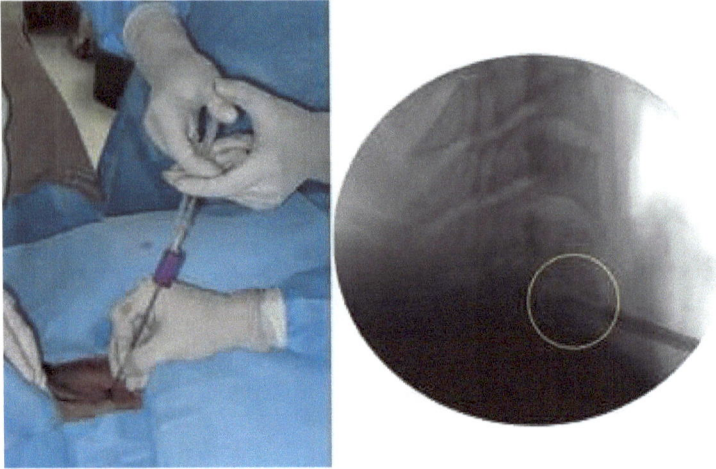

**Fig. (4).** The access needle is safely introduced into the surgical level under fluoroscopic guidance.

Once the needle is into the disc, if the surgeon chooses to do, discography and discogenic test are performed. The purpose of the discogenic tests is to verify that the drive is positive (> 5 points in VAS) and the symptoms consistent with familiar concordant pain. Also, to demonstrate the anatomical outlines of the disc, any internal disruptive dye patterns and leakage of dye suggesting the location of annular tears, as well as extruded disc material and their relationship to the posterior longitudinal ligament and the uncovertebral joint complex. The dilator is then replaced with a trephine and advanced with a rotating hand motion until the annulotomy is accomplished.

Once the guidewire's position is confirmed, the needle is removed, and the set of dilators and cannulas for the endoscope are placed over the annulus of the disc. With the endoscope is positioned, it is frequently necessary to achieve a better visualization and improve dissection through the anterior cervical prevertebral fascia with the use of a bipolar radiofrequency probe. The later also helps with the coagulation of small vessels, thus improving the endoscopic differentiation of anatomical structures. Through the endoscope's working channel, the discectomy instruments, such as grasping forceps, are inserted to perform a mechanic discectomy. Finally, osteophytes located in the foraminal window are endoscopically removed using a shaver. At times, due to the size of the osteophytes compressing the neural structures, it is necessary the use a chisel

(Fig. **5**). Complete decompression is then verified by directly visualizing the released cervical nerve root (Fig. **6**).

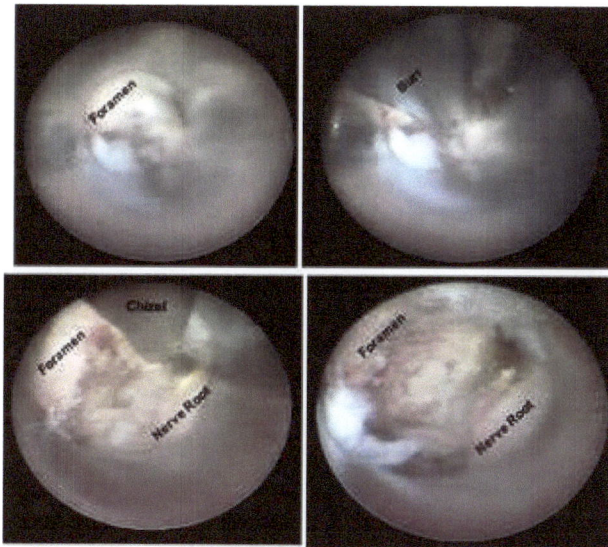

**Fig. (5).** Intraoperative endoscopic views taken during the foraminoplasty done with a burr and a chisel.

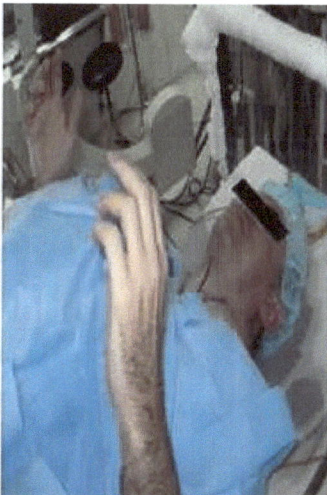

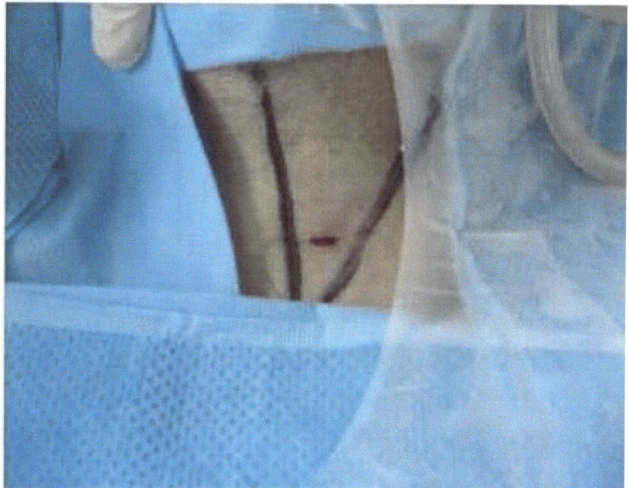

**Fig. (6).** Post-surgical arms mobility evaluation and incision wound (left), Intraoperative endoscopic views after completion of the foraminoplasty showing the decompressed exiting cervical nerve root (right).

## LEARNING CURVE

Although the injury of vital structures, with this approach, is extremely uncommon, it is imperative to consider the presence of relevant anatomic structures in the anterior neck zone. The surgeon must be mindful of the applied surgical anatomy in the anterior cervical area. An essential key factor in achieving successful clinical outcomes is to initiate appropriate training. The learning curve of the procedure is steep, and the outcomes are directly related to the surgeon skills. We recommended beginning performing of, between 20 – 30 cases, of the same technique on the lumbar area, later to complete 10 to 15 cases of non-endoscopic cervical technique, such as cervical thermodiscoplasty and then, under the supervision of an experienced surgeon to perform the endoscopic procedure for non-extruded hernias. Also, we strongly suggest attending cadaver labs and workshops in training centers. Patient selection and surgeon skill level is of the utmost importance to achieve good results with the procedure. This team of authors recommends incorporation of advanced technologies into the surgeon's clinical program. It should be considered and integrated into surgical residency and fellowship spine training programs. It is a timely fit with the ongoing demand by patients and payers alike for less complicated, cost-effective, and reliable solutions to treat cervical radiculopathy.

## CLINICAL OUTCOMES

The endoscopic technique, through an anterior approach for cervical radiculopathy, was introduced in Latin America by the senior author in October 1997. Until 2018 a total of 232 procedures on 169 patients (1,4 levels per patient). The main indication for the procedure was degenerative disc herniation disease and disc hernia in 94.39% (219/232) of patients. An additional 13 patients (4.9%) had procedures for treatment of lateral cervical canal stenosis. Macnab criteria, Visual Analogue Scale (VAS), and Neck Disability Index were used to evaluate clinical outcomes. At one-year follow-up, 90% of patients were rated to have had *Excellent* and *Good* Macnab outcomes, whereas *Fair* and *Poor* results were reported by 7%, and 3% of patients, respectively. Finally, the VAS score (1 no pain – 10 worst pain possible) on average was reported, preoperatively 8, and 2 at final postoperative follow-up. There were no intraoperative or postoperative complications or reoperations associated with the procedure in this cervical stenosis series.

## DISCUSSION

Currently, the most widely used surgical treatment for lateral cervical stenosis remains to be the open technique, either posterior or anterior approach, with or without fusion [15, 25]. These procedures have a proven track record for more than thirty years as a safe and effective means to treat cervical radiculopathy. Henderson *et al.* published a review of 846 surgeries showing a 96% improvement in the radicular symptoms with a posterior laminoforaminotomy for cervical radiculopathy [26]. More recent studies reported results with open techniques between 64% [27] and 93.6% [28]. Regarding endoscopic cervical approach, anterior and posterior cervical decompression were popularized by Ruetten *et al.* [29 - 31] further their research, they compared it to open surgery in two separate studies. In the anterior cervical endoscopic study group, 88,5% of patients were improved.

In our series, differences in the clinical results obtained using both techniques were not statistically significant. Comparable results were reported by Saringer *et al.* [23] They reported 16 patients with unilateral radiculopathy (n = 7: disc; n = 9 osteophytes) treated with endoscopic anterior cervical foraminotomy, with an average follow-up time of 13.8 months. The improvement rate was above 96% without presenting complications or reoperations at the final follow up. In that study, high overall satisfaction was reported by 87.6 of the patients, and 93.8% returned to similar preoperative activities within 3.8 weeks. Fessler *et al.* reported excellent and good resolution of symptoms in 92% in a series of 25 patients [32].

The literature suggests that results obtained with the different versions of anterior cervical discectomy and foraminotomy techniques are similar to those achieved by open, mini-open anterior and anterior- and posterior endoscopic approaches. Nevertheless, the inherent benefits of MIS could be a deciding factor for surgeons on which technique to pursue.

## CONCLUSIONS

Clinical outcomes obtained by the anterior endoscopic cervical technique in the treatment of stenosis are similar to open conventional methods in terms of improvement and symptoms resolution. Endoscopic anterior approach outcomes are not significantly different from those reported with open or mini-open techniques. Considering the low complication rate and other advantages of MIS in terms of decreased length of stay, blood loss, postoperative pain, and narcotic utilization, as well as shorter operative times, it is clear that anterior endoscopic cervical foraminotomy may prove to an attractive alternative to open and other MIS techniques [33, 34].

### CONSENT FOR PUBLICATION

Not applicable.

### CONFLICT OF INTEREST

This manuscript is not meant for or intended to push any other agenda other than reporting the clinical outcome data following endoscopic spinal decompression. The motive for compiling this clinically relevant information is by no means created and/or correlated to directly enrich anyone due to its publication. The authors are accountable for all aspects of the work in ensuring that questions related to the accuracy or integrity of any part of the work are appropriately investigated and resolved. The authors are consultants to Elliquence, LLC, and the first three authors are shareholders of Ortomac, SA.

## ACKNOWLEDGEMENTS

Declared none.

## REFERENCES

[1]     Smith GW, Robinson RA. The treatment of certain cervical-spine disorders by anterior removal of the intervertebral disc and interbody fusion. J Bone Joint Surg Am 1958; 40-A(3): 607-24.
[http://dx.doi.org/10.2106/00004623-195840030-00009] [PMID: 13539086]

[2]     Yang SD, Zhu YB, Yan SZ, Di J, Yang DL, Ding WY. Anterior cervical discectomy and fusion surgery *versus* total disc replacement: A comparative study with minimum of 10-year follow-up. Sci Rep 2017; 7(1): 16443.
[http://dx.doi.org/10.1038/s41598-017-16670-1] [PMID: 29180636]

[3]     Li XC, Huang CM, Zhong CF, Liang RW, Luo SJ. Minimally invasive procedure reduces adjacent segment degeneration and disease: New benefit-based global meta-analysis. PLoS One 2017; 12(2): e0171546.
[http://dx.doi.org/10.1371/journal.pone.0171546] [PMID: 28207762]

[4]     Laxer EB, Brigham CD, Darden BV, *et al.* Adjacent segment degeneration following ProDisc-C total disc replacement (TDR) and anterior cervical discectomy and fusion (ACDF): does surgeon bias effect radiographic interpretation? Eur Spine J 2017; 26(4): 1199-204.
[http://dx.doi.org/10.1007/s00586-016-4780-1] [PMID: 27650387]

[5]     Shriver MF, Lubelski D, Sharma AM, Steinmetz MP, Benzel EC, Mroz TE. Adjacent segment degeneration and disease following cervical arthroplasty: a systematic review and meta-analysis. Spine J 2016; 16(2): 168-81.
[http://dx.doi.org/10.1016/j.spinee.2015.10.032] [PMID: 26515401]

[6]     Yee TJ, Terman SW, La Marca F, Park P. Comparison of adjacent segment disease after minimally invasive or open transforaminal lumbar interbody fusion. J Clin Neurosci 2014; 21(10): 1796-801.
[http://dx.doi.org/10.1016/j.jocn.2014.03.010] [PMID: 24880486]

[7]     Verma K, Gandhi SD, Maltenfort M, *et al.* Rate of adjacent segment disease in cervical disc arthroplasty *versus* single-level fusion: meta-analysis of prospective studies. Spine 2013; 38(26): 2253-7.
[http://dx.doi.org/10.1097/BRS.0000000000000052] [PMID: 24335631]

[8]     Liu CY, Xia T, Tian JW. New progress in adjacent segment degeneration/disease. Orthop Surg 2010; 2(3): 182-6.
[http://dx.doi.org/10.1111/j.1757-7861.2010.00084.x] [PMID: 22009946]

[9]     Roh JS, Teng AL, Yoo JU, Davis J, Furey C, Bohlman HH. Degenerative disorders of the lumbar and cervical spine. Orthop Clin North Am 2005; 36(3): 255-62.
[http://dx.doi.org/10.1016/j.ocl.2005.01.007] [PMID: 15950685]

[10]    Woods BI, Hilibrand AS. Cervical radiculopathy: epidemiology, etiology, diagnosis, and treatment. J Spinal Disord Tech 2015; 28(5): E251-9.
[http://dx.doi.org/10.1097/BSD.0000000000000284] [PMID: 25985461]

[11]    Childress MA. Spine Conditions: Cervical Spine Conditions. FP Essent 2017; 461: 11-4.

[PMID: 29019639]

[12]    Childress MA, Becker BA. Nonoperative Management of Cervical Radiculopathy. Am Fam Physician 2016; 93(9): 746-54.
[PMID: 27175952]

[13]    Pingel A, Castein J, Kandziora F. Posterior stabilization of the cervical spine with lateral mass screws. Eur Spine J 2015; 24 (Suppl. 8): S947-8.
[http://dx.doi.org/10.1007/s00586-015-4237-y] [PMID: 26438171]

[14]    Pingel A, Kandziora F. Anterior decompression and fusion for cervical spinal canal stenosis. Eur Spine J 2013; 22(3): 673-4.
[http://dx.doi.org/10.1007/s00586-013-2708-6] [PMID: 23423161]

[15]    Pingel A, Kandziora F. Anterior decompression and fusion for cervical neuroforaminal stenosis. Eur Spine J 2013; 22(3): 671-2.
[http://dx.doi.org/10.1007/s00586-013-2709-5] [PMID: 23417749]

[16]    Schubert M, Merk S. Retrospective evaluation of efficiency and safety of an anterior percutaneous approach for cervical discectomy. Asian Spine J 2014; 8(4): 412-20.
[http://dx.doi.org/10.4184/asj.2014.8.4.412] [PMID: 25187857]

[17]    Tzaan WC. Anterior percutaneous endoscopic cervical discectomy for cervical intervertebral disc herniation: outcome, complications, and technique. J Spinal Disord Tech 2011; 24(7): 421-31.
[http://dx.doi.org/10.1097/BSD.0b013e31820ef328] [PMID: 21430567]

[18]    Ahn Y, Keum HJ, Shin SH. Percutaneous endoscopic cervical discectomy *versus* anterior cervical discectomy and fusion: a comparative cohort study with a five-year follow-up. J Clin Med 2020; 9(2): E371.
[http://dx.doi.org/10.3390/jcm9020371] [PMID: 32013206]

[19]    Ahn Y, Lee SH, Shin SW. Percutaneous endoscopic cervical discectomy: clinical outcome and radiographic changes. Photomed Laser Surg 2005; 23(4): 362-8.
[http://dx.doi.org/10.1089/pho.2005.23.362] [PMID: 16144477]

[20]    Ramírez León JF, Rugeles Ortíz JG, Martínez CR, Alonso Cuéllar GO, Lewandrowski KU. Surgical treatment of cervical radiculopathy using an anterior cervical endoscopic decompression. J Spine Surg 2020; 6 (Suppl. 1): S179-85.
[http://dx.doi.org/10.21037/jss.2019.09.24] [PMID: 32195426]

[21]    Kong W, Xin Z, Du Q, Cao G, Liao W. Anterior percutaneous full-endoscopic transcorporeal decompression of the spinal cord for single-segment cervical spondylotic myelopathy: The technical interpretation and 2 years of clinical follow-up. J Orthop Surg Res 2019; 14(1): 461.
[http://dx.doi.org/10.1186/s13018-019-1474-5] [PMID: 31870395]

[22]    Kong W, Ao J, Cao G, Xia T, Liu L, Liao W. Local Spinal Cord Decompression Through a Full Endoscopic Percutaneous Transcorporeal Approach for Cervicothoracic Ossification of the Posterior Longitudinal Ligament at the T1-T2 Level. World Neurosurg 2018; 112: 287-93.
[http://dx.doi.org/10.1016/j.wneu.2018.01.099] [PMID: 29410033]

[23]    Saringer WF, Reddy B, Nöbauer-Huhmann I, *et al.* Endoscopic anterior cervical foraminotomy for unilateral radiculopathy: anatomical morphometric analysis and preliminary clinical experience. J Neurosurg 2003; 98(2) (Suppl.): 171-80.
[PMID: 12650402]

[24]    Ramirez Leon JF, Rugeles Ortiz JG, Ramirez C, Osorio JA, Prada N, Alonso Cuellar GO. Anterior percutaneous cervical discectomy. Two-year follow-up of a blunt technique procedure. Coluna/Columna 2017; 16(4): 261-4.
[http://dx.doi.org/10.1590/s1808-185120171604182181]

[25]    Ruetten S, Komp M, Merk H, Godolias G. Full-endoscopic anterior decompression *versus* conventional anterior decompression and fusion in cervical disc herniations. Int Orthop 2009; 33(6):

1677-82.
[http://dx.doi.org/10.1007/s00264-008-0684-y] [PMID: 19015851]

[26] Henderson CM, Hennessy RG, Shuey HM Jr, Shackelford EG. Posterior-lateral foraminotomy as an exclusive operative technique for cervical radiculopathy: a review of 846 consecutively operated cases. Neurosurgery 1983; 13(5): 504-12.
[http://dx.doi.org/10.1227/00006123-198311000-00004] [PMID: 6316196]

[27] Schöggl A, Reddy M, Saringer W, Ungersböck K. Social and economic outcome after posterior microforaminotomy for cervical spondylotic radiculopathy. Wien Klin Wochenschr 2002; 114(5-6): 200-4.
[PMID: 12238309]

[28] Korinth MC, Krüger A, Oertel MF, Gilsbach JM. Posterior foraminotomy or anterior discectomy with polymethyl methacrylate interbody stabilization for cervical soft disc disease: results in 292 patients with monoradiculopathy. Spine 2006; 31(11): 1207-14.
[http://dx.doi.org/10.1097/01.brs.0000217604.02663.59] [PMID: 16688033]

[29] Ruetten S, Komp M, Merk H, Godolias G. Full-endoscopic cervical posterior foraminotomy for the operation of lateral disc herniations using 5.9-mm endoscopes: a prospective, randomized, controlled study. Spine 2008; 33(9): 940-8.
[http://dx.doi.org/10.1097/BRS.0b013e31816c8b67] [PMID: 18427313]

[30] Komp M, Oezdemir S, Hahn P, Ruetten S. Full-endoscopic posterior foraminotomy surgery for cervical disc herniations. Oper Orthop Traumatol 2018; 30(1): 13-24.
[http://dx.doi.org/10.1007/s00064-017-0529-1] [PMID: 29318337]

[31] Ruetten S, Komp M, Merk H, Godolias G. A new full-endoscopic technique for cervical posterior foraminotomy in the treatment of lateral disc herniations using 6.9-mm endoscopes: prospective 2-year results of 87 patients. Minim Invasive Neurosurg 2007; 50(4): 219-26.
[http://dx.doi.org/10.1055/s-2007-985860] [PMID: 17948181]

[32] Fessler RG, Khoo LT. Minimally invasive cervical microendoscopic foraminotomy: an initial clinical experience. Neurosurgery 2002; 51(5) (Suppl.): S37-45.
[http://dx.doi.org/10.1097/00006123-200211002-00006] [PMID: 12234428]

[33] Clark JG, Abdullah KG, Steinmetz MP, Benzel EC, Mroz TE. Minimally Invasive *versus* Open Cervical Foraminotomy: A Systematic Review. Global Spine J 2011; 1(1): 9-14.
[http://dx.doi.org/10.1055/s-0031-1296050] [PMID: 24353931]

[34] Dowling A. Endoscopic anterior cervical discectomy. London: JP Brothers 2013.

# CHAPTER 9

# Posterior Full Endoscopic Cervical Discectomy & Foraminotomy

**Álvaro Dowling[1,2], Kai-Uwe Lewandrowski[3,4,5,*] and Hyeun Sung Kim[6,7,8,9,10]**

[1] *Endoscopic Spine Clinic, Santiago, Chile*

[2] *Department of Orthopaedic Surgery, USP, Ribeirão Preto, Brazil*

[3] *Center for Advanced Spine Care of Southern Arizona and Surgical Institute of Tucson, Tucson, AZ, USA*

[4] *Department of Orthopaedic Surgery, UNIRIO, Rio de Janeiro, Brazil*

[5] *Department of Orthoapedic Surgery, Fundación Universitaria Sanitas, Bogotá, D.C., Colombia, USA*

[6] *Department of Neurosurgery, Nanoori Gangnam Hospital, Seoul, Republic of Korea*

[7] *A President of the Korean Research Society of the Endoscopic Spine Surgery (KOSESS), South Korea*

[8] *A Faculty of the KOrean Minimally Invasive Spine Surgery Society (KOMISS), South Korea*

[9] *A Chairman of the Nanoori Hospital Group Scientific Team, South Korea*

[10] *An Adjunct Professor of the Medical College of the Chosun University, Gwangju, South Korea*

**Abstract:** Cervical radiculopathy is a common disabling condition resulting from advanced degeneration of the cervical spine. Posterior Endoscopic Cervical Discectomy (PECD) surgery preserves soft tissue and accomplishes a form of foraminal decompression with a lower propensity to postoperative instability. The authors described the technique in detail with an illustrative case example and intraoperative endoscopic images. The targeting point is the "V" point made up by the lateral margin of interlaminar space and medial border of facet joint junction. This confluence of the medial junction of the superior and inferior facet can easily be recognized on AP view where it has the appearance of a V. Furthermore; the authors present the results of a prospective clinical PECD study of 29 levels in 25 patients where they analyzed the radiological and clinical outcome with the trans v point PECD technique. Most of the PECD surgeries were carried out at the C5/6 and C6/7 levels. The mean follow up was 29.6 months. There was a 4% complication rate because of motor deficits, which had been resolved after one year. The majority of patients

*  **Corresponding author Kai-Uwe Lewandrowski:** Center for Advanced Spine Care of Southern Arizona and Surgical Institute of Tucson, Tucson, AZ, USA, Department of Orthopaedic Surgery, UNIRIO, Rio de Janeiro, Brazil and Department of Orthoapedic Surgery, Fundación Universitaria Sanitas, Bogotá, D.C., Colombia, USA; Tel: +1 520 204-1495; Fax: +1 623 218-1215; E-mail: business@tucsonspine.com

showed significant improvements in VAS and ODI scores, and 96% achieved good and excellent results by Macnab's criteria. Retrospective evaluation of the radiological and CT data showed sagittal foraminal area increase and craniocaudal foraminal length increases. PECD produced the largest foraminal length increase preferentially in the ventrodorsal direction. Based on our observations, PECD is a good option in the posterior foraminotomy of the cervical spine. Clinical and radiological outcomes are favorable.

**Keywords:** Cervical radiculopathy, Full endoscopic discectomy, Posterior cervical foraminotomy.

## INTRODUCTION

Spurling and Scoville introduced posterior cervical foraminotomy (PCF) first in the mid-20th century [1]. Conventional posterior foraminotomy is traditionally performed through an open approach with a midline incision for bilateral decompression or paraspinal incisions for unilateral decompression. In 2001, micro-endoscopic laminoforaminotomy reports appeared introducing minimally invasive spinal surgery techniques to avoid more extended hospital stays, general anesthesia (GA), more significant operative blood loss, longer recovery and rehabilitation times, increased soft tissue damage, higher risk of operative complications, and minimizing pain associated with the procedure [2 - 4]. Percutaneous, minimally invasive, and endoscopic approaches are attractive alternatives to open surgery [5].

Nowadays, the posterior full-endoscopic cervical discectomy (PECD) with or without foraminotomy is a well-established procedure, with many authors having reported favorable clinical outcomes [6, 7]. This chapter's authors still thought that it is worth reviewing the most contemporary techniques by giving some illustrative examples of their clinical practice to complete this exhaustive text on cervical spinal endoscopy. For the novice endoscopic spine surgeon, PECD is likely the most facile endoscopic surgery technique of the cervical spine to learn and less risky than anterior cervical full-endoscopic surgery. It is a useful technique in any endoscopic spine surgeon's hands, for which reason the authors presented their contemporary version of PECD in this chapter.

## CLINICAL PRESENTATION

Cervical radiculopathy with unrelenting radiating upper extremity, shoulder, upper back or neck shoulder and arm pain radiating into the hand is the hallmark symptom caused by a stenotic process in the cervical neuroforamen [8]. Shoulder-related pathology from rotator cuff tears or other internal shoulder derangements, including a detachment of the long head of the biceps anchor attachment from the glenoid, should be excluded [9]. Another important differential diagnosis to consider is double-crush peripheral nerve compression syndromes in the upper extremities and cause similar symptoms [9]. The patients' pain from cervical radiculopathy is typically described as sharp, tingling, dull, aching, or burning. Decreased sensation or dysesthesias often precede the classic radiculopathy pain [9]. Provocative testing, such as the incitement of the Spurling sign, may aid in the diagnosis [10]. Patients complain of more pain when turning the head toward the painful side or by reporting pain relief by elevating the arm above the shoulder and placing it onto the head – a shoulder-abduction relief sign which is thought to be more representative of a soft herniation. Some authors suggested a negative shoulder-abduction relief sign in a patient with a positive Spurling sign may indicate the cervical neuroforamen's bony encroachment. Typically, patients presenting to the endoscopic spine surgeon with these complaints have already undergone conservative management with non-steroidal anti-inflammatories (NSAIDs) and physical therapy (PT). However, the authors recommend that each patient undergo a minimum of 6 weeks of conservative treatment, additionally including analgesics, activity modification, short-term cervical bracing, facet blocks, and in select cases, cervical transforaminal epidural steroid injections before considering them for surgery. Auxiliary electrodiagnostic studies such as electromyography (EMG) and nerve conduction studies (NCS) may aid in diagnosing [11]. Detailed history taking, physical examination, and clinical judgment are critical in determining the predominant pain generator's location in the cervical spine, as is a careful evaluation of advanced imaging studies, including magnetic resonance imaging (MRI) or the computed tomography (CT) scans [12].

## ADVANTAGES OF ENDOSCOPICALLY VISUALIZED POSTERIOR FORAMINOTOMY

There are some obvious and perhaps not so obvious advantages of using the endoscopic surgery technique. Since the endoscopic working cannula is inserted after the introduction of progressive dilation tubes it can be freely maneuvered or held by an assistant while the surgeon freely inserts the endoscope with his/her non-dominant hand and controls the suction and endoscopic instruments with their dominant hand. Typically, nothing is fixed to any equipment or mounting arm and the endoscope is freely maneuvered inside the working cannula. It is the authors' experience that this operative technique allows for:

1. Exclusive visual angles,
2. Better illumination of deep structures, and
3. Verification of the nerve root trajectory.

In other words, from a small, directly posteriorly placed skin incision, a larger operational area at the posterior cervical spine can be accessed and visualized without having to create a surgical access commensurate with the size of the operative field.

## INDICATIONS & CONTRAINDICATIONS

Surgical indications for PECDF are radiculopathies due to lateral or extraforaminal herniation, degenerative pathology with foraminal bony stenosis, or spondylotic stenosis with root symptoms. The authors recommend the PECDF for patients meeting the following inclusion criteria:

- Unilateral radiculopathy due to bony foraminal stenosis at one or more level,
- Foraminal stenosis due to posterolateral disc herniation causing radiculopathy,
- Patients with contraindications to an anterior approach,
- Persistent radiculopathy after anterior approach surgery,
- Radiculopathies due to lateral or extraforaminal herniation.

Contraindications include central stenosis with myelopathy, tumors, and central or infections. However, surgeons' skill levels may vary, and what may appear as an absolute contraindication to some surgeons may be a relative contraindication to others. An example of that is the endoscopic decompression of the stenotic cervical spinal canal described by one team of authors in this text for cervical spondylotic myelopathy (CSM). Therefore, the authors caution the prospective endoscopic spine surgeon contemplating PECDF for their patients to hesitate and to carefully consider the following situations as relative contraindications commensurate with their abilities:

- Central stenosis with myelopathy (relative)
- Tumors
- Central or posterolateral hernias with mono-radicular symptoms

## POSITIONING & ANESTHESIA

The patient is placed in the prone position on the operating table, and the neck is fixed to a horseshoe-shaped head holder or a foam cushion using tape in a neutral surgical position (Fig. **1**). Typically, the procedure can be done under local anesthesia and sedation, particularly if a single-level unilateral PECDF is contemplated. Placement of an endotracheal (ET) tube or a laryngeal mask airway (LMA) under balanced general anesthesia described in a separate chapter in this text should be considered for lengthy or multilevel procedures. The novice surgeon may consider such balanced general anesthesia with a secured airway if a longer case duration is expected. Patients' comfort throughout the procedure is also considered if it is carried out under monitored anesthesia care (MAC) with local anesthetic injection and sedation [13]. For example, the military position (cervical extension with capital flexion) may facilitate the foraminal decompression but could be very uncomfortable for the patient, mainly under MAC. On the flipside of general anesthesia stands the ability to communicate with a patient under MAC. Some experienced endoscopic spine surgeons have argued that there is no better safety net for the surgeon than communicating with the patient during surgery. It surpasses the reliability of intraoperative neuromonitoring. To debate these opposing points of view herein is beyond the scope of this chapter. However, each surgeon needs to choose the appropriate type of surgery and anesthesia for each patient's painful cervical spine condition in the context of his or her abilities, available equipment, and technical support. The entire decision-making process is a compromise.

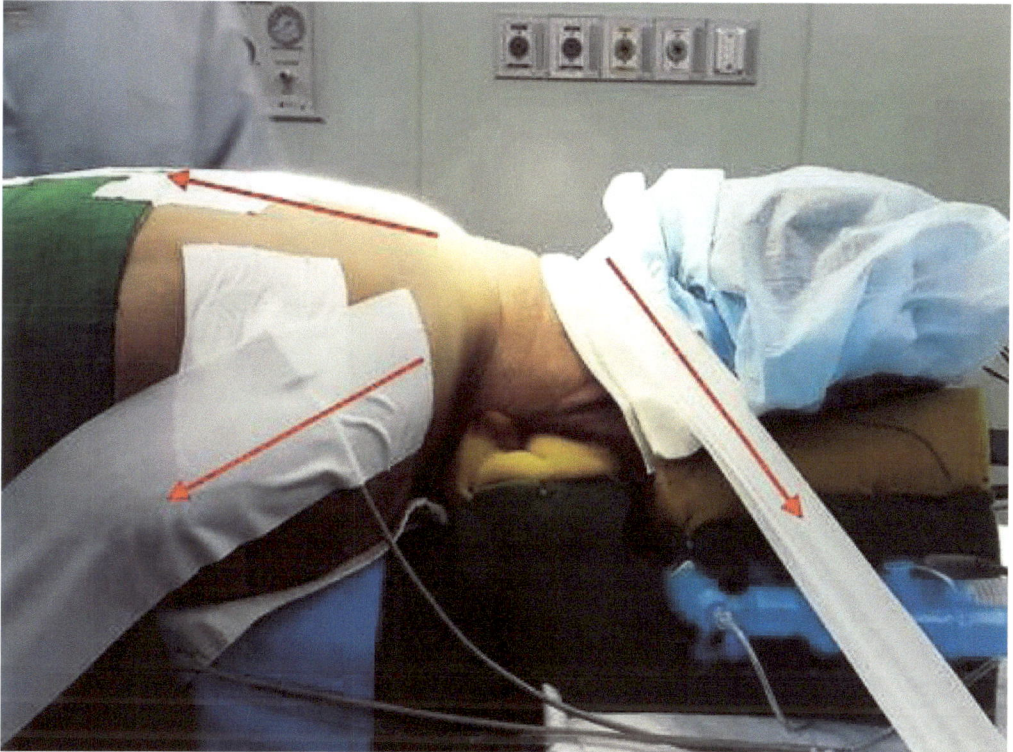

**Fig. (1).** The patient is positioned in prone position in a face cushion under general anesthesia. The shoulders and head are taped back to maintain the cervical spine in neutral.

## OR SETUP

The first author's preference is to stand behind the patient's head. The fluoroscopic

C-arm base is placed on the opposite side to the surgical approach, with fluoroscopic and endoscopic monitors in front. That way, the surgeon can directly look at them when needed. Equipment location should be chosen to allow the surgeon to work comfortably. The anesthesiologist is seated behind and to the surgeon's side, where he/she can see the patient's face, monitor their vital signs, and communicate through a small microphone and headset with the patient, who may be comforted by communication or music during the procedure. The neck should be checked a final time to ensure safe positioning and to allow adequate jugular venous drainage and airway flow if under MAC. The airway should be secured if the patient is under general anesthesia. Prone LMA is becoming more and more accepted by anesthesiologists – particularly by those accustomed to working in an outpatient ambulatory surgery center setting where rapid case turnover and patient discharge are expected. We did not use neuromonitoring during any of the procedures.

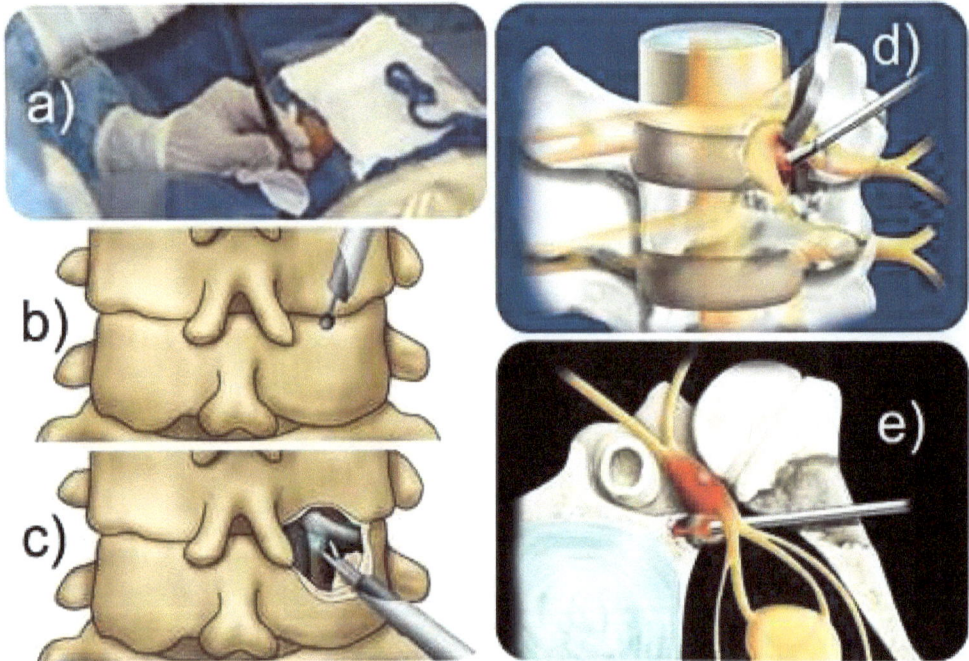

**Fig. (2).** Surgical technique for endoscopic posterior cervical foraminotomy. **(a)** K-wire insertion and following an initial 9-mm incision. Dilation tube insertion. The endoscope is introduced through the working cannula. Soft-tissue vaporization may be executed with radiofrequency through the working cannula assisted with endoscopic instruments. **(b-c)** The foraminotomy is performed once the laminar V point has been identified at the medial aspect of the facet joint complex. **(d)** Power drills, and rongeurs are used to perform the keyhole foraminotomy similar to those in open procedures. **(e)** A laser can be used to remove calcified disc or bony overgrowth causing compression of the exiting cervical nerve root (Illustration d and e courtesy of Mauricio Sepúlveda).

## SURGICAL TECHNIQUE

Once the patient is adequately position and under anesthesia, a series of lateral and AP fluoroscopy images are used to target the appropriate spinal level and to insert the trocar in the inferior pedicle. Then, a less than 1 cm incision is made over the verified surgical level and serial dilation tubes are inserted. Finally, a 7.5 mm working cannula is inserted over the surgical facet joint complex and the foraminotomy may commence. Fluoroscopy images may be taken throughout the procedure to confirm the position of the working cannula and any trajectory adjustments (Fig. **2**). The first author prefers a 30-degree short glass-rod endoscope to which an CCD video camera is attached. From this point, the surgeon visualizes every step of the procedure on a high-definition video. Instruments may be introduced through the central working channel of the cervical endoscope. Initially, a laser or bipolar radiofequency probe (RF) is used to clean of any soft-tissue to expose the facet joint. The RF may also be useful for hemostasis by coagulation. A bur is used to polish the laminar surfaces and the facet and to initiate the foraminotomy decompression (Fig. **2**).

The bony resection is then started with a 2 to 3.5 mm Kerrison rongeurs (Fig. **2**). In cases of significant cervical facet hypertrophy, a more extensive lateral resection may be warranted. The decompression is then turned medially by resecting a small portion of the inferior lamina to the pedicle inferiorly with power drills or Kerrison rongeurs. Care must be taken not to damage the dura. Foraminal lesions often require greater cephalad than caudal exposure. It is crucial to preserve at least 50% of the facet to maintain its biomechanical integrity. When adequate exposure of the nerve root has been achieved a small nerve hook gently retracts it away superiorly from the underlying disc.

The disc can be removed with small endoscopic rongeurs or a laser at times particularly if there is a calcified disc or bony overgrowth from adjacent structures (Fig. **2**). The foramen is inspected one final time to ensure full decompression. The nerve root should present a full color recovery, a strong dural pulsations. Before removal of the working cannula, hemostasis is achieved with bipolar vascular cauterization. The wound is closed with a simple horizontal mattress stitch using a resorbable monofilament suture. An exemplary case is shown in Fig. (**3**).

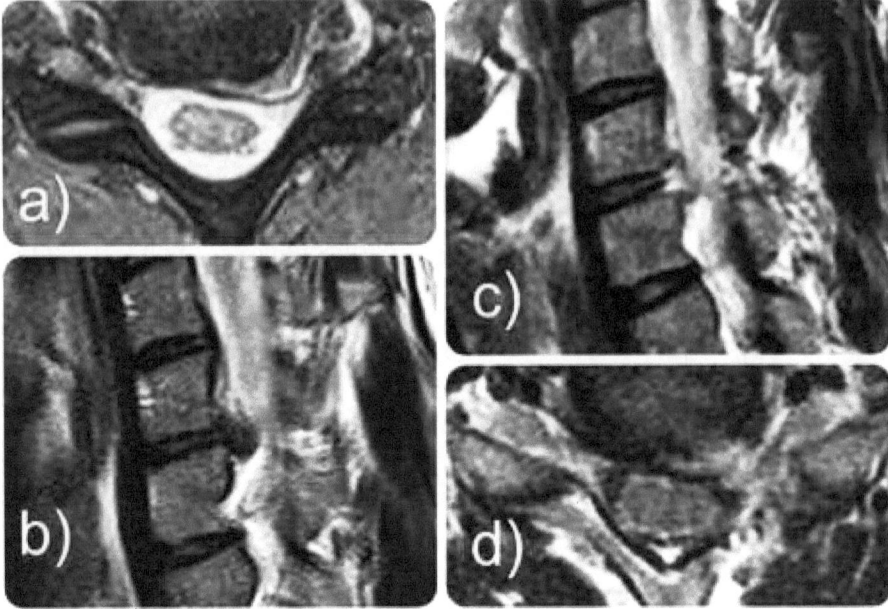

**Fig. (3).** Preoperative axial **(a)** and sagittal **(b)** T2-weighted MRI images of a 45-year-old male with a lateral C5/6 disc herniation which was treated with PECD. The respective postoperative MRI scans demonstrating adequate decompression are shown in panel **(c)** and **(d)**.

## The Trans-"V-point" Foraminotomy Technique

The skin marking is done under guidance of anteroposterior (AP) and lateral view cervical fluoroscopy. The target point is the lateral margin of interlaminar space and medial border of facet joint junction - the "v" point [14]. The confluence of the medial junction of superior and inferior facet) on AP view has the appearance of a V. Fluoroscopic lateral view was performed to confirm facet joint of the correct level. The incision was made at the "v" point and obturator was inserted and docked, tip position was confirmed with fluoroscopy. A 30-degree viewing angle, 7.3 mm outer diameter, and 4.7 mm working channel (Joimax GmbH, Karlsruhe, Germany) is used for the procedure under continuous normal saline irrigation of pressure of 25 mmHg. Hemostasis and soft tissue dissection was done with the radiofrequency probe (Ellman's bipolar radiofrequency electrocoagulator – Elliquence, Baldwin, New York, USA) and endoscopic forceps. Once V point was identified and double check on fluoroscopy, medial aspect of lateral mass and facet joint was drilled with a long straight high speed drill (Primado High-Speed Drill System – NSK, Nakanishi, Japan) to create a working window depending on the size of herniated material and degree of foraminal stenosis which is typically an area of 3-5 mm in diameter where bone is removed from lateral inferior aspect of upper lamina followed by about 3mm of the medial inferior portion of upper facet from the lamina-facet border ("V" point) to gain access to the nerve root. We then asked anesthetist to tilt patient away from surgeon to drilled on the medial superior articular facet of lower vertebra and resected the medial aspect of superior articular facet of caudal vertebra lying on dorsal aspect of the nerve root, it would lead to the proximal portion of nerve root which lied closely superior to the pedicle. After posterior foraminotomy was complete and exposure of the exiting nerve root and medial third of spinal cord both of which were closely related to the pedicle of caudal vertebra were inspected. This marked the completion of what the authors termed as "V" point foraminotomy (Fig. 4).

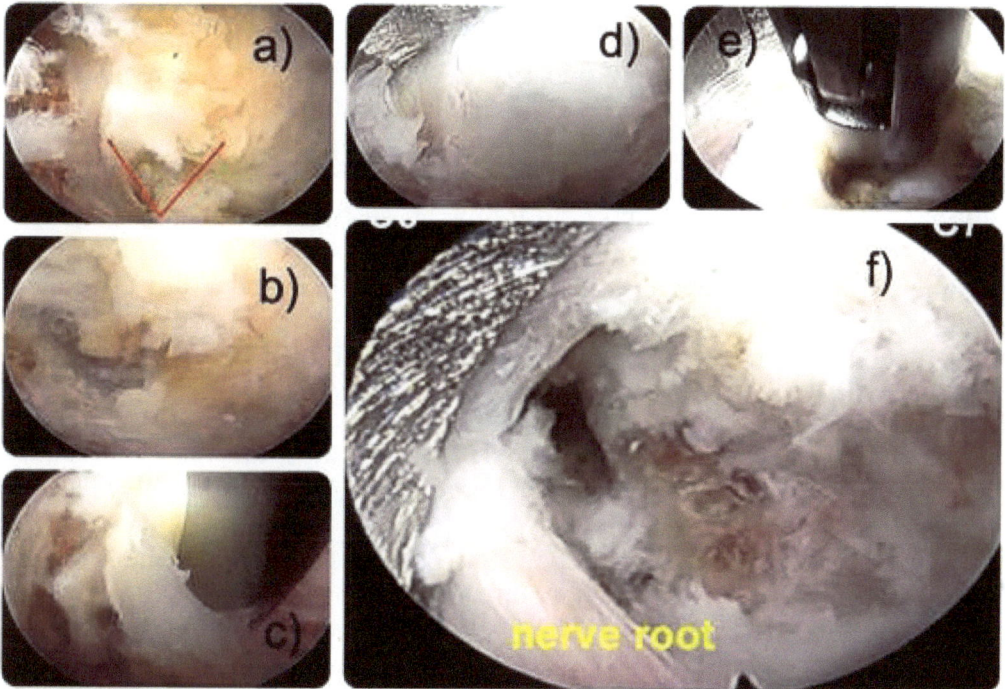

**Fig. (4).** Intraoperative endoscopic views obtained during posterior endoscopic cervical discectomy showing the identification of the laminar V point (**a**). The foraminotomy can be accomplished with drilling (**b**), and use of a chisel to enlarge the foraminotomy site (**c**). The disc is exposed by rotating the working cannula over it in such way as to retract the cervical nerve root (**d**). A pituitary rongeur is used to decompress the disc herniation (**e**) until the decompression is complete (**f**).

## Posterior Cervical Disectomy with Neural Retraction

After foraminotomy was completed, the working channel was rotated with open beveled facing away from the axilla of the spinal cord and exiting nerve root retracting, the exiting nerve root gently medially and exposing the prolapsed disc. Endoscopic forceps and Kerisson rongeurs were used to retrieved the prolapsed disc. Radiofrequency was used to help in hemostasis and gentle release of the adhesion of the neural elements to disc facilitating the retrieval of the prolapsed disc. Uncovertebral hypertrophy was taken down with a cutter. The pedicle was left intact and disc was approached through gentle retraction of exiting nerve root with working channel maneuver, we did not retract the spinal cord as it could lead to significant neurological sequelae. Drain was inserted and closed in layers with dermabond to skin.

## CLINICAL SERIES

The authors employed the posterior endoscopic cervical discectomy technique in a prospective clinical and retrospective radiological evaluation of patients with 29 levels of cervical radiculopathy in illustrative series of 25 patients [14]. They underwent point posterior endoscopic cervical discectomy from November 2016 to December 2018 employing the V point targeting technique. Clinical outcomes of Visual Analog Scale [15], Oswestry Disability Index [16] and Macnab's score [17, 18] was evaluated preoperatively, at 1 week, 3 months postoperatively and at final follow-up. Preoperative and final follow up post-operative imaging with x-rays for evaluation of cervical stability was done. Computer Tomography evaluation of foraminal length in ventro-dorsal, cephalad-caudal dimensions and area in sagittal view was performed. Preoperative and post-operative CT 3D reconstruction area of decompression evaluation performed was performed.

Of the 29 levels of Posterior Endoscopic Cervical Decompression (PECD), the most common levels are C5/6 and C6/7. The mean follow up was 29.6 months. There was 4% complication in terms of motor deficits which had resolved after 1 year. There was significant clinical improvement in Visual Analog Scale, Oswestry Disability Index and Mac Nab's criteria. Prospective comparative study between preoperative and final follow up mean improvement in VAS score was $5.08 \pm 1.75$, and ODI was $45.1 \pm 13.3$., 96% of the patients achieved good and excellent results by MacNab's criteria. Retrospective evaluation of the radiological data showed 1) sagittal area increased $21.4 \pm 11.2$ $mm_2$, 2) CT Cranio- Caudal length increased 1.21 mm $\pm$ 1.30 mm and 3) CT ventrodorsal length increased $2.09 \pm 1.35mm$ and 4) and 3D CT scan reconstruction decompression area increased $536 \pm 176$ $mm^2$, $p<0.05$. As a result of these favorable clinical results, the authors concluded that the trans "V" point approach (Fig. **4**) for posterior endoscopic cervical foraminotomy and discectomy is a good option in posterior endoscopic decompression of cervical spine. The radiographic postoperative follow-up data clearly demonstrated the ability of PECD to adequately decompress the compressed cervical neuroforamina. There was 4% complication in terms of motor deficits which had resolved after 1 year.

## DISCUSSION

Cervical radiculopathy is a common disabling degenerative condition of the cervical spine with nerve root dysfunction [1]. Recently, more professionals work remotely on computers, laptops, and other portable devices that may contribute to a higher incidence of cervical radiculopathy and posture-related accelerated cervical degeneration. The natural history of cervical radiculopathy due to disc herniation is often benign, and symptoms may resolve on their own or with supportive care measures directed at subsiding the inflammatory cytokines from the prolapsed intervertebral disc [19]. Mechanical compression may remain over time despite symptomatic relief with management. Spontaneous symptom resolution may occur over 2 to 3 years in 83% of the patients [20]. However, a subset of patients suffer significant disabling symptoms despite conservative management [20]. Surgical treatment is recommended after patients have failed at least six weeks of conservative therapy for cervical radiculopathy without myelopathy [1]. However, many patients go through several rounds of acute on chronic episodes before they are seriously considering surgical treatment.

While reviewing the pros and cons of the various surgical approaches to the cervical spine would be beyond the scope of this chapter on posterior endoscopic cervical discectomy (PECD), it is evident that the approach-related trauma and the overall burden to patients associated with the outpatient PECD are much lower than with traditional anterior approaches and their treatment options including anterior cervical discectomy and fusion (ACDF). Not every patient is ready to make such big decisions even if motion preservation with a cervical artificial disc replacement (ADR) is proposed [21]. The PECD has the advantage of a motion preservation surgery since it does not involve sacrificing an intervertebral disc and indirect decompression and establishing the foraminal height *via* an implant [22 - 25]. Additional negative fallout from such aggressive surgical treatments may include adjacent segment disease and pseudoarthrosis with the latter being the most typical postoperative complications of ACDF. Furthermore, anterior cervical surgery's overall complication rate ranges from 13.2 to 19.3%, making the PECD an attractive alternative [26]. However, one of the concerns associated with PECD is excessive resection of the facet joint, leading to focal instability [27].

During the preoperative evaluation, the preoperative advanced imaging studies, including MRI and CT scans, should be carefully analyzed for obstruction in the access to the surgical cervical disc. The presence of osseous and bony compression involving the median and paramedian region should be noted. Two-thirds of the soft disc should be lateral to the thecal sac of the cervical spinal cord to improve the chances of success in posterior cervical foraminotomy and discectomy. As outlined earlier in this chapter, the contraindications are patients with predominant pure axial neck pain from advanced degeneration of the intervertebral disc or facet joints in the cervical spine. Besides, patients with radiological cervical instability should not be selected for the PECD procedure. Relative contraindications are central disc and calcified disc [28, 29]. While there are limited studies on radiological evaluation of the effect of PECD on the stability of the cervical spine following posterior cervical foraminotomy and discectomy, it seems intuitive that PECD is a lesser destabilizing procedure even though most of the PECD studies assessing clinical and radiographic outcomes focused on the preservation of disc height, range of motion of cervical spine and preservation of cervical stability. These studies corroborated the author's notion of PECD being producing few problems with postoperative instability and degenerative disease progression by showing good radiological results within those parameters measured [30]. The limitations of clinical and radiological evaluation studies were that there was no measurement of the amount of decompression achieved comparing pre and postoperative data. However, this information gap was closed by the clinical series data described by the authors herein.

While the concept of preserving neck motion seems more reasonable by performing a PECD, it comes at a price of neck pain in some patients, which at its heart is one of the main reasons why many surgeons preferred an anterior procedure over the posterior procedure in the treatment of cervical radiculopathy [27, 31]. To prevent postoperative kyphosis, instability, and axial neck pain, preserving the cervical soft tissue and ligamentous structures is the key. The development of endoscopic techniques and, in particular, PECD aim to preserve posterior structures and yet achieve the similar goals of conventional posterior cervical foraminotomy [32]. This approach has been corroborated by several other authors in their clinical series, where they have achieved good clinical outcomes [33, 34].

Our feasibility study also showed the extent of the foraminal decompression with PECD. We found that using a CT scan, there was a statistically significant increase in foraminal enlargement in both sagittal and coronal parameters. However, there was more decompression in the ventral to dorsal direction with the PECD technique than cranial to the caudal direction, at least in the sagittal plane. Twice, the amount of bone was resected lengthwise, measuring, on average, 2.1 mm in the ventral to dorsal direction and 1.2 mm in the cranial to caudal direction. Overall, the PECD decompression produced a mean increase of 21.5 mm$^2$ of the foramen area in the sagittal image planes. Employing 3D CT reconstructions, the foraminal decompression effect was more accurately assessed with a much wider area of increase in medial to lateral direction with a mean increase of 537 mm$^2$ compared to preoperative imaging. Since there is a more significant decompression effect in the ventral to dorsal direction with the PECD technique, an excessive medial to lateral resection of the facet joint complex is not necessary to accomplish pain relief. While no CT-based comparison foraminal decompression data between PECD and open or other minimally invasive decompression techniques, it is clear that the preferential ventral to dorsal decompression effect is another benefit of the PECD compared to these other posterior decompression techniques. This observation made by the authors in their feasibility clinical series presented herein provides the theoretical explanation and rationale as to why lower instability and kyphosis rates should be expected in more extensive clinical trials, which will hopefully be conducted soon. This team of authors is highly motivated to conduct such studies as the lower propensity of PECD to produce lower instability rates may be the key to lower axial neck pain rates in posterior cervical foraminotomy patients.

A study by Raynor *et al.* reported that to decompress the exiting nerve root by 5 mm, 50% of the facets needed to be sacrificed to expose the root [35]. To decompress it by 8-10 mm, 70% of the facet joint had to be decompressed. However, he demonstrated biomechanical failure in 70% facetectomized specimen at 159 lbs load but none in 50% facetectomized specimens loaded up to 208 lbs. Hence, the recommendation was generally to decompress less than 50% of the facet joint [35]. The authors trans "V" PECD aims to medialize the access to the exiting cervical nerve root and thus further diminish the necessary medial facet joint resection to access the painful nerve root. We propose performing it through the same stepwise choreography described herein. It can help identify critical structures and provide adequate target decompression while achieving good radiological and clinical outcomes without a high percentage of patients with postoperative instability-related problems. None of these problems were observed in any of the patients who we followed up for the mean of 29 months.

Complication rate of the surgery in the authors' feasibility study was 4% which is comparable to other minimally invasive posterior cervical foraminotomy literature [36 - 38]. The most common complications in the literature related to posterior cervical foraminotomy are wound issues, neuropraxia and durotomy. PECD has good potential in decreasing wound related complications in view of preservation of soft tissue and avoidance of prolonged retraction of any particular cervical muscle group due to constant mobility of endoscope [36]. Neuropraxia is an unavoidable sequelae with the PECD that should be expected. Patients should be educated and prepared for this annoying condition. Although the authors of this chapter have had relatively few problems in their patients, many of them are very experienced veterans of endoscopic spine surgery and operate with the spinal endoscope at a very high skill level over many years. Therefore, the novice surgeon should be prepared to manage such neuropraxia- or dysesthesia-related

postoperative problems may arise. The careful and skillful use of the beveled working cannula as a retractor for the exiting nerve is advisable. More advanced endoscopic techniques include the creation of a subneural space by drilling on the pedicle and vertebra body which is described in another chapter of this text on cervical endoscopy. Such additional subneural decompression may facilitate access to the disc without excessive neural retraction. However, further study of this technique is warranted [39]. Incidental durotomy can be a problem in any endoscopic procedure. A patch blocking repair technique for small incidental dura tear is a common strategy in treatment of endoscopic dural tear [40]. However, one needs to be careful when pushing the patch against spinal cord to avoid cord injury. The question arises if the unexperienced surgeon should change the surgical strategy to a different open or other minimally invasive spinal surgery technique if an incidental durotomy of the cervical spinal cord is encountered. In the authors' opinion, durotomy in the cervical spinal cord definitively increases the risk of the surgery and high vigilance of the surgical team needs to be applied.

## CONCLUSIONS

The PECD is one of the most commonly performed endoscopic minimally invasive surgical techniques for treating symptomatic cervical disc herniation in the lateral canal and the neuroforamen. Minimum two-year clinical outcome data with the PECD are favorable and par with open or other forms of minimally invasive spinal surgery techniques. To minimize decompression-related instability, the authors recommend using Trans "V" point Posterior Endoscopic Cervical Decompression by Foraminotomy and Discectomy (TV PECD). The radiological assessment of foraminal was statistically significant compared to preoperative values. The absence of postoperative instability was attributed to the preferential ventral to dorsal decompression accomplished with the PECD technique. PECD should be learned from master surgeons to shorten the learning curve, which can be considerable, mainly if the surgeon is unfamiliar with spinal endoscopy overall.

## CONSENT FOR PUBLICATION

Not applicable.

## CONFLICT OF INTEREST

The author declares no conflict of interest, financial or otherwise.

## ACKNOWLEDGEMENTS

Declared none.

# REFERENCES

[1]     Woods BI, Hilibrand AS. Cervical radiculopathy: epidemiology, etiology, diagnosis, and treatment. J Spinal Disord Tech 2015; 28(5): E251-9.
[http://dx.doi.org/10.1097/BSD.0000000000000284] [PMID: 25985461]

[2]     Adamson TE. Microendoscopic posterior cervical laminoforaminotomy for unilateral radiculopathy: results of a new technique in 100 cases. J Neurosurg 2001; 95(1) (Suppl.): 51-7.
[PMID: 11453432]

[3]     Knight MT, Goswami A, Patko JT. Cervical percutaneous laser disc decompression: preliminary results of an ongoing prospective outcome study. J Clin Laser Med Surg 2001; 19(1): 3-8.
[http://dx.doi.org/10.1089/104454701750066875] [PMID: 11547816]

[4]     Taşçioğlu AO, Attar A, Taşçioğlu B. Microsurgical anterior cervical foraminotomy (uncinatectomy) for cervical disc herniation. Report of three cases. J Neurosurg 2001; 94(1) (Suppl.): 121-5.
[PMID: 11147846]

[5]     Yabuki S, Kikuchi S. Endoscopic partial laminectomy for cervical myelopathy. J Neurosurg Spine 2005; 2(2): 170-4.
[http://dx.doi.org/10.3171/spi.2005.2.2.0170] [PMID: 15739529]

[6]     Saringer WF, Reddy B, Nöbauer-Huhmann I, *et al.* Endoscopic anterior cervical foraminotomy for unilateral radiculopathy: anatomical morphometric analysis and preliminary clinical experience. J Neurosurg 2003; 98(2) (Suppl.): 171-80.
[PMID: 12650402]

[7]     Yuchi CX, Sun G, Chen C, *et al.* Comparison of the Biomechanical Changes After Percutaneous Full-Endoscopic Anterior Cervical Discectomy *versus* Posterior Cervical Foraminotomy at C5-C6: A Finite Element-Based Study. World Neurosurg 2019; 128: e905-11.
[http://dx.doi.org/10.1016/j.wneu.2019.05.025] [PMID: 31096026]

[8]     Ramírez León JF, Rugeles Ortíz JG, Martínez CR, Alonso Cuéllar GO, Lewandrowski KU. Surgical treatment of cervical radiculopathy using an anterior cervical endoscopic decompression. J Spine Surg 2020; 6 (Suppl. 1): S179-85.
[http://dx.doi.org/10.21037/jss.2019.09.24] [PMID: 32195426]

[9]     Childress MA, Becker BA. Nonoperative Management of Cervical Radiculopathy. Am Fam Physician 2016; 93(9): 746-54.
[PMID: 27175952]

[10]   Cvetanovich GL, Hsu AR, Frank RM, An HS, Andersson GB. Spontaneous resorption of a large cervical herniated nucleus pulposus. Am J Orthop 2014; 43(7): E140-5.
[PMID: 25046190]

[11]   Hattori S, Kawai K, Mabuchi Y, Shibayama M. The relationship between magnetic resonance imaging and quantitative electromyography findings in patients with compressive cervical myelopathy. Spine 2010; 35(8): E290-4.
[http://dx.doi.org/10.1097/BRS.0b013e3181c84700] [PMID: 20354473]

[12]   Park HJ, Kim SS, Lee SY, *et al.* A practical MRI grading system for cervical foraminal stenosis based on oblique sagittal images. Br J Radiol 2013; 86(1025): 20120515.
[http://dx.doi.org/10.1259/bjr.20120515] [PMID: 23410800]

[13]   Ghisi D, Fanelli A, Tosi M, Nuzzi M, Fanelli G. Monitored anesthesia care. Minerva Anestesiol 2005; 71(9): 533-8.
[PMID: 16166913]

[14]   Wu PH, Kim HS, Lee YJ, *et al.* Posterior endoscopic cervical foramiotomy and discectomy: clinical and radiological computer tomography evaluation on the bony effect of decompression with 2 years follow-up. Eur Spine J 2021; 30(2): 534-46.
[http://dx.doi.org/10.1007/s00586-020-06637-8] [PMID: 33078265]

[15]  Reed CC, Wolf WA, Cotton CC, Dellon ES. A visual analogue scale and a Likert scale are simple and responsive tools for assessing dysphagia in eosinophilic oesophagitis. Aliment Pharmacol Ther 2017; 45(11): 1443-8.
[http://dx.doi.org/10.1111/apt.14061] [PMID: 28370355]

[16]  Fairbank J. Use of Oswestry Disability Index (ODI). Spine 1995; 20(13): 1535-7.
[http://dx.doi.org/10.1097/00007632-199507000-00020] [PMID: 8623078]

[17]  Macnab I. Negative disc exploration. An analysis of the causes of nerve-root involvement in sixty-eight patients. J Bone Joint Surg Am 1971; 53(5): 891-903.
[http://dx.doi.org/10.2106/00004623-197153050-00004] [PMID: 4326746]

[18]  Macnab I. The surgery of lumbar disc degeneration. Surg Annu 1976; 8: 447-80.
[PMID: 936011]

[19]  Lee MJ, Dettori JR, Standaert CJ, Brodt ED, Chapman JR. The natural history of degeneration of the lumbar and cervical spines: a systematic review. Spine 2012; 37(22) (Suppl.): S18-30.
[http://dx.doi.org/10.1097/BRS.0b013e31826cac62] [PMID: 22872220]

[20]  Wong JJ, Côté P, Quesnele JJ, Stern PJ, Mior SA. The course and prognostic factors of symptomatic cervical disc herniation with radiculopathy: a systematic review of the literature. Spine J 2014; 14(8): 1781-9.
[http://dx.doi.org/10.1016/j.spinee.2014.02.032] [PMID: 24614255]

[21]  Richards O, Choi D, Timothy J. Cervical arthroplasty: the beginning, the middle, the end? Br J Neurosurg 2012; 26(1): 2-6.
[http://dx.doi.org/10.3109/02688697.2011.595846] [PMID: 21815734]

[22]  Lee DG, Park CK, Lee DC. Clinical and radiological results of posterior cervical foraminotomy at two or three levels: a 3-year follow-up. Acta Neurochir (Wien) 2017; 159(12): 2369-77.
[http://dx.doi.org/10.1007/s00701-017-3360-4] [PMID: 29063273]

[23]  Papavero L, Kothe R. Correction to: Minimally invasive posterior cervical foraminotomy for treatment of radiculopathy : an effective, time-tested, and cost-efficient motion-preservation technique. Oper Orthop Traumatol 2018; 30(1): 46.
[http://dx.doi.org/10.1007/s00064-017-0526-4] [PMID: 29270676]

[24]  Papavero L, Kothe R. Minimally invasive posterior cervical foraminotomy for treatment of radiculopathy : An effective, time-tested, and cost-efficient motion-preservation technique. Oper Orthop Traumatol 2018; 30(1): 36-45.
[http://dx.doi.org/10.1007/s00064-017-0516-6] [PMID: 28929274]

[25]  Selvanathan SK, Beagrie C, Thomson S, *et al.* Anterior cervical discectomy and fusion *versus* posterior cervical foraminotomy in the treatment of brachialgia: the Leeds spinal unit experience (2008-2013). Acta Neurochir (Wien) 2015; 157(9): 1595-600.
[http://dx.doi.org/10.1007/s00701-015-2491-8] [PMID: 26144567]

[26]  Epstein NE. A Review of Complication Rates for Anterior Cervical Diskectomy and Fusion (ACDF). Surg Neurol Int 2019; 10: 100.
[http://dx.doi.org/10.25259/SNI-191-2019] [PMID: 31528438]

[27]  Jödicke A, Daentzer D, Kästner S, Asamoto S, Böker DK. Risk factors for outcome and complications of dorsal foraminotomy in cervical disc herniation. Surg Neurol 2003; 60(2): 124-9.
[http://dx.doi.org/10.1016/S0090-3019(03)00267-2] [PMID: 12900115]

[28]  Peto I, Scheiwe C, Kogias E, Hubbe U. Minimally invasive posterior cervical foraminotomy: freiburg experience with 34 patients. Clin Spine Surg 2017; 30(10): E1419-25.
[http://dx.doi.org/10.1097/BSD.0000000000000517] [PMID: 28234772]

[29]  Witzmann A, Hejazi N, Krasznai L. Posterior cervical foraminotomy. A follow-up study of 67 surgically treated patients with compressive radiculopathy. Neurosurg Rev 2000; 23(4): 213-7.
[http://dx.doi.org/10.1007/PL00011957] [PMID: 11153550]

[30]    Kwon YJ. Long-term clinical and radiologic outcomes of minimally invasive posterior cervical foraminotomy. J Korean Neurosurg Soc 2014; 56(3): 224-9.
[http://dx.doi.org/10.3340/jkns.2014.56.3.224] [PMID: 25368765]

[31]    Abe M, Takata Y, Higashino K, *et al.* Foraminoplastic transforaminal percutaneous endoscopic discectomy at the lumbosacral junction under local anesthesia in an elite rugby player. J Med Invest 2015; 62(3-4): 238-41.
[http://dx.doi.org/10.2152/jmi.62.238] [PMID: 26399355]

[32]    Chang JC, Park HK, Choi SK. Posterior cervical inclinatory foraminotomy for spondylotic radiculopathy preliminary. J Korean Neurosurg Soc 2011; 49(5): 308-13.
[http://dx.doi.org/10.3340/jkns.2011.49.5.308] [PMID: 21716632]

[33]    Lee SH, Erken HY, Bae J. Percutaneous transforaminal endoscopic lumbar interbody fusion: clinical and radiological results of mean 46-month follow-up. BioMed Res Int 2017; 2017: 3731983.
[PMID: 28337448]

[34]    Ruetten S, Komp M, Merk H, Godolias G. Full-endoscopic cervical posterior foraminotomy for the operation of lateral disc herniations using 5.9-mm endoscopes: a prospective, randomized, controlled study. Spine 2008; 33(9): 940-8.
[http://dx.doi.org/10.1097/BRS.0b013e31816c8b67] [PMID: 18427313]

[35]    Raynor RB, Pugh J, Shapiro I. Cervical facetectomy and its effect on spine strength. J Neurosurg 1985; 63(2): 278-82.
[http://dx.doi.org/10.3171/jns.1985.63.2.0278] [PMID: 4020449]

[36]    Sahai N, Changoor S, Dunn CJ, *et al.* Minimally invasive posterior cervical foraminotomy as an alternative to anterior cervical discectomy and fusion for unilateral cervical radiculopathy: a systematic review and meta-analysis. Spine 2019; 44(24): 1731-9.
[http://dx.doi.org/10.1097/BRS.0000000000003156] [PMID: 31343619]

[37]    Skovrlj B, Gologorsky Y, Haque R, Fessler RG, Qureshi SA. Complications, outcomes, and need for fusion after minimally invasive posterior cervical foraminotomy and microdiscectomy. Spine J 2014; 14(10): 2405-11.
[http://dx.doi.org/10.1016/j.spinee.2014.01.048] [PMID: 24486472]

[38]    Komp M, Oezdemir S, Hahn P, Ruetten S. Full-endoscopic posterior foraminotomy surgery for cervical disc herniations. Oper Orthop Traumatol 2018; 30(1): 13-24.
[http://dx.doi.org/10.1007/s00064-017-0529-1] [PMID: 29318337]

[39]    Xiao CM, Yu KX, Deng R, *et al.* Modified k-hole percutaneous endoscopic surgery for cervical foraminal stenosis: partial pediculectomy approach. Pain Physician 2019; 22(5): E407-16.
[PMID: 31561650]

[40]    Kim HS, Raorane HD, Hung WP, Heo DH, Sharma SB, Jang IT. Incidental durotomy during endoscopic stenotic lumbar decompression (ESLD): incidence, classification and proposed management strategies. World Neurosurg 2020; 139: e13-22.
[http://dx.doi.org/10.1016/j.wneu.2020.01.242]

# CHAPTER 10

# Posterior Endoscopic Decompression for Cervical Spondylotic Myelopathy

**Yuan Heng**[1]**, Zhang Xi-feng**[2]**, Zhang Lei-ming**[3]**, Yan Yu-qiu**[4]**, Liu Yan-kang**[1,5] and **Kai-Uwe Lewandrowski**[5,6,7,*]

[1] *Shanxi Medical University, Taiyuan 030001, China*

[2] *Department of Orthopedics, First Medical Center, PLA General Hospital, Beijing 100853, China*

[3] *Department of Neurosurgery, the Sixth Medical Center, PLA General Hospital, Beijing 100048, China*

[4] *Minimally Invasive Spinal Surgery, Beijing Yuhe Integrated Traditional Chinese and Western Medicine Rehabilitation Hospital, Beijing 100039, China*

[5] *Center for Advanced Spine Care of Southern Arizona and Surgical Institute of Tucson, Tucson, AZ, USA*

[6] *Department of Orthopaedic Surgery, UNIRIO, Rio de Janeiro, Brazil*

[7] *Department of Orthoapedic Surgery, Fundación Universitaria Sanitas, Bogotá, D.C., Colombia, USA*

**Abstract:** The authors describe the technique and clinical outcomes with the posterior endoscopic cervical spinal cord compression to treat cervical spondylotic myelopathy. A total of twenty-two cervical spondylotic myelopathy patients were treated with endoscopic spine surgery fusion from January 2015 to June 2017 at the Medical School of Chinese PLA. The operation time, intraoperative blood loss, and hospitalization stay were recorded and compared. Japanese Orthopaedic Association (JOA) scores before the operation, three months, and one year after operation were recorded and analyzed. There were twenty-two cases in the spinal endoscopy group. There were significant differences in preoperative JOA scores three months after surgery and one year after surgery. The JOA scores were significantly increased after surgery, and the symptoms gradually improved postoperatively. Clinical outcomes were Excellent in 81.8% of patients. The efficacy and safety of endoscopic spinal surgery for single-level cervical spondylotic myelopathy were established. The operation time, the intraoperative blood loss, and the hospitalization stay were reduced compared to historical numbers for competing decompression and fusion procedures.

---

*** Corresponding author Kai-Uwe Lewandrowski:** Center for Advanced Spine Care of Southern Arizona and Surgical Institute of Tucson, Tucson, AZ, USA, Department of Orthopaedic Surgery, UNIRIO, Rio de Janeiro, Brazil and Department of Orthoapedic Surgery, Fundación Universitaria Sanitas, Bogotá, D.C., Colombia, USA; Tel: +1 520 204-1495; Fax: +1 623 218-1215; E-mail: business@tucsonspine.com

**Keywords:** Cervical spondylotic myelopathy, Decompression, Gait imbalance, Laminectomy, Motion preservation, Non-fusion, Posterior cervical approach, Spinal cord compression, Spinal endoscopy, Upper motor neuron dysfunction.

## INTRODUCTION

Cervical spondylotic myelopathy (CSM) is spinal cord dysfunction caused by spinal cord degeneration. Compressive pathology may cause reduced blood supply and further contribute to the deterioration of the cervical myelon [1 - 3]. CSM has a high incidence among middle-aged and older adults over age 55 [4]. Patients with mild clinical symptoms may be successfully treated with physical therapy, massage, intermittent soft cervical collar bracing. Non-steroidal anti-inflammatory drugs also play a minor role [5, 6]. For patients with severe clinical signs of progressive deterioration of neurological function, surgery is recommended [7].

Anterior cervical decompression and fusion (ACDF) [8 - 13] and posterior cervical decompressions *via* laminectomy-, or laminoplasty technique with or without fusion remains the mainstream of surgical CSM treatment. The efficacy and safety of these [14 - 17] types of procedures have been established in short- [1, 2], and long- [18 - 23] term studies, mainly when applied in patients with multilevel disease. However, these surgeries are associated with significant morbidity due to soft tissue trauma from open incisions, muscle atrophy from prolonged retraction, increased blood loss, and implant-related problems. These disadvantages are of particular relevance to posterior decompressive procedures. The anterior approach exploiting the access to the anterior cervical spine afforded by blunt dissection of the tracheoesophageal groove carries the risk of dysphagia [24], recurrent laryngeal nerve palsy, Horner syndrome, vagal nerve injury, tracheoesophageal- and vascular damage, postoperative hematoma [25], intervertebral disc infection, or postoperative headaches [10, 26 - 33]. In addition, ACDF is associated with adjacent segment disease (ASD) [34, 35].

Endoscopic surgery may be an alternative to open decompression, particularly if the compressive pathology extends only over one or two levels. A few authors have demonstrated the feasibility, indications, complications, and clinical efficacy of endoscopic spinal surgery for this disease [36 - 39]. In this chapter, the authors describe the technical steps of a one- or two-level posterior endoscopic decompression in 22 patients who underwent surgical treatment and complete follow-up in the General Hospital of the People's Liberation Army for the past three years for symptomatic CSM.

## CLINICAL SERIES

There were 22 patients treated with spinal endoscopy, 14 males (63.6%), eight females (36.4%) with an average age of 42.41±7.06 years. Among them, 16 patients had single-level compressive lesions, and six patients had two-level compressive lesions. Two patients had a history of trauma, 14 patients suffered from upper limb motor dysfunction, 15 patients displayed lower limb motor dysfunction, and another nine patients suffered from combined upper and lower limb dysfunction. The preoperative workup included routine plain film x-ray, CT, and MRI studies of the cervical spine. The compressive pathology was often constituted by different degrees of disc herniation (15 patients), posterior marginal hypertrophy (2 patients), and ligamentum flavum hypertrophy (2 cases). Three patients had and spinal cord degeneration with evidence of myelomalacia on preoperative MRI scanning. Patients were enrolled in this consecutive cohort study if they had preserved motor function in the limbs, decreased or lost sensory function, positive pathological upper motor neuron signs, a preoperative JOA score ≤ of 12 points, neck and shoulder pain, and upper limb pain VAS > 6 points. Only patients with advanced imaging studies showed corroborating compressive pathology, including cervical degenerative disease, spinal stenosis, and spinal cord compression, consistent with the correlative clinical symptoms and signs. Moreover, the authors limited patient selection for the endoscopic spinal cord decompression with single- or two-level cervical spinal stenosis. Patients with bony cervical spinal stenosis, severe vertebral posterior marginal osteophyte formation, posterior longitudinal ligament ossification, congenital developmental cervical spinal stenosis, large cervical disc herniation, cervical intervertebral disc prolapse, and apparent cervical segmental instability and significant focal kyphosis were excluded.

## ENDOSCOPIC SURGICAL TECHNIQUE

Surgeries were performed under local anesthesia with the patient in a prone position with the neck flexed and fixed in tongues. Placing the head in capital flexion and cervical extension should facilitate access to the posterior elements. The surgical level and skin entry point were identified with the fluoroscopy unit placed in the anterior-posterior plane. The skin is prepped in standard surgical fashion, and a layer-by-layer infiltration with local anesthesia is applied. An 18G spinal needle was advanced to the trailing edge of the lamina of the surgical level. The trajectory of the guidewire is checked in both fluoroscopic planes. A skin incision is made around the guidewire, and serial dilators are advanced over it. The endoscopic working cannular is then placed at the surgical cervical lamina medical trailing edge to the facet joint complex. Typically, around a 7-mm working cannula was used to introduce the endoscope and directly visualize the cervical spine's posterior elements. The surgical decompression was facilitated by rongeurs, Kerrisons, and a high-speed drill.

A radiofrequency probe was used to ablate the remaining fibrous tissue around the surgical decompression area. A good start for the decompression is the lamina V point, comprised of the lower edge of the upper lamina and the rostral margin of the lower lamina as they converge onto the cervical facet joint. First, a standard foraminotomy is performed. Then, an endoscopic laminectomy is performed using the same endoscopic high-speed drills, rongers, and forceps. The ligamentum flavum was only removed if it was part of the compressive pathology. It was intentionally left to protect the spinal cord if decompression of the contralateral side was contemplated. During these maneuvers, the endoscope is maneuvered left and right and directed over the top to decompress the contralateral lateral cervical canal.

Sometimes, portions of the spinous process have to be removed to accommodate the endoscopic working channel. This can be achieved with rongeurs or a motorized bur. The contralateral decompression entails removing portions of the rostral and caudal lamina similarly as on the initial access side. The decompression is assessed by probing the increased canal volume under fluoroscopic image control. Only when needed to complete the decompression, the ligamentum flavum and the dural sac were separated using a dissecting nerve hook to facilitate removal of the portions of the ligamentum flavum. Laterally, the nuclear material from the intervertebral disc was removed to complete the anterior canal decompression. Typically, the entire decompression, regardless of whether unilateral or bilateral, can be accomplished from a single access portal. In the authors' experience, bilateral endoscopic decompression can be achieved in a reasonable amount of time for up to 3 levels. Before withdrawing the endoscope and its working cannula, the wounds and decompression sites should be checked for hemostasis. Wound closure can be accomplished with a single horizontal mattress stitch for skin closure.

## POSTOPERATIVE REHABILITATION

After surgery, patients are immediately allowed to ambulate as soon as they have recovered from anesthesia, sometimes as early as 4 hours after surgery. All patients are placed in a soft cervical collar. Postoperatively, patients were admitted to the hospital for routine intravenous infusion of mannitol and dexamethasone rehydration treatment, analgesic administration for pain control, and reduced risk of postoperative spinal cord irritation from surgical manipulation and continuous intraoperative use of irrigation fluid during the endoscopy. Patients without excessive postoperative incisional pain or any other problems or obvious complications were typically discharged to their homes after a short 24-hour overnight observation stay. They were sent home with their neck support and instructed to wear it for about 6-8 weeks or at a minimum to their first follow-up visit with their treating surgeon.

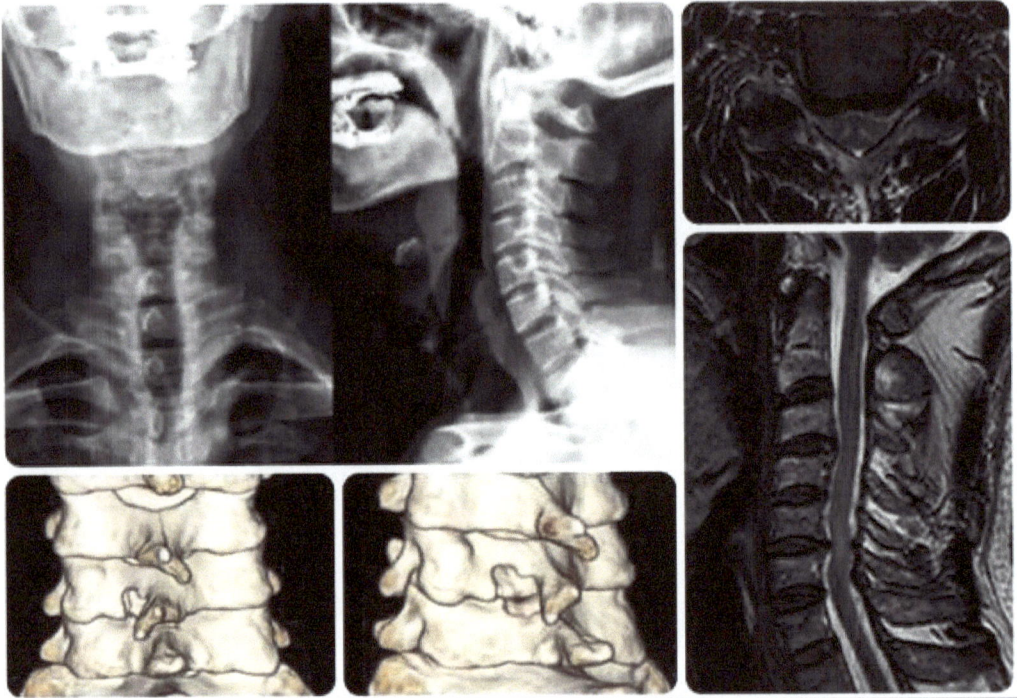

**Fig. (1).**  Preoperative X-rays and MRI scan of the cervical spine of a 59-year-old male patient with CSM. Images confirm loss of physiological curvature of the cervical spine and narrowing of the C5-6 intervertebral space. There is also hypertrophy of an infolded ligamentum flavum without calcification.

## EXEMPLARY CASES

This 59-years-old male patient with a chief complaint of neck pain for nine years, accompanied by pain in both hands and unstable walking for three months. His physical examination showed ataxic gait, loss of physiological curvature of the cervical spine, cervical spinous process space, and bilateral trapezius area was tender. The patient had an antalgic gait. There was no significant loss of sensation in both upper limbs, by partial limitation of cervical spine movement, without spasticity, with 5/5 motor strength and normal muscle tone. Both patella tendon reflexes were hyperactive, and there were bilateral Hoffman signs. Preoperative imaging studies did not show any instability or spondylolisthesis of the cervical spine (Fig. **1**). A magnetic resonance scan of the cervical spine showed cervical spinal canal stenosis secondary to a herniated disc at C5/6 and hypertrophy of the yellow ligament. In this case of C5-6 cervical spondylotic myelopathy, we performed a minimally invasive endoscopic laminectomy and decompression under local anesthesia. During the entire operation, the patient is completely awake and pain-free and can communicate with the doctor throughout the operation. The operation time was short with minimal intraoperative bleeding, and the 7-mm incision was closed with only one stitch. The treatment was effective as the patient noticed immediate pain relief following the endoscopic decompression. Additional illustrative case examples are shown in Figs. (2 - 4).

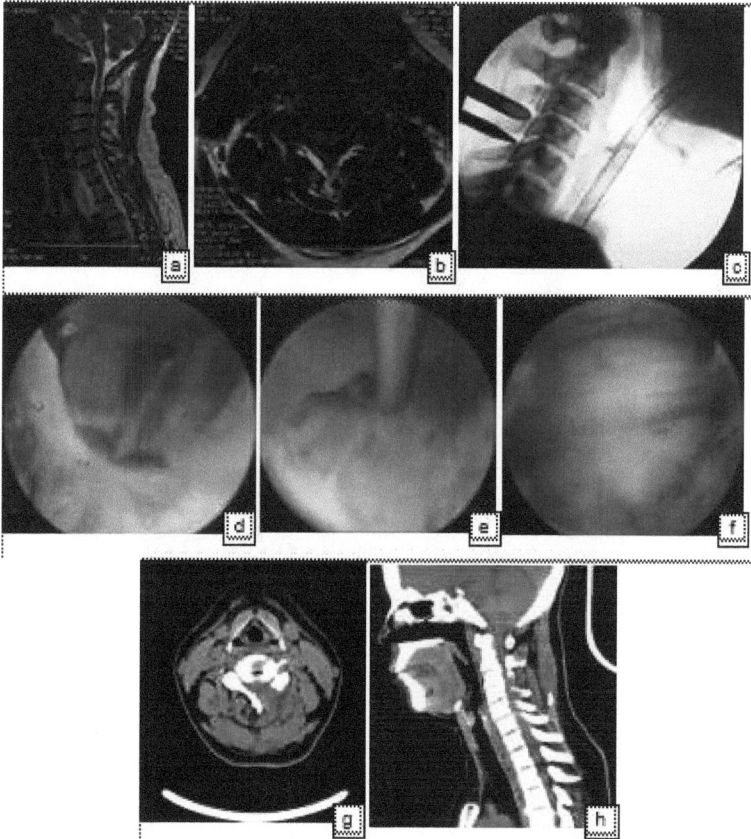

**Fig. (2).** An illustrative case of a symptomatic 46-year old male patient suffering from CSM is shown. The patient underwent C4-6 two-level posterior endoscopic decompression. The preoperative MRI scan (**a, b**) showed C4-6 compressive pathology consisting of disc herniation and a thickened infolded ligamentum flavum. The endoscopic working cannula position was confirmed on intraoperative fluoroscopic images (**c**). The decompression was facilitated with endoscopic burs (**d, e**). The endoscopic nerve hook (e) was used to free the yellow ligament margin. Ultimately, the dural sack of the cervical spinal cord was decompressed entirely (**f**). The postoperative axial (**g**), and sagittal (CT) demonstrate the extent of the decompression.

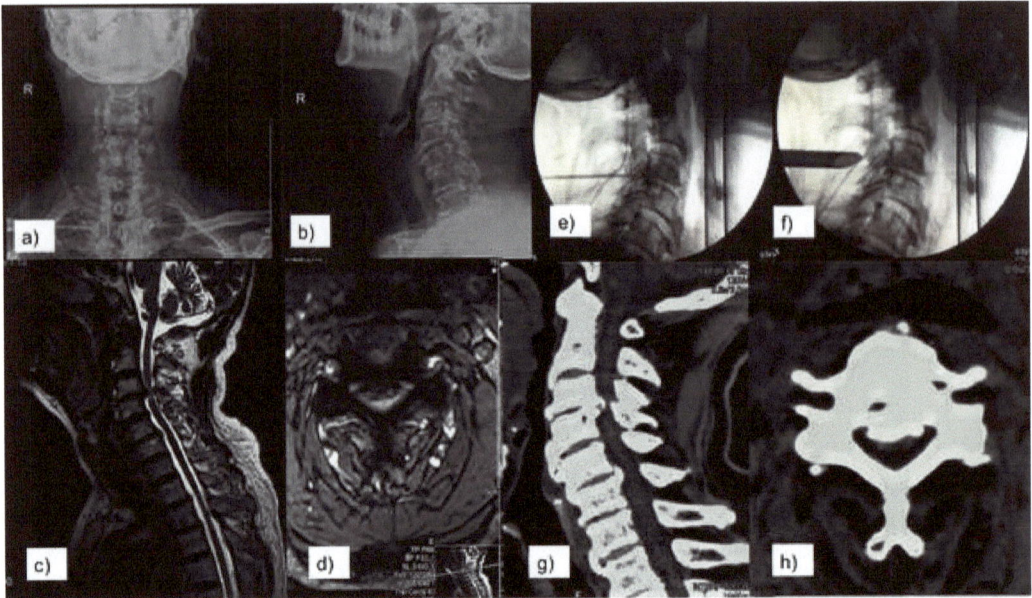

**Fig. (3).** An exemplary case of a symptomatic 76-year old CSM patient is shown. The patient was treated with posterior cervical endoscopic decompression at C3/4 **(a-d)**. The position of the working cannula is offered in several intraoperative fluoroscopic images **(e-f)**. The patient's preoperative CT sagittal and axial scans are shown in panels **g** and **h**.

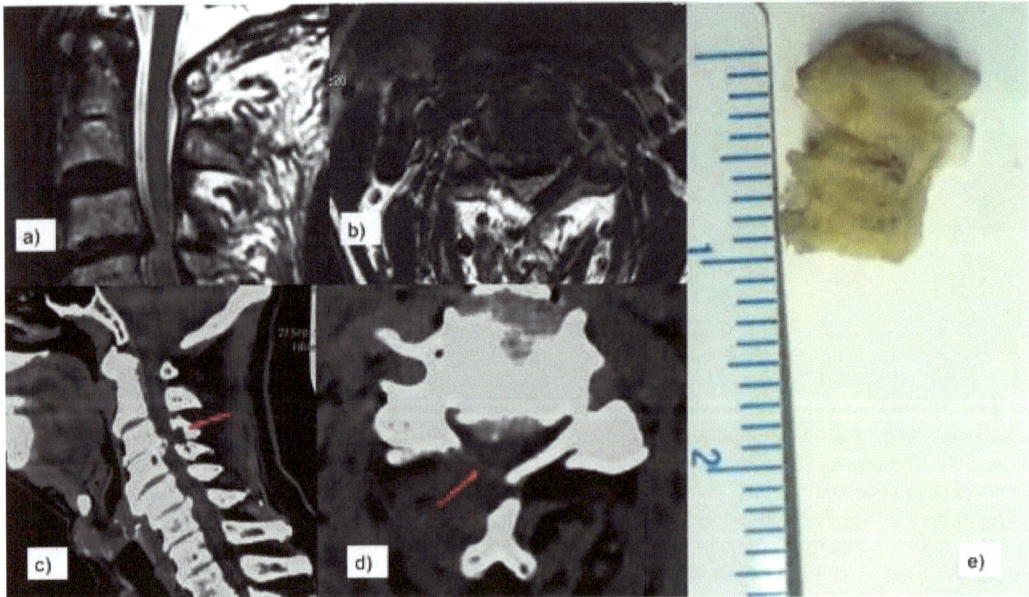

**Fig. (4).** Postoperative MRI **(a-b)** and CT **(c-d)** images of the same case described in Fig. **(2)** are shown. They show adequate decompression following the posterior endoscopic decompression. A large piece of the infolded ligamentum flavum was resected **(e)**.

## CLINICAL OUTCOMES

The primary outcome measures were the Macnab score. Secondary outcome measures were:

- The operation time.
- The intraoperative blood loss.
- Length of hospital stay.
- Surgery-related complications.
- The number of reoperations.

Moreover, the JOA scores were determined preoperatively and at three months and one year after surgery. The JOA improvement rate was calculated at these respective follow-up times. The improvement rate = (postoperative JOA - preoperative JOA) / (17 - preoperative JOA). The clinical efficacy was determined by assigning patients according to their improvement rate one year postoperatively into four grades. Improvement rates were grouped by the treating surgeon into the followed four categories according to modified Macnab criteria (6): 80% improvement rate, 50% improvement rate, 25% improvement rate, and <25% improvement rate. Descriptive statistics were performed on the primary outcome variables using SPSS 26.0 statistical software. The data count was expressed as a percentage or mean with the range and standard deviation. Crosstabulation testing was done using the Chi-Square test with a significance level of 0.05 as the acceptable p-value (Table **1**).

**Table 1. Clinical data and descriptive statistics.**

| N, % | Spinal Endoscopy Patients (n=22) |
|---|---|
| Age | $42.41 \pm 7.06$ |
| Gender (male, female) | 14(63.6%), 12 (36.4%) |
| Level Distribution | - |
| $C_{3-4}$ | 2(9.1%) |
| $C_{3-5}$ | 1(4.5%) |
| $C_{4-5}$ | 3(13.6%) |
| $C_{4-6}$ | 2(9.1%) |
| $C_{5-6}$ | 9(40.9%) |
| $C_{5-7}$ | 3(13.6%) |
| $C_{6-7}$ | 2(9.1%) |
| Clinical feature | - |
| Upper limb motor function | 14(63.6%) |

*(Table 1) cont.....*

| N, % | Spinal Endoscopy Patients (n=22) |
|---|---|
| Lower limb motor function | 15(68.2%) |
| Sensory function | 9(40.9%) |
| Bladder function | 0(0.0) |
| Reoperation | 1(4.5%) |

At one year postoperatively, the primary outcome measures in the cervical endoscopy patients were: Excellent in 11 patients (50%), Good in 7 patients (31.8%), Fair in 3 patients (13.6%), and Poor in 1 case (4.5%). Hence, Excellent and Good outcomes were achieved in 81.8% of patients (Table 2). ANOVA and simple effect tests were performed on the JOA scores on the cervical endoscopy patients' pre-and postoperative scores, which showed significant differences between the preoperative- and postoperative JOA scores at three months after surgery and one year after surgery (Table 3). The postoperative JOA scores in the cervical endoscopy patients were significantly increased after surgery, and the symptoms gradually improved postoperatively. The secondary outcome measures, including the average operation time, intraoperative blood loss, and length of hospital stay, are listed in Table 4.

Table 2. Primary Macnab outcome parameters at one-year after the endoscopic spinal cord decompression.

| - | Excellent | Good | Fair | Poor |
|---|---|---|---|---|
| Spinal endoscopy patients | 11(50.0%) | 7(31.8%) | 3(13.6%) | 1(4.5%) |

Table 3. Comparison of the JOA score and improvement rate before and after the endoscopic spinal cord decompression.

| - | JOA Rating JOA score | | | JOA Improvement Rate | |
|---|---|---|---|---|---|
| | Preop | Three Months Postop | One Year Postop | Three Months Postop | One Year Postop |
| Spinal endoscopy patients | 9.53±1.06 | 14.27±0.92 | 14.61±1.03 | 62.99±13.14 | 67.59±14.80 |
| $P$ | - | 0.0174 | 0.0042 | 0.0259 | 0.0114 |

Table 4. Secondary perioperative outcome parameter.

| | Operation Lasting Time/ Min | Intraoperative Blood Loss / ml | Hospitalization Stay/ d |
|---|---|---|---|
| Spinal endoscopy patients | 70.23±10.91 | 30.00±7.30 | 4.23±1.11 |

## DISCUSSION

Endoscopic spinal cord decompression for symptomatic spinal cord compression (CSM) is feasible. Most of the time, there is anterior compressive pathology in the form of osteophytes and disc bulges. Posterior compressive pathology arises from a thickened and infolding ligamentum flavum and may lead to spinal cord compression due to stenosis and ultimately produce the symptoms of florid CSM. In the authors' opinion, decompression is the crucial part of the operation – fusion is secondary. One could argue that fusion provides more reliable results. On the other hand, spinal endoscopy without fusion may be practical and constitute a more simplified treatment. Even for myelopathy, a cervical discectomy may be sufficient to relieve the symptoms. In comparison, there are few reports on the alternative posterior endoscopic resection of the lamina and the often-hypertrophied ligamentum flavum [37, 40 - 43]. There has been one additional cadaver study to establish the feasibility [44]. The purpose of the authors' study was to establish the feasibility of the endoscopic posterior cervical decompression in CSM patients and to perform an analysis of clinical outcomes.

Anterior cervical spinal cord decompression is typically done with anterior cervical discectomy and fusion (ACDF). It is widely accepted as the gold standard operation. ACDF works well if the predominant compressive pathology is anteriorly due to disc herniations and any associated osteophytes. The procedure is aimed at the restoration of spinal cord function. However, anterior decompression and fusion of the cervical spinal canal *via* ACDF only removes any compressive pathology closed the intervertebral disc space. A much more aggressive decompression *via* corpectomy is required to decompress the anterior longitudinal ligament and osteophytes behind the posterior cervical vertebral body if these structures are involved in spinal cord compression. In comparison, the endoscopic approach allows directly visualized decompression of the posterior spinal canal with a substantial volumetric expansion. The latter is minimal with ACDF [45]. The posterior enlargement of the spinal canal allows for posterior expansion of the cervical spinal cord.

The posterior endoscopic cervical spinal cord decompression requires a high skill level. For this reason, the indications for the procedure are narrow is required of the surgeon to remove the posterior lamina and the thickened folded ligamentum flavum. Posterior enlargement of the spinal canal's volume is contraindicated in patients with large disc herniation, ossification of the posterior longitudinal ligament, and large posterior vertebral body osteophytes. Endoscopic decompression is less burdensome for elderly CSM patients with medical comorbidities and an attractive alternative to open surgery. Nonetheless, the authors recommend only consider posterior endoscopic spinal cord decompression when the predominant pathology is posterior. Anterior endoscopic spinal decompression is not recommended from posterior access due to the high-risk nature of the procedure. Hands-on training in cadaver courses and side-b--side mentoring with a master surgeon is highly recommended.

A non-fusion surgery significantly reduces operative time and intraoperative blood loss. The small endoscopic approach may also reduce the risk of postoperative infection and maintains the integrity of the posterior interspinous ligament – an important anatomical tension band. The overall reduced tissue trauma with the endoscopic spinal surgery results in decreased incision pain and rapid postoperative recovery. The authors perform the procedure on an inpatient basis with a short hospital stay. Conceivably, it could be done in an ambulatory surgery center setting after some observation since serious peri- and postoperative complications are uncommon. The improved visualization due to reduced bleeding and magnification under continuous irrigation allows for accurate and precise identification of the spinal cord and cervical nerve roots. The authors have had no dural tears or nerve root injuries [46]. Neither were there any patients with postoperative kyphosis and axial neck pain, which is frequently seen with posterior cervical laminectomy. Future studies will investigate whether the endoscopic posterior cervical spinal decompression results in lower fusion requirements postoperatively with the motion-preserving endoscopic decompression surgery.

The learning curve is steep with the endoscopic procedure. The use of high-speed power drills and other endoscopic instruments through a minor surgical access corridor can be dangerous. Endoscopic removal of the upper and lower lamina and the medial portion of the articular pillar of the cervical facet joints requires a significant skill level. The novice surgeon should team up with a master surgeon to guide him or her through the individual learning steps. First, one should focus on thinning out the lamina. Then, one could move on to removing the remaining laminar bone with endoscopic rongeurs. In the final step of the training program, the training surgeon should learn how to complete the spinal cord decompression under close supervision. The authors of this chapter have implemented such a training program at their institution to prevent injury to the spinal cord and nerve roots. Only the central portion of the ligamentum flavum is removed as its lateral portion can protect the spinal cord and nerve roots when the base of the spinous process and the contralateral lamina are treated with a power drill. When removing the ligamentum flavum, the ligamentum flavum is dissected off the nerve root to free it entirely and to avoid dural tears and adhesions with the spinal cord. The facet joint resection should not exceed 50% of the joint pillar.

Otherwise, axial neck and shoulders pain may ensue postoperatively. Conceivably, it could prompt instability and even compromise of the vertebral artery and other serious consequences.

## CONCLUSIONS

Favorable short and medium-term clinical outcomes can be achieved with the posterior endoscopic spinal canal decompression for the treatment of CSM. The authors' feasibility study presented in this chapter suffered from a short follow-up of only 12 months and a small patient sample. Patient selection bias may have impacted the outcomes as well since all patients came from one institution. They also did not consider the duration and severity of preoperative symptoms and upper motor neuron signs, neurological status in the analysis of postoperative symptom resolution, and overall prognosis. In skilled hands, endoscopic cervical spinal cord decompression is an attractive alternative to ACDF or open or other types of following MIS procedures with higher approach-related morbidity. However, the indications are narrow. Notably, the novice surgeon should limit the scope of this surgery to one or two levels. Posterior endoscopic spinal cord decompression in CSM patients has the apparent advantages of reduced operative time, intraoperative blood loss, and length of stay at the hospital. The technique warrants further clinical investigation to investigate its efficacy in the long run.

## CONSENT FOR PUBLICATION

Not applicable.

## CONFLICT OF INTEREST

The author declares no conflict of interest, financial or otherwise.

## ACKNOWLEDGEMENTS

Declared none.

## REFERENCES

[1]     Epstein NE. Laminectomy for cervical myelopathy. Spinal Cord 2003; 41(6): 317-27.
        [http://dx.doi.org/10.1038/sj.sc.3101477] [PMID: 12746738]

[2]     Blizzard DJ, Caputo AM, Sheets CZ, *et al.* Laminoplasty *versus* laminectomy with fusion for the treatment of spondylotic cervical myelopathy: short-term follow-up. Eur Spine J 2017; 26(1): 85-93.
        [http://dx.doi.org/10.1007/s00586-016-4746-3] [PMID: 27554354]

[3]     Qi Q, Huang S, Ling Z, *et al.* A New Diagnostic Medium for Cervical Spondylotic Myelopathy: Dynamic Somatosensory Evoked Potentials. World Neurosurg 2020; 133: e225-32.
        [http://dx.doi.org/10.1016/j.wneu.2019.08.205] [PMID: 31493599]

[4]     Young WF. Cervical spondylotic myelopathy: a common cause of spinal cord dysfunction in older persons. Am Fam Physician 2000; 62(5): 1064-70-73.

[5]    Bernhardt M, Hynes RA, Blume HW, White AA III. Cervical spondylotic myelopathy. J Bone Joint Surg Am 1993; 75(1): 119-28.
[http://dx.doi.org/10.2106/00004623-199301000-00016] [PMID: 8419381]

[6]    Law MD Jr, Bernhardt M, White AA III. Evaluation and management of cervical spondylotic myelopathy. Instr Course Lect 1995; 44: 99-110.
[PMID: 7797896]

[7]    Law MD Jr, Bernhardt M, White AA III. Cervical spondylotic myelopathy: a review of surgical indications and decision making. Yale J Biol Med 1993; 66(3): 165-77.
[PMID: 8209553]

[8]    Kang L, Lin D, Ding Z, Liang B, Lian K. Artificial disk replacement combined with midlevel ACDF *versus* multilevel fusion for cervical disk disease involving 3 levels. Orthopedics 2013; 36(1): e88-94.
[http://dx.doi.org/10.3928/01477447-20121217-24] [PMID: 23276359]

[9]    Laxer EB, Brigham CD, Darden BV, *et al.* Adjacent segment degeneration following ProDisc-C total disc replacement (TDR) and anterior cervical discectomy and fusion (ACDF): does surgeon bias effect radiographic interpretation? Eur Spine J 2017; 26(4): 1199-204.
[http://dx.doi.org/10.1007/s00586-016-4780-1] [PMID: 27650387]

[10]   Lee HC, Chen CH, Wu CY, Guo JH, Chen YS. Comparison of radiological outcomes and complications between single-level and multilevel anterior cervical discectomy and fusion (ACDF) by using a polyetheretherketone (PEEK) cage-plate fusion system. Medicine (Baltimore) 2019; 98(5): e14277.
[http://dx.doi.org/10.1097/MD.0000000000014277] [PMID: 30702590]

[11]   Sasso R. Cervical arthroplasty compares favourably to ACDF at half-decade follow-up. Evid Based Med 2016; 21(1): 15.
[http://dx.doi.org/10.1136/ebmed-2015-110239] [PMID: 26537354]

[12]   Xie L, Liu M, Ding F, Li P, Ma D. Cervical disc arthroplasty (CDA) *versus* anterior cervical discectomy and fusion (ACDF) in symptomatic cervical degenerative disc diseases (CDDDs): an updated meta-analysis of prospective randomized controlled trials (RCTs). Springerplus 2016; 5(1): 1188.
[http://dx.doi.org/10.1186/s40064-016-2851-8] [PMID: 27516926]

[13]   Zheng B, Hao D, Guo H, He B. ACDF *vs* TDR for patients with cervical spondylosis - an 8 year follow up study. BMC Surg 2017; 17(1): 113.
[http://dx.doi.org/10.1186/s12893-017-0316-9] [PMID: 29183306]

[14]   Hitchon PW, Woodroffe RW, Noeller JA, Helland L, Hramakova N, Nourski KV. Anterior and posterior approaches for cervical myelopathy: clinical and radiographic outcomes. Spine 2019; 44(9): 615-23.
[http://dx.doi.org/10.1097/BRS.0000000000002912] [PMID: 30724826]

[15]   Yuan X, Wei C, Xu W, Gan X, Cao S, Luo J. Comparison of laminectomy and fusion *vs* laminoplasty in the treatment of multilevel cervical spondylotic myelopathy: A meta-analysis. Medicine (Baltimore) 2019; 98(13): e14971.
[http://dx.doi.org/10.1097/MD.0000000000014971] [PMID: 30921202]

[16]   Dobran M, Mancini F, Paracino R, *et al.* Laminectomy *versus* open-door laminoplasty for cervical spondylotic myelopathy: a clinical outcome analysis. Surg Neurol Int 2020; 11: 73.
[http://dx.doi.org/10.25259/SNI_85_2020] [PMID: 32363068]

[17]   Li Q, Han X, Wang R, Zhang Y, Liu P, Dong Q. Clinical recovery after 5 level of posterior decompression spine surgeries in patients with cervical spondylotic myelopathy: a retrospective cohort study. Asian J Surg 2020; 43(5): 613-24.
[http://dx.doi.org/10.1016/j.asjsur.2019.08.003] [PMID: 31481282]

[18]   Kato Y, Iwasaki M, Fuji T, Yonenobu K, Ochi T. Long-term follow-up results of laminectomy for

cervical myelopathy caused by ossification of the posterior longitudinal ligament. J Neurosurg 1998; 89(2): 217-23.
[http://dx.doi.org/10.3171/jns.1998.89.2.0217] [PMID: 9688116]

[19]   Chen Y, Guo Y, Chen D, Wang X, Lu X, Yuan W. Long-term outcome of laminectomy and instrumented fusion for cervical ossification of the posterior longitudinal ligament. Int Orthop 2009; 33(4): 1075-80.
[http://dx.doi.org/10.1007/s00264-008-0609-9] [PMID: 18685849]

[20]   Asthagiri AR, Mehta GU, Butman JA, Baggenstos M, Oldfield EH, Lonser RR. Long-term stability after multilevel cervical laminectomy for spinal cord tumor resection in von Hippel-Lindau disease. J Neurosurg Spine 2011; 14(4): 444-52.
[http://dx.doi.org/10.3171/2010.11.SPINE10429] [PMID: 21275550]

[21]   Lee SE, Chung CK, Jahng TA, Kim HJ. Long-term outcome of laminectomy for cervical ossification of the posterior longitudinal ligament. J Neurosurg Spine 2013; 18(5): 465-71.
[http://dx.doi.org/10.3171/2013.1.SPINE12779] [PMID: 23452249]

[22]   Laiginhas AR, Silva PA, Pereira P, Vaz R. Long-term clinical and radiological follow-up after laminectomy for cervical spondylotic myelopathy. Surg Neurol Int 2015; 6: 162.
[http://dx.doi.org/10.4103/2152-7806.167211] [PMID: 26543671]

[23]   Houten JK, Weinstein GR, Collins M. Long-term fate of C3-7 arthrodesis: 4-level ACDF *versus* Cervical Laminectomy and Fusion. J Neurosurg Sci 2018.
[PMID: 30290695]

[24]   Ebot J, Domingo R, Nottmeier E. Post-operative dysphagia in patients undergoing a four level anterior cervical discectomy and fusion (ACDF). J Clin Neurosci 2020; 72: 211-3.
[http://dx.doi.org/10.1016/j.jocn.2019.12.002] [PMID: 31839384]

[25]   Epstein NE. A review of complication rates for Anterior Cervical Diskectomy and Fusion (ACDF). Surg Neurol Int 2019; 10: 100.
[http://dx.doi.org/10.25259/SNI-191-2019] [PMID: 31528438]

[26]   Arshi A, Wang C, Park HY, *et al.* Ambulatory anterior cervical discectomy and fusion is associated with a higher risk of revision surgery and perioperative complications: an analysis of a large nationwide database. Spine J 2018; 18(7): 1180-7.
[http://dx.doi.org/10.1016/j.spinee.2017.11.012] [PMID: 29155340]

[27]   Kelly MP, Eliasberg CD, Riley MS, Ajiboye RM, SooHoo NF. Reoperation and complications after anterior cervical discectomy and fusion and cervical disc arthroplasty: a study of 52,395 cases. Eur Spine J 2018; 27(6): 1432-9.
[http://dx.doi.org/10.1007/s00586-018-5570-8] [PMID: 29605899]

[28]   Khanna R, Kim RB, Lam SK, Cybulski GR, Smith ZA, Dahdaleh NS. Comparing short-term complications of inpatient *versus* outpatient single-level anterior cervical discectomy and fusion: an analysis of 6940 patients using the ACS-NSQIP database. Clin Spine Surg 2018; 31(1): 43-7.
[http://dx.doi.org/10.1097/BSD.0000000000000499] [PMID: 28079682]

[29]   Rumalla K, Smith KA, Arnold PM. Cervical total disc replacement and anterior cervical discectomy and fusion: reoperation rates, complications, and hospital resource utilization in 72 688 patients in the United States. Neurosurgery 2018; 82(4): 441-53.
[http://dx.doi.org/10.1093/neuros/nyx289] [PMID: 28973385]

[30]   Kashkoush A, Mehta A, Agarwal N, *et al.* Perioperative neurological complications following anterior cervical discectomy and fusion: clinical impact on 317, 789 patients from the National Inpatient Sample. World Neurosurg 2019; 128: e107-15.
[http://dx.doi.org/10.1016/j.wneu.2019.04.037] [PMID: 30980979]

[31]   Al Eissa S, Konbaz F, Aldeghaither S, *et al.* Anterior cervical discectomy and fusion complications and thirty-day mortality and morbidity. Cureus 2020; 12(4): e7643.
[http://dx.doi.org/10.7759/cureus.7643] [PMID: 32411545]

[32]  Narain AS, Hijji FY, Haws BE, *et al.* Risk factors for medical and surgical complications after 1--level anterior cervical discectomy and fusion procedures. Int J Spine Surg 2020; 14(3): 286-93.
[http://dx.doi.org/10.14444/7038] [PMID: 32699749]

[33]  Ranson WA, Neifert SN, Cheung ZB, Mikhail CM, Caridi JM, Cho SK. Predicting in-hospital complications after anterior cervical discectomy and fusion: a comparison of the elixhauser and charlson comorbidity indices. World Neurosurg 2020; 134: e487-96.
[http://dx.doi.org/10.1016/j.wneu.2019.10.102] [PMID: 31669536]

[34]  Verma K, Gandhi SD, Maltenfort M, *et al.* Rate of adjacent segment disease in cervical disc arthroplasty *versus* single-level fusion: meta-analysis of prospective studies. Spine 2013; 38(26): 2253-7.
[http://dx.doi.org/10.1097/BRS.0000000000000052] [PMID: 24335631]

[35]  Shriver MF, Lubelski D, Sharma AM, Steinmetz MP, Benzel EC, Mroz TE. Adjacent segment degeneration and disease following cervical arthroplasty: a systematic review and meta-analysis. Spine J 2016; 16(2): 168-81.
[http://dx.doi.org/10.1016/j.spinee.2015.10.032] [PMID: 26515401]

[36]  Dahdaleh NS, Wong AP, Smith ZA, Wong RH, Lam SK, Fessler RG. Microendoscopic decompression for cervical spondylotic myelopathy. Neurosurg Focus 2013; 35(1): E8.
[http://dx.doi.org/10.3171/2013.3.FOCUS135] [PMID: 23815253]

[37]  Yadav YR, Parihar V, Ratre S, Kher Y, Bhatele PR. Endoscopic decompression of cervical spondylotic myelopathy using posterior approach. Neurol India 2014; 62(6): 640-5.
[http://dx.doi.org/10.4103/0028-3886.149388] [PMID: 25591677]

[38]  Minamide A, Yoshida M, Simpson AK, *et al.* Microendoscopic laminotomy *versus* conventional laminoplasty for cervical spondylotic myelopathy: 5-year follow-up study. J Neurosurg Spine 2017; 27(4): 403-9.
[http://dx.doi.org/10.3171/2017.2.SPINE16939] [PMID: 28708041]

[39]  Yuan H, Zhang X, Zhang LM, Yan YQ, Liu YK, Lewandrowski KU. Comparative study of curative effect of spinal endoscopic surgery and anterior cervical decompression for cervical spondylotic myelopathy. J Spine Surg 2020; 6 (Suppl. 1): S186-96.
[http://dx.doi.org/10.21037/jss.2019.11.15] [PMID: 32195427]

[40]  Lin Y, Rao S, Li Y, Zhao S, Chen B. Posterior percutaneous full-endoscopic cervical laminectomy and decompression for cervical stenosis with myelopathy: a technical note. World Neurosurg 2019; S1878-8750 (19): 30051-8.
[http://dx.doi.org/10.1016/j.wneu.2018.12.180] [PMID: 30648610]

[41]  Yabuki S, Kikuchi S. Endoscopic partial laminectomy for cervical myelopathy. J Neurosurg Spine 2005; 2(2): 170-4.
[http://dx.doi.org/10.3171/spi.2005.2.2.0170] [PMID: 15739529]

[42]  Yabuki S, Kikuchi S. Endoscopic surgery for cervical myelopathy due to calcification of the ligamentum flavum. J Spinal Disord Tech 2008; 21(7): 518-23.
[http://dx.doi.org/10.1097/BSD.0b013e31815a6151] [PMID: 18836365]

[43]  Zhang C, Li D, Wang C, Yan X. Cervical endoscopic laminoplasty for cervical myelopathy. Spine 2016; 41 (Suppl. 19): B44-51.
[http://dx.doi.org/10.1097/BRS.0000000000001816] [PMID: 27656783]

[44]  Eicker SO, Klingenhöfer M, Stummer W, Steiger HJ, Hänggi D. Full-endoscopic cervical arcocristectomy for the treatment of spinal stenosis: results of a cadaver study. Eur Spine J 2012; 21(12): 2487-91.
[http://dx.doi.org/10.1007/s00586-012-2392-y] [PMID: 22706668]

[45]  Ruetten S. Full-endoscopic operations of the spine in disk herniations and spinal stenosis. Surg Technol Int 2011; 21: 284-98.

[PMID: 22505003]

[46]   Shin DA, Kim KN, Shin HC, Yoon DH. The efficacy of microendoscopic discectomy in reducing iatrogenic muscle injury. J Neurosurg Spine 2008; 8(1): 39-43.
[http://dx.doi.org/10.3171/SPI-08/01/039] [PMID: 18173345]

# CHAPTER 11

# Full Endoscopic Partial Pediculotomy, Partial Vertebrotomy Technique For Cervical Degenerative Spinal Disease

**Pang Hung Wu**[1,6]**, Hyeun Sung Kim**[1,2,3,4,5,*] **and Il-Tae Jang**[1]

[1] *Department of Neurosurgery, Nanoori Gangnam Hospital, Seoul, Republic of Korea*

[2] *A President of the Korean Research Society of the Endoscopic Spine Surgery (KOSESS), South Korea*

[3] *A Faculty of the KOrean Minimally Invasive Spine Surgery Society (KOMISS), South Korea*

[4] *A Chairman of the Nanoori Hospital Group Scientific Team, South Korea*

[5] *An Adjunct Professor of the Medical College of the Chosun University, Gwangju, South Korea*

[6] *Departments of Orthopaedic Surgery, National University Health System, Jurong Health Campus, Singapore*

**Abstract:** The challenges of decompression surgeries performed in the cervical spine for degenerative spinal disease are 1) the avoidance of injuries to vital structures, 2) prevention of neurological deterioration, or deficit 3) preservation of cervical segmental stability to avoid post-decompression kyphosis 4) adequate decompression of neural structures. Endoscopic spine surgery optimizes two essential aspects of minimally invasive spine surgery: optimal visualization and minimal soft tissue damage. Despite using a small diameter endoscope, the proximity of exiting nerve root, spinal cord, and pedicle to the intervertebral disc make posterior endoscopic cervical foraminotomy and discectomy difficult. To remove the disc without significant neural retraction, our technique of full endoscopic partial pediculotomy, partial vertebrotomy posterior endoscopic cervical foraminotomy and discectomy (PECFD) allows the creation of a subneural working space for the endoscopic equipment to reach the prolapsed disc or hypertrophic uncovertebral joint. This chapter describes this technique and its clinical pearls to perform PPPV PECFD safely and efficiently.

**Keywords:** Cervical radiculopathy, Degeneration, Full endoscopic partial pediculotomy, Partial vertebrotomy technique.

---

* **Corresponding author Hyeun Sung Kim:** Department of Neurosurgery, Nanoori Gangnam Hospital, Seoul, Republic of Korea, A President of the Korean Research Society of the Endoscopic Spine Surgery (KOSESS), South Korea, A Faculty of the Korean Minimally Invasive Spine Surgery Society (KOMISS), South Korea and A Chairman of the Nanoori Hospital Group Scientific Team, South Korea; E-mail: neurospinekim@gmail.com

# INTRODUCTION

The incidence of cervical degenerative spinal disease increases with age. Most adults aged above 40 years have severe cervical degeneration in one or more of the levels in MRI based population studies [1]. Fortunately, most of the patients are usually asymptomatic. Cervical degenerative spinal disease typically presents as degenerative disc disease and facet arthropathy with axial neck pain. As the degeneration progresses, the compression of the uncovertebral joint, bulging or prolapsing intervertebral disc, facet hypertrophy, and buckling of ligamentum flavum and posterior longitudinal ligament on the exiting nerve root can lead to cervical radiculopathy. The cervical spinal cord's compression can lead to myelopathy [2]. Conservative management includes physiotherapy, spinal injection, and immobilization by cervical collars. Cervical traction is helpful in most of the patients with cervical radiculopathy patients [3]. There is no clear consensus of surgical indications with cervical radiculopathy. Often a protracted failure of conservative management with progressive neurologic deficits and signs of evolving myelopathy indicates operative management [4]. Anterior cervical and posterior cervical approaches for radiculopathy have both achieved good clinical results at an average of 12-43 months after surgery [5]. Posterior cervical foraminotomy has a low risk of index level fusion rate and adjacent segment disease requiring around 1%, respectively [6]. However, posterior cervical foraminotomy significantly decreased the risk of recurrent laryngeal nerve palsy, dysphagia, trachea-esophageal injuries, and preserved cervical motion. The disadvantage in traditional open posterior cervical foraminotomy is extensive soft tissue dissection to expose the laminofacet junction of the index level (V point) [7]. Since endoscopic spine surgery started its development in the lumbar spine, technical and technological improvement has extended its indications to most of the lumbar degenerative conditions and more recently to cervical spine neurodegenerative diseases as well [8].

The full endoscopic cervical approach can be divided into an anterior and posterior procedure. Anterior Endoscopic Cervical Discectomy is an effective method with excellent clinical outcomes [9]. However, there is an inherent danger of significant organ injuries such as a carotid artery, esophagus, and trachea injuries with these vital structures close to the docking point. Posterior endoscopic cervical foraminotomy and discectomy have the benefits of directly docking onto the V point by serial dilation to minimize soft tissue damage. It is possible to treat a large percentage of degenerative cervical diseases [10]. Improved vision by optical lens magnification at the endoscope's distal tip with direct delivery of instruments through the working channel of endoscope under endoscopic vision improves safety in decompression posterior cervical bony and soft tissue [11]. Cervical exiting nerve root and cervical spinal cord injuries are dreaded complications of posterior approaches. There are advantages in minimizing the neural elements retraction in posterior endoscopic cervical foraminotomy and discectomy (PECFD).

In this chapter, we elaborate on the technique of full endoscopic partial pediculotomy, partial vertebrotomy posterior endoscopic cervical foraminotomy and discectomy (PPPV PECFD) which is done to create sufficient space to occupy a small endoscopic working cannula and decreases the amount of retraction of neural elements necessary to remove the prolapsed disc and decompress the uncovertebral joint of the index level.

## RATIONALE

### Anatomical Relationship of Cervical Disc, Pedicle & Exiting Nerve Root

The exiting cervical nerve root exits the spinal canal above their number vertebra, *i.e.*, C5 nerve root passes above the C5 pedicle and passes through the C4/5 intervertebral foramen. The exiting cervical nerve root commonly arises from its corresponding spinal cord and traverses just above their numbered pedicle. The cervical disc's lateral margin is closely associated with the superior and medial aspect of the pedicle (Fig. 1).

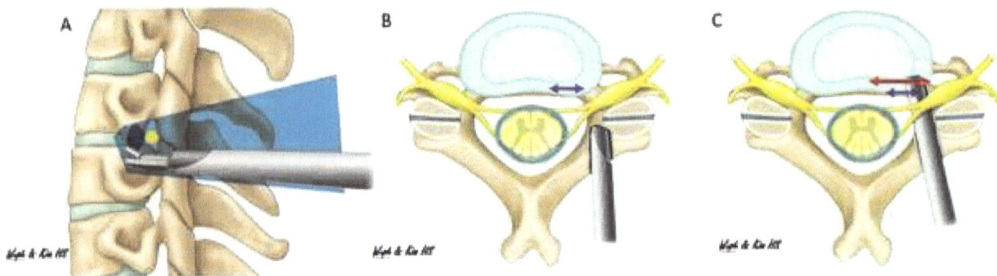

**Fig. (1).** Illustrative drawing of Partial Pediculotomy Partial Vertebrotomy Posterior endoscopic cervical foraminotomy and discectomy (PPPV PECFD). **(1a)**: Sagittal View and the amount of decompression in blue shadow. **(1b)**: Purple double arrow showed the amount of disc exposure in traditional PECFD. **(1c)**: Red double arrow showed the amount of disc exposure in PPPV PECFD.

## Current Limitation of Posterior Endoscopic Cervical Foraminotomy and Discectomy

The intimate relationship of the cervical nerve roots with the bony confines of the cervical spinal canal coupled with low tolerance of retraction for cervical neural elements poses significant challenges to retrieving prolapsed cervical disc and the uncovertebral joint decompression. The incidence of neurological complications of posterior cervical surgeries was reported to be around 0.18%, [12] while C5 palsy around 3.4% [13]. The occurrence of these neurological complications is debilitating to the patients and is associated with poor outcomes. While the surgeon can decompress more of the facet joint to expose the exiting nerve root, there is a limitation of the lateral extent of the facet decompression without compromising the spinal segment's stability. Raynor *et al.* demonstrated that the limit of facetectomy was around 50% of the facet before instability [14]. There is insufficient working space for endoscopic instruments and exposure of the intervertebral disc with a limited facetectomy. There is a tendency to retract the exiting nerve root to gain more access to the uncovertebral joint and intervertebral disc, which might increase the risk of nerve root dysesthesia and palsy.

## Concept of Subneural Space Creation for Endoscopic Instruments

The principle of creation of safe working space is key to successful endoscopic spine surgery. With the understanding of the limitation of cervical facet resection, we seek to create working space by drilling the pedicle and caudal vertebra body. Our team creates a subneural working space of 3-5mm diameter by drilling the superior and medial aspect of the pedicle to provide safe access to the uncovertebral joint and lateral third of the intervertebral disc (Fig. **1a**). We found in our study with a follow up of 13.7+/- 6.4 months that doing PPPV PECFD does not cause cervical instability [10].

## Concepts of Creation of Sub-Corporeal Space

With the current limitation of access to prolapsed disc, traditional PECFD indicates that two-third of the soft disc is lateral to the thecal sac of the cervical spinal cord. (Fig. **1b**) We found that if we can reach more medial portion of the disc between the lateral two third and half of the soft disc lateral to the thecal sac when we drill the caudal vertebral of the corresponding disc to create a 3-5 mm diameter of subneural working space without the need for any spinal cord retraction (Fig. **1c**).

## Preoperative Evaluation

The patients typically presented with clinical presentations were persistent and protracted cervical radiculopathy, with failed conservative treatment for more than six weeks. The patients may have motor and sensory impairment. We performed preoperative anteroposterior, lateral, flexion, and extension plain radiographs (XR), Computer Tomography (CT), Magnetic Resonance Imaging (MRI) were done in our institution. MRI and CT scan showed concordant cervical foraminal nerve root compression by cervical foraminal stenosis secondary to degenerative disc and uncovertebral joint hypertrophy and osteophyte in the facet joint and soft herniated cervical intervertebral disc. The disc material and uncal hypertrophy should be present in the lateral aspect of the cervical intervertebral disc. Half of the bulk of disc material is lateral to the thecal sac on the MRI axial view. We included patients who had more medial than the typical 2/3 of the bulk of disc being lateral to the thecal sac due to our PPPV PECFD technique. Certain categories of patients with contraindications for posterior cervical spine decompression are not suitable for PPPV PECFD. They are calcified central disc, instability of the cervical spine, significant cervical kyphosis of more than 10 degrees clinically if we excluded patients with predominant axial neck pain without radiculopathy, and cervical myelopathy.

## Anesthesia and Positioning

Our patients underwent general anesthesia, and a single dose of intravenous antibiotics was given. We did not need Mayfield. The patient's face was placed in a commercial anesthesia pillow foam supporting bony prominence with space created for eyes, nose, and mouth. He was positioned prone on Wilson frame with a shoulder strapped and neck flexed in a slight reverse Trendelenburg position using 3 points plaster traction technique on the head, shoulder, and back to increase interlaminar space of cervical spine [15]. The head attachment was tilted down slightly, allowing cervical spine flexion and secured with plaster. The patient's arms were tucked longitudinally and padded next to the patient. The hips and knees were flexed slightly.

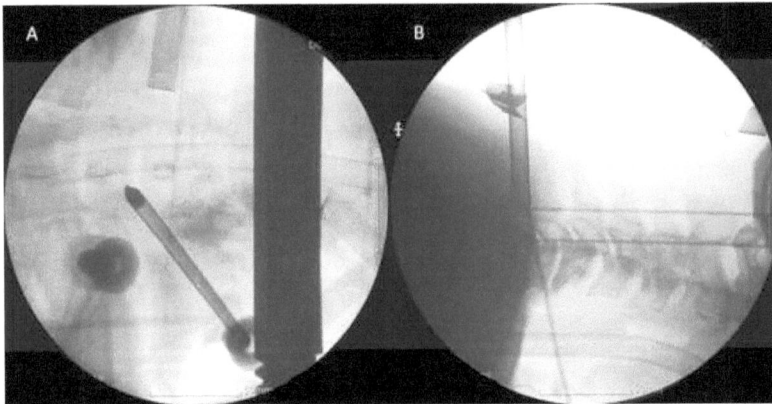

**Fig. (2).** Intraoperative anteroposterior and lateral fluoroscopic pictures of left C6/7 PPPV PECFD.

## SURGICAL STEPS

## Identification of Level and Safe Docking of the Endoscope

The skin was marked to the cervical spine's corresponding surgical level defined under the fluoroscopic guidance of anteroposterior (AP) and lateral view. The intersection of intervertebral disc space and the medial border of the facet joint junction on the AP view and the lateral view of the surgical level was then targeted by correlating the intraoperative view of the "V" point as defined by the V-shaped confluence of cephalad and caudal laminar facet junction [12]. At the "V"-point, we made a transverse 8-mm incision and placed the endoscopic working cannula after serial dilation with various obturators at the target area. The position of the tip of the working cannula was confirmed with fluoroscopy (Fig. **2**). We used an endoscope with a 7.3 mm outer diameter, and a 4.7 mm working channel. The authors' endoscope of choice was 171-mm long and had a 30-degree viewing angle. The procedure was performed under continuous irrigation with normal saline at hydraulic pressures not exceeding 25 mm Hg.

## Superficial Soft Tissue Dissection & Bone Drilling

We used a radiofrequency probe and endoscopic forceps for hemostasis and soft tissue dissection to expose the capsule of the facet joint and cephalad and caudal lateral part of the bony lamina to expose the " V" point (Fig. **3A**). We drilled the lateral portion of the cephalad lamina and medial third to half of the cephalad facet (Fig. **3B**). That would help to expose the deep "V" point of laminofacet junction (Fig. **3C**).

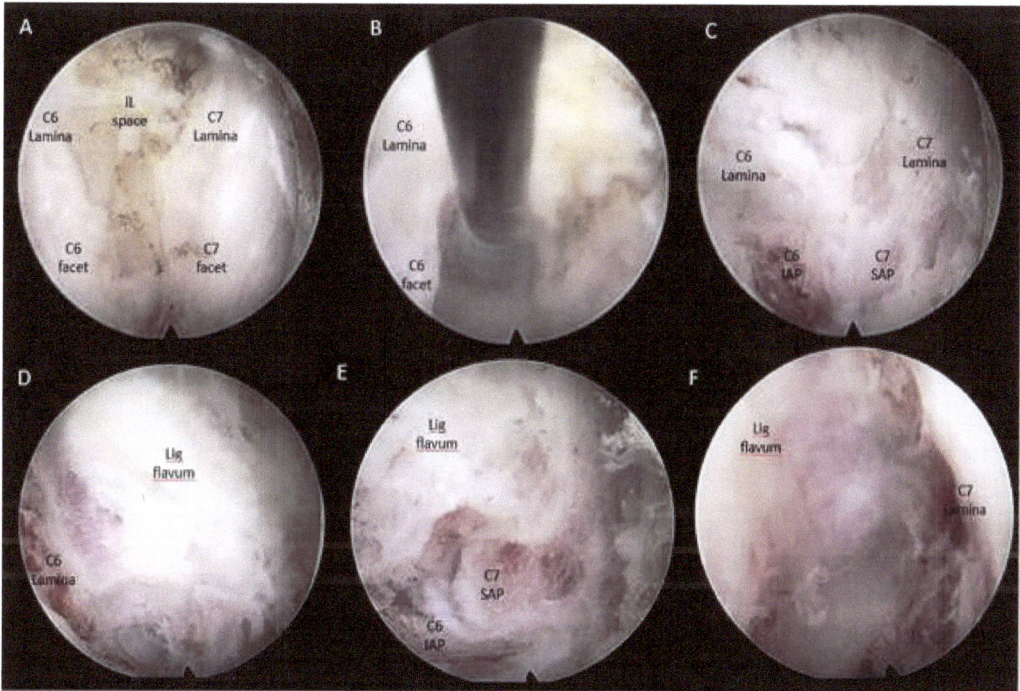

**Fig. (3).** Superficial Dissection And Surgical Steps of Partial Pediculotomy Partial Vertebrotomy Posterior endoscopic cervical foraminotomy and discectomy (PPPV PECFD).

## Deep Bony Dissection

We continued deeper bony drilling to thin out the cephalad lateral lamina (Fig. **3D**). We then shifted our focus of drilling on the medial facet joint (Fig. **3E**). Then, we drilled the medial third to half of the facet joint and caudal lamina (Fig. **3F**) until the lateral ligamentum flavum was detached from the lateral canal wall.

## Partial Pediculotomy

At this stage of the procedure, the pedicle was exposed. Then, we drilled below the cervical nerve root to create a 3-5mm deep subneural space (Fig. **4A**). Care should be taken only to drill out the superomedial quadrant of the pedicle by no more than 3-5 mm corresponding to the diameter of the diamond burr. One drill bit width can be used to intraoperatively gauge the amount of pedicle removed. This adjunct procedure created an extra working space, which could minimize neural retraction without causing any significant instability.

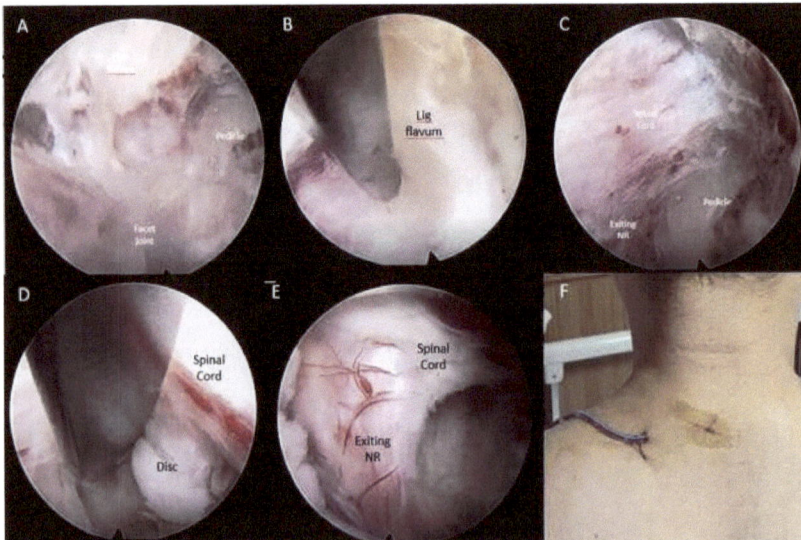

**Fig. (4).** Deep Dissection And Surgical Steps of Partial Pediculotomy Partial Vertebrotomy Posterior endoscopic cervical foraminotomy and discectomy (PPPV PECFD) and post-operative clinical photograph.

## Exposure of Neural Elements

We used a blunt bent probe to lift off the ligamentum flavum to expose and retrieve the thin flavum with endoscopic forceps (Figs. **4B** and **4C**). That would expose exiting nerve root, and spinal cord in close relationship with the pedicle's drilled superior medial portion. We exposed the disc space at the axilla of the neural elements closely related to the pedicle's superomedial aspect. The partial pediculotomy provided space for a blunt probe to retrieve the herniated disc (Fig.

4D).

## Decompression of Uncovertebral Joint in Cases of Foraminal Stenosis

For patients with uncovertebral hypertrophy leading to foraminal stenosis, retractor tube (working cannula) was placed directly over the uncovertebral joint. The partial pediculotomy allowed more space for retractor tube placement. We rotated the beveled tube with opening away from neural elements, and we drilled the uncovertebral joint with an endoscopic drill.

## Partial Vertebrotomy (Optional)

To gain access to the more medial disc, we could drill the caudal vertebra (partial vertebrotomy) with the tubular retractor being angled at the subneural space at 45 degrees and placed underneath the root without any neural retraction.

## Discectomy

The disc could be retrieved by using a blunt probe, nerve hooks. With increased subneural space, the disc typically would move into the area of least tissue resistance within the endoscopic surgical field to be removed by endoscopic forceps. Completion of decompression revealed by good pulsation of neural elements under irrigation fluid (Fig. **4E**).

## Hemostasis & Closure

Using radiofrequency ablation and hemostatic agents, bleeding was controlled meticulously. We used a drain for all our cases of PPPV PECFD. The drain was left in place to drain the blood and irrigation fluid for the first two postoperative days (Fig. **4F**).

## POTENTIAL RISKS

The potential risks of the procedure include wrong level surgery, excessive facet resection leading to cervical segmental instability, pedicle fracture, vertebral body fracture, vertebral artery injury with excessive drilling of the pedicle in a ventral and lateral direction, exiting nerve root injury (dysesthesia, motor, and sensory deficit), spinal cord injury, recurrence of stenosis, and the progression of degeneration leading to further deterioration of cervical myeloradiculopathy. However, from our evaluation of the technique in our cohort of patients, the complications listed are not common [10].

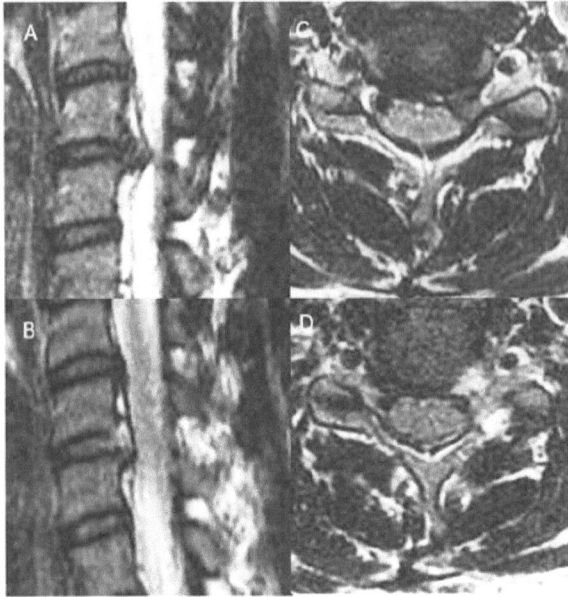

**Fig. (5). A and B:** Postoperative Sagittal MRI of the illustrative patient who had undergone left C6/7 PPPV PECFD. **C and D:** Pre and postoperative Axial MRI of the illustrative patient who had undergone left C6/7 PPPV PECFD. There was complete removal of prolapsed disc with partial pedicle and partial vertebra resected.

## POSTOPERATIVE AND REHABILITATION PROTOCOL

The patient can be prescribed with a soft Aspen collar for comfort and soft tissue recovery. They are mobilized the same day and can be discharged from the hospital when the drain is removed. The drain is typically removed on post-operative day one (Fig. **5**).

## CLINICAL SERIES

The authors employed the partial pediculolectomy and vertebrotomy technique to create space for the operating surgeon to decompress the prolapsed disc abutting the spinal cord and nerve root. The creation of subneural space ventral to the nerve root for safe retrieval rather than directly pulling the disc off the neural elements is the authors' preferred endoscopic technique. Traditional posterior cervical decompression technique carries the increased risk of dura tear and neurological deficit. In the authors' clinical series, partial vertebrotomy was employed to gain gain access to a more medial position. In addition, we found that we could readily retrieve prolapsed disc which had half the bulk of the disc material lateral to the thecal sac rather than 2/3 of the bulk of the disc. As we used endoscopic drill extensively and even underneath and ventral to the spinal cord and nerve root, we were able to treat calcified prolapsed disc by directly drilling on them. The neural elements were protected by the working cannula and the instruments were safely delivered through the working channel in the endoscope directly to the targeted calcified disc. With this technique, we could gain access to the disc without any spinal cord retraction and with less exiting nerve root retraction. Hence, we expected a decreased rate of neural injuries. In our clinical series, we found no complication and recurrence in our retrospective cohort of 36 levels of PPPV PECFD in 30 patients during the study period from January 2017 to December 2019. Preoperative, post-operative radiographic evaluation of stability, computer tomography evaluation of foraminal dimensions and area in sagittal view was performed. 3D reconstruction area of decompression evaluations were performed. Clinical outcomes of Visual Analog Scale (VAS), Oswestry Disability Index(ODI) and MacNab's score were evaluated. At preoperative, 1 week postoperative, and 3months postoperative and final follow up, the mean Visual Analog Scale had significant improvement with scores of 7.6, 3.0, 2.1, and 1.7, respectively (P<0.05). The mean Oswestry Disability Index with scores of 73.9, 28.1, 23.3, and 21.5, respectively (P<0.05). All patients achieved excellent and good Macnab outcomes. Radiological follow up studies showed PPPV PECFD had significant increase in decompression in the neuroforaminal volume corroborated by improvements in all CT measured parameters [10].

## DISCUSSION

Posterior cervical foraminotomy has the advantage of motion preservation compared to anterior cervical discectomy and fusion. It does not require any prosthetic implants, unlike the disc replacement. It is a good option for radiculopathy secondary to a prolapsed disc and foraminal stenosis. Conventional posterior cervical foraminotomy required significant soft tissue dissection from the midline incision. Tubular posterior cervical foraminotomy has the added advantage of working through a tube placed directly on the laminofacet junction. However, as the surgeon's vision is obtained from a microscope placed around 30-50cm away from the skin surface, the soft tissue in the line of vision needs to be dissected and sacrificed to perform the procedure. There is also considerable difficulty removing the prolapsed disc after foraminotomy as the instruments used in MIS tubular surgery are significantly large. At the same time, retraction is not possible for the spinal cord. Further confounded by the visualization around the disc is notoriously tricky due to the abundance of epidural vessels in the cervical disc region. Despite these difficulties, there is an improved hospital length of stay, blood loss and perioperative pain score in the tubular group of patients [5].

Endoscopic spine surgery is perhaps the least invasive form of surgery among minimally invasive spine surgery. The presence of an optical lens at the distal end of the endoscope coupled with irrigation and working channel addressed the shortcoming of tubular and open microscopic posterior cervical foraminotomy. However, there is a significant learning curve that exists for performing endoscopic spine surgery and, in particular, with PECFD. The operative proficiency is estimated to be 22 cases [13]. There is also a concern of insufficient decompression and residual disc protrusion, which could continue to cause compressive symptoms to the patients. A wider laminotomy and facetectomy would theoretically help in preventing residual compressive symptoms. However, there is a limit to cervical facet joint resection without causing instability. Raynor *et al.* found that when 70% of the facet was removed, fracture occurred in the anatomical specimen at 159 lb compressive load. In comparison, specimens which had 50% of the facet joint complex removed could withstand 208 lbs of axial load [14]. Therefore, we should preserve as many aspects as possible while we aimed to remove the prolapsed cervical disc. Hence, we further modified the traditional endoscopic cervical foraminotomy and discectomy by doing partial pediculotomy and partial vertebrotomy.

## TECHNICAL PEARLS

In the authors' opinion, there are the following surgical pearls of the procedures:

1. Preoperative evaluation should aim at better understanding the extent of medial superior pedicle and lateral superior vertebral body removal required to perform the discectomy safely. Partial vertebrotomy is indicated in patients where half of the bulk of herniated disc are located medial to lateral margin of thecal sac.
2. The "V" point should be clearly visualized under endoscopic vision and checked with intraoperative fluoroscopy to confirm its correct position at the desired surgical level.
3. The cephalad lamina and lateral mass should be carefully drilled with an endoscopic drill to expose the underlying medial aspect of the facet joint which we termed as bony " V" point.
4. Drilling should be limited to medial half of the pedicle hence to avoid a potential injury to the vertebra artery which lies ventral to lateral half of the pedicle in the transverse foramen.
5. The exiting nerve root should be identified by elevating and removing loose ligamentum flavum off it. The location and relationship of the exiting nerve root also defines to the medial pedicle may be used it as a key landmark and defines the extent of partial pediculotomy and partial vertebrotomy required to create the subneural space aimed at avoiding retraction.
6. The surgeon must not retract the spinal cord and limit the retraction of the exiting nerve root. If the need for greater mobilization of the exiting nerve root

is deemed necessary, the authors recommend more bone drilling to enlarge the subneural space rather than attempting to retract more.

7. Meticulous hemostasis should always be achieved with bipolar pulsed radiofrequency. The authors prefer placement of a drain to prevent postoperative wound hematoma or symptomatic collections of the irrigation fluid.

## CONCLUSIONS

Partial pediculotomy, partial vertebrotomy approach for posterior endoscopic cervical foraminotomy and discectomy is a technically challenging but rewarding surgery with potential benefits of less neural retraction. The authors conclude that it could be applied to more complex spinal pathologies, thus, expanding the clinical indications.

## CONSENT FOR PUBLICATION

Not applicable.

## CONFLICT OF INTEREST

The author declares no conflict of interest, financial or otherwise.

## ACKNOWLEDGEMENTS

Declared none.

## REFERENCES

[1]     Siivola SM, Levoska S, Tervonen O, Ilkko E, Vanharanta H, Keinänen-Kiukaanniemi S. MRI changes of cervical spine in asymptomatic and symptomatic young adults. European spine journal : official publication of the European Spine Society, the European Spinal Deformity Society, and the European Section of the Cervical Spine Research Society 2002; 11(4): 63-358.
        [http://dx.doi.org/10.1007/s00586-001-0370-x]

[2]     Kato S, Fehlings M. Degenerative cervical myelopathy. Curr Rev Musculoskelet Med 2016; 9(3): 263-71.
        [http://dx.doi.org/10.1007/s12178-016-9348-5] [PMID: 27250040]

[3]     Wong JJ, Côté P, Quesnele JJ, Stern PJ, Mior SA. The course and prognostic factors of symptomatic cervical disc herniation with radiculopathy: a systematic review of the literature. Spine J 2014; 14(8): 1781-9.
        [http://dx.doi.org/10.1016/j.spinee.2014.02.032] [PMID: 24614255]

[4]     Iyer S, Kim HJ. Cervical radiculopathy. Curr Rev Musculoskelet Med 2016; 9(3): 272-80.
        [http://dx.doi.org/10.1007/s12178-016-9349-4] [PMID: 27250042]

[5]     Hussain I, Schmidt FA, Kirnaz S, Wipplinger C, Schwartz TH, Härtl R. MIS approaches in the cervical spine. Journal of spine surgery (Hong Kong) 2019; 5(Suppl 1): S74-83.
        [http://dx.doi.org/10.21037/jss.2019.04.21]

[6]     Skovrlj B, Gologorsky Y, Haque R, Fessler RG, Qureshi SA. Complications, outcomes, and need for

fusion after minimally invasive posterior cervical foraminotomy and microdiscectomy. Spine J 2014; 14(10): 2405-11.
[http://dx.doi.org/10.1016/j.spinee.2014.01.048] [PMID: 24486472]

[7]     Adamson TE. Microendoscopic posterior cervical laminoforaminotomy for unilateral radiculopathy: results of a new technique in 100 cases. J Neurosurg 2001; 95(1) (Suppl.): 51-7.
[PMID: 11453432]

[8]     Wu PH, Kim HS, Jang I-T. A Narrative Review of Development of Full-Endoscopic Lumbar Spine Surgery. Neurospine 2020; 17 (Suppl. 1): S20-33.
[http://dx.doi.org/10.14245/ns.2040116.058] [PMID: 32746515]

[9]     Quillo-Olvera J, Lin GX, Kim JS. Percutaneous endoscopic cervical discectomy: a technical review. Ann Transl Med 2018; 6(6): 100.
[http://dx.doi.org/10.21037/atm.2018.02.09] [PMID: 29707549]

[10]    Kim HS, Wu PH, Lee YJ, *et al.* Safe route for cervical approach: partial pediculotomy, partial vertebrotomy approach for posterior endoscopic cervical foraminotomy and discectomy. World Neurosurg 2020; 140: e273-82.
[http://dx.doi.org/10.1016/j.wneu.2020.05.033]

[11]    Kim HS, Wu PH, Jang I-T. Development of endoscopic spine surgery for healthy life: to provide spine care for better, for worse, for richer, for poorer, in sickness and in health. Neurospine 2020; 17 (Suppl. 1): S3-8.
[http://dx.doi.org/10.14245/ns.2040188.094] [PMID: 32746510]

[12]    Quillo-Olvera J, Lin G-X, Kim J-S. Percutaneous endoscopic cervical discectomy: a technical review. Ann Transl Med 2018; 6(6): 100.
[http://dx.doi.org/10.21037/atm.2018.02.09] [PMID: 29707549]

[13]    Zhang C, Wu J, Zheng W, Li C, Zhou Y. Posterior endoscopic cervical decompression: review and technical note. Neurospine 2020; 17 (Suppl. 1): S74-80.
[http://dx.doi.org/10.14245/ns.2040166.083] [PMID: 32746520]

[14]    Raynor RB, Pugh J, Shapiro I. Cervical facetectomy and its effect on spine strength. J Neurosurg 1985; 63(2): 278-82.
[http://dx.doi.org/10.3171/jns.1985.63.2.0278] [PMID: 4020449]

# CHAPTER 12

# Full Endoscopic Anterior Cervical Decompression & Fusion With Iliac Crest Dowel Graft

**Stefan Hellinger**[1,*]

[1] *Department of Orthopedic and Spine Surgery, Arabellaklinik, Munich, Germany*

**Abstract:** Isolated discogenic cervical pain syndromes are somewhat difficult to treat. Many of these patients have underlying painful degenerative conditions of the cervical spine that do not meet accepted criteria for surgical treatments. Hence, many of these patients remain untreated or undergo interventional pain management procedures to meliorate the pain. The author presents a simple endoscopic outpatient method intended to treat a small subsection of this patient population complaining of isolated neck pain without any arm pain. Often these patients have end-stage degenerative cervical disc disease with near complete collapse with minimal associated foraminal stenosis. The author presents an endoscopic interbody fusion technique he has developed for these types for patients using an autograft bone dowel harvested from the iliac crest.

**Keywords:** Autograft, Cervical spine, Degenerative disc disease, Discogenic pain, Dowel graft, Endoscopic, Iliac crest graft, Minimally invasive, Outpatient surgery, Percutaneous.

## INTRODUCTION

The incidence of cervical discogenic pain symptoms in the general population is high [1 - 7]. In Germany, insurance claims analysis estimated that one in five patients visit their orthopedic surgeon for symptomatic cervical disc syndromes [8]. The treatment of cervical discogenic diseases makes high is challenging both in terms of diagnostic work-up and treatment [9]. Advances in medical imaging and neurological testing have enhanced the diagnostic accuracy in identifying those patients with isolated discogenic neck pain without cervical radiculopathy [10 - 15]. Typically, patients with isolated discogenic neck pain without neurological symptoms are initially denied effective surgical treatments since the

---

[*] **Corresponding author Stefan Hellinger:** Department of Orthopedic and Spine Surgery, Arabellaklinik, Munich, Germany; E-mail: hellinger@gmx.de

**Kai-Uwe Lewandrowski, Jorge Felipe Ramírez León, Anthony Yeung, Hyeun-Sung Kim, Xifeng Zhang, Gun Choi, Stefan Hellinger and Álvaro Dowling (Eds.)**

literature on beneficial therapies is not as favorable as for cervical disc herniations causing radiculopathy or spinal cord dysfunction [6].

The most common cause of cervical pain syndromes is a degenerative change in the intervertebral disc. The disease may be accompanied by painful displacement of disc tissue causing mechanical compression, inflammation, and vascular compromise of neural structures [1, 16, 17]. A myriad of well-understood symptoms may arise: a) pain in the neck and head region, b) radiating into the arms, and hands, and at its worst cervical myelopathy [16]. More subtle causes of neck pain stemming from the cervical intervertebral disc may relate to tears in the dorsal annulus fibrosus. Additional sources of cervical pain may arise from the vertebral bodies, the periosteum, joint- and ligament complexes both in the anterior and posterior columns [1]. Thankfully, over 80 percent of patients with these symptoms experience spontaneous resolution with supportive medical and interventional care measures including physical therapy, non-steroidal anti-inflammatories, spinal injections, acupuncture, massage- or chiropractic care, and activity modification [18, 19].

In this chapter, the author attempted to highlight a full endoscopic technique of performing an anterior cervical decompression fusion with an iliac crest bone dowel intended to treat those patients with failed conservative therapies and a conclusive diagnostic work-up for isolated cervical discogenic pain. The concept of using the full-endoscopic technique is based both on reducing the burden associated with more traditional cervical disc surgery, and by offering a more simplified method of treating the condition in an ambulatory surgery setting to reduce operation related morbidity, and cost.

## HISTORICAL CONSIDERATIONS

The development of surgical procedures for intervertebral disc treatment began in 1908 with the transdural removal of disc tissue with the aid of laminectomy by Oppenheimer and Krause. Extradural extirpation of a herniated disc proposed by Mixter and Barr in 1934 [20]. Stookey began looking at cervical intervertebral disc displacements [21]. The intervention was developed on the lumbar spine, progressing from laminectomy to hemilaminectomy, and then to fenestrotomy and finally endoscopy (Hijikata 1989) [22]. The first operation on the cervical spine was performed by Elsberg in 1922, also transdurally [23]. As of 1958, anterior approaches were introduced by Cloward [24], Smith, and Robinson [25], and these are still standard procedures in the surgical treatment of cervical pathologies. Ultimately, these decompression techniques have been combined with the fusion of the segment by a bone graft.

While time-proven, anterior cervical discectomy and fusion (ACDF) continues to be plagued by the problems of access morbidity such as injury to the recurrent laryngeal nerve (RLN) or swallowing problems [26]. Apfelbaum reported RLN lesions between 11%-15% [27]. The desire to reduce access-related morbidity prompted the application of alternative treatments such as the posterior cervical foraminotomy. In revisiting the past, surgeons with a preference for the anterior approach ask whether cervical interbody fusion is necessary? Cervical artificial disc replacement has been offered as an alternative with the intent of reducing reoperation rates for adjacent segment disease by preserving motion [28 - 33]. However, this procedure suffers from similar access related problems. Dating back to 1960, Hirsch *et al.* reported his results with anterior cervical discectomy without fusion or an implant [34]. Cervical chemonucleolysis was introduced by Smith in 1964 [35]. Similarly, automated discectomy (Onik 1985) [36], percutaneous laser disc decompression, and nucleotomy [37] and the use of radiofrequency (Coblation 2003) [38] added to the spectrum of percutaneous cervical surgeries. Many studies reported clinical outcomes comparable to fusion [39]. Additional studies corroborated these results by offering limited disc removal in favor of a more targeted and selective procedure [40, 41].

## THE OBJECTIVE

The aim is to miniaturize the anterior cervical surgery further. Non-endoscopic percutaneous procedures were previously used in select patients with excellent results and a complication rate of less than 1 percent (Hellinger 2004) [42, 43]. Incorporation of endoscopy into the percutaneous techniques was for the author a natural progression of his development strategies for simplified, less burdensome ambulatory anterior cervical surgeries. Pioneers of the endoscopy of the cervical spine were Lee [44 - 46], Chiu [37, 47], and Fontanella [48]. These authors reported their outcomes with their minimal access anterior cervical surgery in the early 1990ies, which hinged about leaving a large proportion of the intervertebral disc, in particular, most of the annulus fibrosus preserved. Removing only the painful pathology selectively in the area of the nucleus pulposus and on the dorsal fibrous ring were symptomatic neural element compression occurred was recommended by these authors and others [49, 50]. They stipulated that the remaining disc tissue preserved some biomechanical function of the degenerated intervertebral disc. Adding the video-endoscopy to these techniques was an easy-to-implement modification not only because of improved visualization but also because of the ability to ablate and shrink diseased tissue with the use of a laser [51]. Consequently, the risk of complications was further reduced while enhancing the efficiency of the treatment, thereby making it suitable for an ambulatory surgery setting. Additional advancements of the endoscopic technique and available instruments increased miniaturization of the cervical endoscopic surgery.

This author's primary objective was to create adequate working space in front of the endoscope while preserving the minimally invasive nature of the approach and minimizing the necessary dissection in the prevertebral cervical compartment. The author employed serial dilation sheaths placing them and thee endoscopic working cannula between the superior and inferior endplate with slight force, thus distracting them and creating a working field of 5 mm or 6 mm providing sufficient visualization and expose of the ventral epidural space. Applying swiveling motion helps to maneuver the endoscope in front of the intervertebral disc by sweeping the prevertebral tissues away – a technique that was advocated by Chiu *et al.* [52 - 54]. Advancing the working cannula into the intervertebral disc space enables the surgeon to perform partial in the painful area and expose and remove portions of the uncovertebral joint deemed necessary under constant irrigation to remove the ablated disc material out of the field of view and to maintain hemostasis. In patients with advanced end-stage cervical degenerative disc disease attempting to preserve cervical motion may be an inappropriate goal. Additional fusion may be necessary for patients with instability or deformity to treat the painful pathology adequately.

## SURGICAL CONCEPTS

The surgical procedure advocated by the authors is based on encouraging outcomes report by Lee *et al.* with the implantation of the WSH Cervical B-Twin as a standalone cervical spacer [55]. Based on these encouraging results with a modern version of the standalone cervical fusion, the author decided to modify the original Cloward procedure for the endoscopic application of a cylindrical iliac crest bone graft. The stipulation was that the introduction of an iliac crest dowel graft between the endplates of a diseased cervical motion segment would facilitate an osseous fusion and induce resorption of uncovertebral spurs originally described by Cloward [24]. The author began this type of full endoscopic anterior cervical decompression and fusion surgery in March of 2006. The first case was a 50-year old female with neck pain, headaches, and left arm pain (VAS score 8) due to end-stage degenerative cervical disc disease with near complete collapse. Preoperative plain films showed mild spondylosis at the symptomatic C4/5 level with listhesis on the dynamic/extension flexion views. The sagittal MRI confirm a left-sided extruded disc herniation. This case is used for an exemplary illustration of the endoscopic technique (Figs. **1** - **4**).

## PROCEDURTAL STEPS

The patient is positioned in a prone position and placed under monitored anesthesia care consisting of a combination of local anesthesia and sedation. The patient's airway was maintained with a laryngeal mask airway (LMA). After standard surgical prepping and draping, the tentative skin incision and entry point for the surgical intervertebral disc level were marked using intraoperative fluoroscopy in the anterior-posterior (AP) and the lateral (LAT) projection (Figs. **5** and **6**). Then, an approximately 5-mm skin incision is made approaching the disc herniation from the opposite side by entering medial to the sternocleidomastoid muscle. The platysma is exposed and traversed by splitting its fibers. The tracheoesophageal groove is used to create a surgical access corridor with blunt dissection facilitating lateral retraction of the carotid sheath. Care should be taken to mobilize the artery and the jugular vein sufficiently to allow for medial retraction of the larynx, trachea, esophagus, and thyroid gland (if visible in the surgical field). The surgeon's index and middle finger are used to apply pressure to the cervical spine's anterior surface, thereby further facilitating dissection of the tracheoesophageal groove. Under frequent fluoroscopic control, an 18G spinal needle is inserted into the intervertebral disc, preferably in its mid-portion *via* the skin incision. The needle's position is checked in the AP and LAT planes several times with the C-arm in the sterile field to verify its appropriate location at the surgical level. Then, a metal guidewire may be placed into the cervical disc, and the spinal needle is withdrawn.

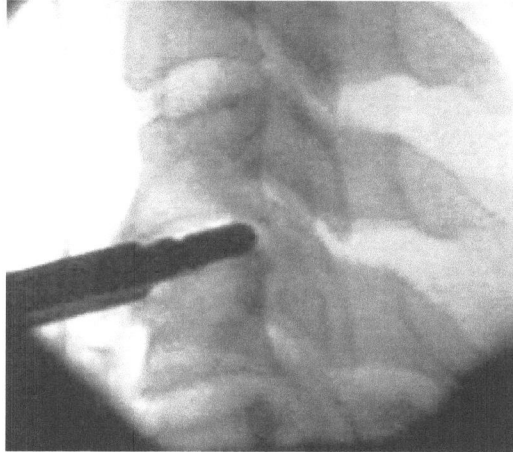

**Fig. (1).** Intraoperative fluoroscopic LAT view during of the endoscopic preparation of the endplates with a power burr at the C4/5 level.

Then, over the guidewire, various obturators can be placed on the intervertebral disc. After the final dilator's placement, a 6,5 mm working cannula is inserted into the intervertebral disc by advancing it beyond anterior annulus. The author prefers a particular sleeve with two narrow lips, which facilitates positioning the working sleeve by tapping it through the anterior fibrous annular ring with a small lightweight hammer under constant rotating motion until its final position between the rostral and distal cervical endplates. The resultant distraction establishes a working space. The working sleeve can now be directed further into the disk space towards the painful pathology. The nuclear decompression procedure is facilitated by using a shaver. A trephine may be useful for the bony uncovertebral decompression if necessary (Fig. **2**). Under direct and continuous endoscopic visualization, the intervertebral disc can be curetted in a wide channel as far as the posterior annular ring. The painful pathological region should be targeted using medial to lateral attack angles previously determined on the advanced preoperative imaging studies. The mechanical discectomy with shavers, trephines, and pituitaries may be followed by a laser-ablation of the prolapsed disc tissue that escaped the prior decompression attempts. When so doing, the working area can be extended as far as the uncovertebral joints are deemed necessary by the operating surgeon by swiveling the endoscope side-to-side until the axillary decompression of the exiting nerve root is adequate. Sometimes, the posterior longitudinal ligament may have to be incised to excise herniated disc fragments trapped between the superficial and deep layers of this ligament. Endoscopic forceps can be used to carefully open the posterior spinal ligament to then finally expose the epidural space.

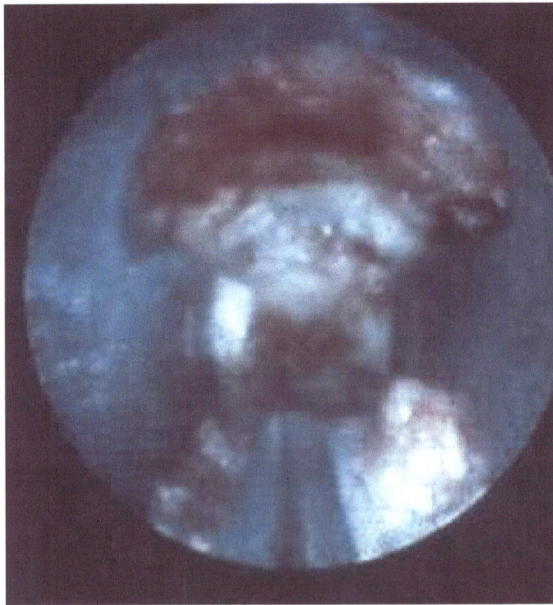

**Fig. (2).**  Endoscopic view of the intervertebral space after endoscopic preparation and control of the uncovertebral decompression with an endoscopic nerve hook.

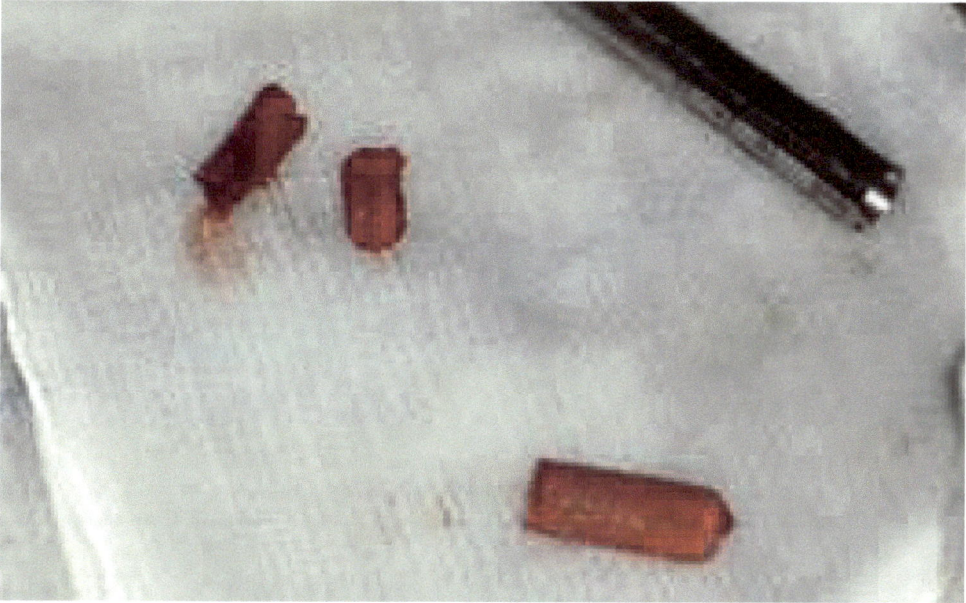

**Fig. (3).** The bone graft is harvested from the iliac crest and fashioned into a compressed cylinder of 6-mm diameter and applied through the endoscopic working cannula in conjunction with an osteoinductive material (Coloss®) to facilitate the uninstrumented cervical interbody fusion.

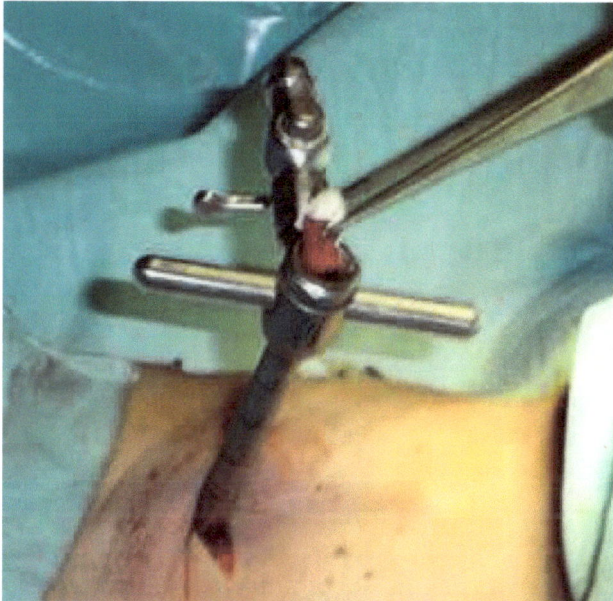

**Fig. (4).** Percutaneous position of the endoscopic cervical working cannula in the C4/5 intervertebral disc space. The cylindrical bone graft dowel is inserted though the working cannula and then impacted under visualization into the intervertebral disc space.

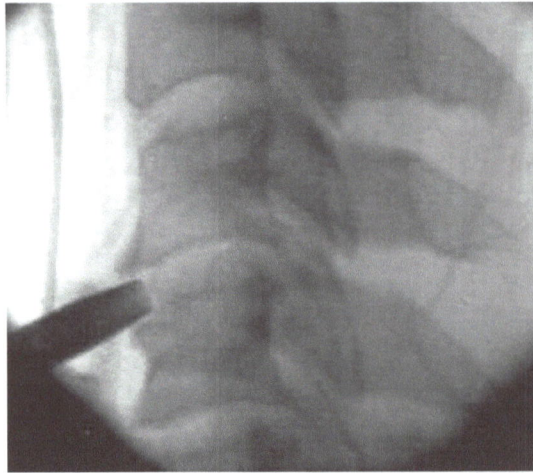

**Fig. (5).** Intraoperative LAT fluoroscopic view showing the endoscopic working cannula placed in between the prepared endplates with the autologous cylindrical dowel craft placed all the way to the posterior annulus and recessed just below the anterior ring appophysis.

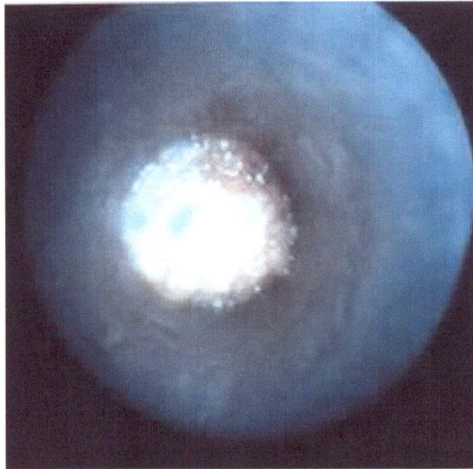

**Fig. (6).** Intraoperative endoscopic view to control the position of the autograft bone cylinder.

Similarly, small osteophytes can be decompressed under fluoroscopic guidance using a ring curette. In select cases and depending on surgeon skill level and preference, it may be appropriate to employ a gas medium at this stage of the operation to facilitate visualization and hemostasis rather than irrigation fluid. The use of the gas medium renders endoscopic images similar to those obtained with microscopy and may be more familiar to the inexperienced endoscopic spine surgeon. At the end of the operation, a final check of the decompression should be carried out. A long endoscopic nerve hook may be useful when passing it out laterally into the decompressed axilla of the exiting nerve root. After adequate decompression has been achieved, the rostral and caudal endplates need to be decorticated, and the graft bed for the round iliac crest dowel has to be prepared. The author's preference is to do that with different mechanical burrs, ideally placing the dowel in the midline.

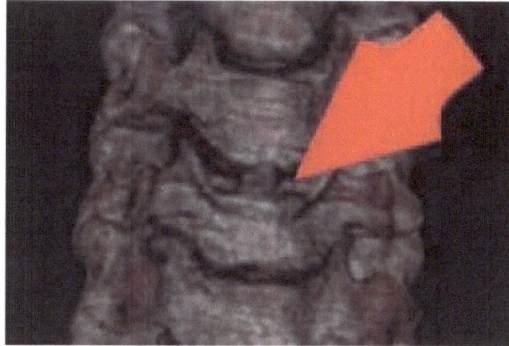

**Fig. (7).** Postoperative three-dimensional computed tomography (CT) scan with a coronal view of the fusion showing the autologous cylindrical bone graft dowel in optimum position in the midline with evidence of good distraction between the rostral and caudal endplate.

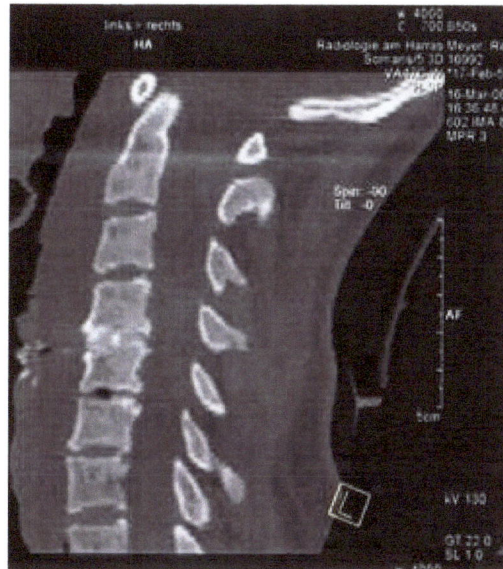

**Fig. (8).** One-year postoperative sagittal CT scan showing the dowel bone graft in maintained position without resorption and near complete osseous fusion at the C4/5 level.

The bone graft is harvested from the iliac crest with a special gauge to create a compressed spongeous cylinder of 6-mm diameter in the checked measured intraoperatively through the endoscopic working channel with a depth gauge (Fig. 3). An osteoinductive material (Coloss®) was used as an adjunct to the autograft dowel fashioned from the iliac crest bone graft. Both autograft and the adjunct were placed in the intervertebral bed through the working cannula under direct endoscopic visualization and frequent fluoroscopic control employing various pushers during the deployment of the bone graft and its advancement into its final position. The graft site was then once more inspected endoscopically and checked for its position of the graft and hemostasis. The endoscopic working sleeve was then removed, slowing also examining the tissues and content of the tracheoesophageal groove for any source of bleeding. After wound closure, a band-aid was applied. The awake patient is then transported to the recovery room from which he or she is typically discharged to their home within an hour of uneventful observation and recovery from anesthesia with a soft cervical collar. Discharge criteria include that the patient is comfortable, has no signs of neurological compromise or deficits, has a stable airway, and can walk independently. Before discharge, the wound is checked one more time for wound hematoma, which suggests a bleeding source that could require prompt surgical reexploration.

Furthermore, the patients' ability to swallow liquid and simple solid foods and the status of the voice are checked and documented before letting the patient leave the ambulatory surgery center. This author recommends that each surgeon implement protocols and establish transfer agreements to nearby local hospitals should any of these problems be found in the patients who underwent the full endoscopic anterior cervical discectomy and autograft fusion surgery described herein. In the example patient referenced earlier in this chapter, in the recovery room, the pain was diminished to VAS 1 concerning her neck pain, and the arm pain denied any arm pain. The postoperative CT scans and X-rays show an optimum positioning of the bone dowel with good distraction of the interspace, which can facilitate the indirect decompression of compromised cervical nerve roots (Figs. **7** and **8**).

## DISCUSSION

A full-endoscopic fusion of the cervical spine with an iliac crest bone dowel is technically feasible with contemporary spinal endoscopes and instruments adopted and modified for the cervical spine. Conceptionally, the technique is comparable to the classic Cloward procedure. However, the authors stipulate that the full endoscopic approach to perform the procedure with a 6.5 mm dowel diminishes the incidence of approach-related complications – a hypothesis the author is currently investigating. This author also recognizes the need further to research the best clinical indication for the procedure and delineate the inclusion- and exclusion criteria for the procedure better. Clearly, it entails less surgical trauma, and considerably reduces surgery-related stress for the patient, while also shortening the period of hospitalization.

Further, the limitations of the procedure will need to be better understood. The author proposes structured prospective and randomized clinical trials comparing the full endoscopic anterior cervical decompression and fusion to those obtained with the traditional open ACDF as a control. There is no question, though, that the full endoscopic version of the procedure has greater appeal to patients and is more conducive to being done in an outpatient surgery setting, such as an ambulatory surgery center, where patient satisfaction is typically higher, and cost savings can be realized.

## CONCLUSION

Full endoscopic anterior cervical decompression and fusion may be indicated in patients with the majority of symptoms revolving around axial discogenic neck pain and minimal radiculopathy. The low-burden nature makes it attractive to surgeons and patients searching for simplified outpatient procedures to treat common degenerative conditions of the cervical spine. Although this minimally invasive cervical fusion negates the use of contemporary implants which have been proven over time to improve outcomes and the reliability of the procedure, it may be appropriate for select patients with end-stage degenerative cervical disc disease where the bony fusion of the painful motion segment eliminates the discogenic pain and any radicular component by resorption of any uncovertebral osteophytes in the process. Although the author's feasibility study is encouraging, such claims cannot be made until further substantiated by relevant clinical research.

## CONSENT FOR PUBLICATION

Not applicable.

## CONFLICT OF INTEREST

The author declares no conflict of interest, financial or otherwise.

## ACKNOWLEDGEMENTS

Declared none.

## REFERENCES

[1]     Moskovich R. Neck pain in the elderly: common causes and management. Geriatrics 1988; 43(4): 65-70.

[2]     Bogduk N. The anatomical basis for spinal pain syndromes. J Manipulative Physiol Ther 1995; 18(9): 603-5.
        [PMID: 8775022]

[3]     Senter BS. Cervical discogenic syndrome: a cause of chronic head and neck pain. J Miss State Med

Assoc 1995; 36(8): 231-4.
[PMID: 7473695]

[4]     Schellhas KP, Smith MD, Gundry CR, Pollei SR. Cervical discogenic pain. Prospective correlation of magnetic resonance imaging and discography in asymptomatic subjects and pain sufferers. Spine 1996; 21(3): 300-11.
[http://dx.doi.org/10.1097/00007632-199602010-00009] [PMID: 8742205]

[5]     Peng B, DePalma MJ. Cervical disc degeneration and neck pain. J Pain Res 2018; 11: 2853-7.
[http://dx.doi.org/10.2147/JPR.S180018] [PMID: 30532580]

[6]     Eloqayli H. Cervical discogenic pain treatment with percutaneous jellified ethanol: preliminary experience. BioMed Res Int 2019; 2019: 2193436.
[http://dx.doi.org/10.1155/2019/2193436] [PMID: 31001552]

[7]     Saini A, Mukhdomi T. Cervical Discogenic Syndrome. Treasure Island, FL: StatPearls 2020.

[8]     Füssel S, Janka M, Schuh A. Chronisches hws-syndrom, was lässt sich wie konservativ behandeln? 2014; 156(10).

[9]     Motimaya A, Arici M, George D, Ramsby G. Diagnostic value of cervical discography in the management of cervical discogenic pain. Conn Med 2000; 64(7): 395-8.
[PMID: 10946476]

[10]    Harada GK, Tao Y, Louie PK, et al. Cervical spine MRI phenotypes and prediction of pain, disability and adjacent segment degeneration/disease after ACDF. J Orthop Res 2021; 39(3): 657-70.
[http://dx.doi.org/10.1002/jor.24658] [PMID: 32159238]

[11]    Jensen RK, Jensen TS, Grøn S, et al. Prevalence of MRI findings in the cervical spine in patients with persistent neck pain based on quantification of narrative MRI reports. Chiropr Man Therap 2019; 27: 13.
[http://dx.doi.org/10.1186/s12998-019-0233-3] [PMID: 30873276]

[12]    Daimon K, Fujiwara H, Nishiwaki Y, et al. A 20-year prospective longitudinal MRI study on cervical spine after whiplash injury: Follow-up of a cross-sectional study. J Orthop Sci 2019; 24(4): 579-83.
[http://dx.doi.org/10.1016/j.jos.2018.11.011] [PMID: 30553607]

[13]    Suleiman LI, Weber KA II, Rosenthal BD, et al. High-resolution magnetization transfer MRI in patients with cervical spondylotic myelopathy. J Clin Neurosci 2018; 51: 57-61.
[http://dx.doi.org/10.1016/j.jocn.2018.02.023] [PMID: 29530383]

[14]    Okada E, Daimon K, Fujiwara H, et al. Twenty-year Longitudinal Follow-up MRI Study of Asymptomatic Volunteers: The Impact of Cervical Alignment on Disk Degeneration. Clin Spine Surg 2018; 31(10): 446-51.
[http://dx.doi.org/10.1097/BSD.0000000000000706] [PMID: 30102637]

[15]    Moll LT, Kindt MW, Stapelfeldt CM, Jensen TS. Degenerative findings on MRI of the cervical spine: an inter- and intra-rater reliability study. Chiropr Man Therap 2018; 26: 43.
[http://dx.doi.org/10.1186/s12998-018-0210-2] [PMID: 30356854]

[16]    Geissinger JD, Davis FM. Cervical disc disease and other causes of upper extremity pain. J Fla Med Assoc 1976; 63(11): 872-5.
[PMID: 1003155]

[17]    Idelberger K. Shoulder pain and shoulder stiffness: causes, differential diagnosis and therapy. MMW Munch Med Wochenschr 1975; 117(10): 373-82.
[PMID: 804599]

[18]    Cvetanovich GL, Hsu AR, Frank RM, An HS, Andersson GB. Spontaneous resorption of a large cervical herniated nucleus pulposus. Am J Orthop 2014; 43(7): E140-5.
[PMID: 25046190]

[19]    Gautschi OP, Stienen MN, Schaller K. Spontaneous regression of lumbar and cervical disc herniations

- a well established phenomenon. Praxis (Bern 1994) 2013; 102(11): 80-675.

[20] Mixter W, Barr J. Rupture of the Intervertebral Disc with Involvement of the Spinal N Engl. J Med 1934; 211: 210-5.

[21] B S. Compression of the spinal cord due to ventral extradural cervical chondromas. Arch Neurol Psychiatry 1928; 20: 275-8.
[http://dx.doi.org/10.1001/archneurpsyc.1928.02210140043003]

[22] Hijikata S. Percutaneous nucleotomy. A new concept technique and 12 years' experience. Clin Orthop Relat Res 1989; (238): 9-23.
[http://dx.doi.org/10.1097/00003086-198901000-00003] [PMID: 2910622]

[23] Elsberg C. Tumors of the spinal cord and the symptoms of irritation and compression of the spinal cord and nerve roots: pathology, symptomatology, diagnosis and treatment. New York: Paul B Hoeber 1922.

[24] Cloward RB. The anterior approach for removal of ruptured cervical disks. J Neurosurg 1958; 15(6): 602-17.
[http://dx.doi.org/10.3171/jns.1958.15.6.0602] [PMID: 13599052]

[25] Smith GW, Robinson RA. The treatment of certain cervical-spine disorders by anterior removal of the intervertebral disc and interbody fusion. J Bone Joint Surg Am 1958; 40-A(3): 607-24.
[http://dx.doi.org/10.2106/00004623-195840030-00009] [PMID: 13539086]

[26] Epstein NE. A Review of Complication Rates for Anterior Cervical Diskectomy and Fusion (ACDF). Surg Neurol Int 2019; 10: 100.
[http://dx.doi.org/10.25259/SNI-191-2019] [PMID: 31528438]

[27] Apfelbaum RI, Kriskovich MD, Haller JR. On the incidence, cause, and prevention of recurrent laryngeal nerve palsies during anterior cervical spine surgery. Spine 2000; 25(22): 2906-12.
[http://dx.doi.org/10.1097/00007632-200011150-00012] [PMID: 11074678]

[28] Zheng B, Hao D, Guo H, He B. ACDF *vs* TDR for patients with cervical spondylosis - an 8 year follow up study. BMC Surg 2017; 17(1): 113.
[http://dx.doi.org/10.1186/s12893-017-0316-9] [PMID: 29183306]

[29] Laxer EB, Brigham CD, Darden BV, *et al.* Adjacent segment degeneration following ProDisc-C total disc replacement (TDR) and anterior cervical discectomy and fusion (ACDF): does surgeon bias effect radiographic interpretation? Eur Spine J 2017; 26(4): 1199-204.
[http://dx.doi.org/10.1007/s00586-016-4780-1] [PMID: 27650387]

[30] Yang Y, Ma L, Liu H, *et al.* Comparison of the incidence of patient-reported post-operative dysphagia between ACDF with a traditional anterior plate and artificial cervical disc replacement. Clin Neurol Neurosurg 2016; 148: 72-8.
[http://dx.doi.org/10.1016/j.clineuro.2016.07.020] [PMID: 27428486]

[31] Sasso R. Cervical arthroplasty compares favourably to ACDF at half-decade follow-up. Evid Based Med 2016; 21(1): 15.
[http://dx.doi.org/10.1136/ebmed-2015-110239] [PMID: 26537354]

[32] Kang L, Lin D, Ding Z, Liang B, Lian K. Artificial disk replacement combined with midlevel ACDF *versus* multilevel fusion for cervical disk disease involving 3 levels. Orthopedics 2013; 36(1): e88-94.
[http://dx.doi.org/10.3928/01477447-20121217-24] [PMID: 23276359]

[33] Gao Y, Liu M, Li T, Huang F, Tang T, Xiang Z. A meta-analysis comparing the results of cervical disc arthroplasty with anterior cervical discectomy and fusion (ACDF) for the treatment of symptomatic cervical disc disease. J Bone Joint Surg Am 2013; 95(6): 555-61.
[http://dx.doi.org/10.2106/JBJS.K.00599] [PMID: 23515991]

[34] Hirsch C. Cervical disk rupture: diagnosis and therapy. Acta Orthop 1960; 30: 172-86.
[http://dx.doi.org/10.3109/17453676109149538]

[35]   Smith L. Enzyme dissolution of the nucleus pulposus in humans. JAMA 1964; 187: 137-40.
[http://dx.doi.org/10.1001/jama.1964.03060150061016]

[36]   Onik G, Helms C, Ginsburb L. Percutaneous lumbar discectomy using a new aspiration probe 1985; 144: 3-290.

[37]   Choy DS, Hellinger J, Tassi GP, Hellinger S. Percutaneous laser disc decompression. Photomed Laser Surg 2007; 25(1): 60.
[PMID: 17352640]

[38]   Hellinger J, Stern S, Hellinger S. Nonendoscopic Nd-YAG 1064 nm PLDN in the treatment of thoracic discogenic pain syndromes. J Clin Laser Med Surg 2003; 21(2): 61-6.
[http://dx.doi.org/10.1089/104454703765035475] [PMID: 12737645]

[39]   Grisoli F, Graziani N, Fabrizi AP, Peragut JC, Vincentelli F, Diaz-Vasquez P. Anterior discectomy without fusion for treatment of cervical lateral soft disc extrusion: a follow-up of 120 cases. Neurosurgery 1989; 24(6): 853-9.
[http://dx.doi.org/10.1227/00006123-198906000-00010] [PMID: 2747859]

[40]   Savitz MH. Anterior cervical discectomy without fusion or instrumentation: 25 years' experience. Mt Sinai J Med 2000; 67(4): 314-7.
[PMID: 11021782]

[41]   Sheth JH, Patankar AP, Shah R. Anterior cervical microdiscectomy: is bone grafting and in-situ fusion with instrumentation required? Br J Neurosurg 2012; 26(1): 12-5.
[http://dx.doi.org/10.3109/02688697.2011.591854] [PMID: 21767123]

[42]   Hellinger J. Technical aspects of the percutaneous cervical and lumbar laser-disc-decompression and -nucleotomy. Neurol Res 1999; 21(1): 99-102.
[http://dx.doi.org/10.1080/01616412.1999.11740902] [PMID: 10048065]

[43]   Hellinger J. Complications of non-endoscopic percutaneous laser disc decompression and nucleotomy with the neodymium: YAG laser 1064 nm. Photomed Laser Surg 2004; 22(5): 418-22.
[http://dx.doi.org/10.1089/pho.2004.22.418] [PMID: 15671715]

[44]   Ahn Y, Lee SH, Lee SC, Shin SW, Chung SE. Factors predicting excellent outcome of percutaneous cervical discectomy: analysis of 111 consecutive cases. Neuroradiology 2004; 46(5): 378-84.
[http://dx.doi.org/10.1007/s00234-004-1197-z] [PMID: 15103434]

[45]   Ahn Y, Lee SH, Shin SW. Percutaneous endoscopic cervical discectomy: clinical outcome and radiographic changes. Photomed Laser Surg 2005; 23(4): 362-8.
[http://dx.doi.org/10.1089/pho.2005.23.362] [PMID: 16144477]

[46]   Lee SH, Ahn Y, Lee JH. Laser-assisted anterior cervical corpectomy *versus* posterior laminoplasty for cervical myelopathic patients with multilevel ossification of the posterior longitudinal ligament. Photomed Laser Surg 2008; 26(2): 119-27.
[http://dx.doi.org/10.1089/pho.2007.2110] [PMID: 18341415]

[47]   Choy DS, Hellinger J, Hellinger S, Tassi GP, Lee SH. 23rd Anniversary of Percutaneous Laser Disc Decompression (PLDD). Photomed Laser Surg 2009; 27(4): 535-8.
[http://dx.doi.org/10.1089/pho.2009.2512] [PMID: 19416003]

[48]   Fontanella A. Endoscopic microsurgery in herniated cervical discs. Neurol Res 1999; 21(1): 31-8.
[http://dx.doi.org/10.1080/01616412.1999.11740888] [PMID: 10048051]

[49]   Knight MT, Goswami A, Patko JT. Comparative outcome of Holmium: YAG and KTP laser disc ablation in degenerative cervical disc disease: results of an ongoing study. Ortop Traumatol Rehabil 2000; 2(2): 39-43.
[PMID: 18034117]

[50]   Knight MT, Goswami A, Patko JT. Cervical percutaneous laser disc decompression: preliminary results of an ongoing prospective outcome study. J Clin Laser Med Surg 2001; 19(1): 3-8.

[http://dx.doi.org/10.1089/104454701750066875] [PMID: 11547816]

[51]  Lee SH, Kang HS. Percutaneous endoscopic laser annuloplasty for discogenic low back pain. World Neurosurg 2010; 73(3): 198-206.
[http://dx.doi.org/10.1016/j.surneu.2009.01.023] [PMID: 20860958]

[52]  Chiu JC, Hansraj KK, Akiyama C, Greenspan M. Percutaneous (endoscopic) decompression discectomy for non-extruded cervical herniated nucleus pulposus. Surg Technol Int 1997; 6: 405-11.
[PMID: 16161004]

[53]  Chiu JC, Clifford TJ, Greenspan M, Richley RC, Lohman G, Sison RB. Percutaneous microdecompressive endoscopic cervical discectomy with laser thermodiskoplasty. Mt Sinai J Med 2000; 67(4): 278-82.
[PMID: 11021777]

[54]  Chiu JC. Endoscopic assisted microdecompression of cervical disc and foramen. Surg Technol Int 2008; 17: 269-79.
[PMID: 18802913]

[55]  Lee SH, Lee JH, Choi WC, Jung B, Mehta R. Anterior minimally invasive approaches for the cervical spine. Orthop Clin North Am 2007; 38(3): 327-37.
[http://dx.doi.org/10.1016/j.ocl.2007.02.007] [PMID: 17629981]

CHAPTER 13

# Percutaneous Endoscopically Assisted Cervical Facet Reduction

**Xifeng Zhang[1], Zhu Zexing[1]** and **Jiang Hongzhen[2,*]**

[1] *Department of Orthopedics, First Medical Center, PLA General Hospital, Beijing 100853, China*

[2] *Minimally Invasive Spinal Surgery, Beijing Yuhe Integrated Traditional Chinese and Western Medicine Rehabilitation Hospital, Beijing 100853, China*

**Abstract:** The authors describe the percutaneous endoscopic release of jumped and locked cervical facet joints under direct visualization as an alternative technique to open posterior decompression and reduction under capital traction. Instead of under general anesthesia, the procedure can be done under local anesthesia allowing the surgeon to communicate verbally with the injured patient while directly visualizing the decompression, release, and spontaneous reduction of the locked facet, thus, lowering the risk of unrecognized grave neurological complications. The author's endoscopic technique affords the surgeon the ability to provide the patient with a more simplified solution to the jumped and locked facet problem, thereby decreasing the overall morbidity and surgical risks associated with a combined anterior and posterior approach typically performed for this condition. The authors present a representative case example to illustrate their technique.

**Keywords:** Cervical facet dislocation, Decompression, Jumped facets, Laminectomy, Locked facets, Posterior cervical approach, Spinal cord compression, Spinal endoscopy, Upper motor neuron dysfunction.

## INTRODUCTION

Dislocations of the cervical spine are the result of flexion-rotation injuries [1]. [2] Typically, they occur between the C3 and T1 level. As a consequence of this injury, the superior facet dislocates forward in relationship to the inferior facet. Fractures of either of the two are common. However, facet dislocation without fracture is also possible since their orientation in the cervical spine is nearly horizontal [3]. This situation has been described with the term 'jumped facets' [4].

* **Corresponding author Jiang Hongzhen:** Minimally Invasive Spinal Surgery, Beijing Yuhe Integrated Traditional Chinese and Western Medicine Rehabilitation Hospital, Beijing 100853, China; Tel: 086-010-5325 9627; E-mail: XifengZhangChina @hotmail.com

If the facets are locked, the injury may be relatively stable. An unstable injury is often associated with spinal cord injury and neurological deficit. Facet dislocation may be unilateral or bilateral. Anterior displacement may be complete or incomplete. Reduction under cervical traction may be employed to reduce the facet dislocation [5]. However, the risk of neurological deficit following closed reduction exists [6], for which reason, surgical reduction is often considered mainly if the initial attempts at closed reduction are unsuccessful [7, 8]. Unstable fracture-dislocations require surgical decompression and stabilization of the cervical spine [3, 5, 7, 9 - 16].

Optimal initial treatment for these injuries is frequently debated in the neurologically intact patient with, particularly when it comes to surgically treatment of less common unilateral facet injuries or facet injuries without overt instability [6, 17]. Decisions for non-operative or surgical treatment are often based on the consulting surgeon's experience and training [7, 18 - 25]. If surgical treatment is contemplated, a shared decision with the injured patient on how to best return to preinjury functioning may improve satisfaction with the clinical outcome [15]. Delayed surgical treatment of facet dislocations presents their own set of challenges [26 - 31], and spontaneous fusion of the facet joint complex may occur in the long-run [32]. Several studies have been published advocating for anterior only [33 - 35], or a posterior only approach [15]. Most authors recommend combined anterior and posterior reduction and fixation techniques with some precise guidelines when to favor one over the other [14, 22, 29, 34, 36, 37].

To date, the literature suggests that there is not a lot of minimally invasive technology application in the surgical treatment of cervical facet injuries. Typically, these injuries are present as a result of high-energy injuries, often from motor vehicular accidents (MVA) through the emergency room in level I trauma centers. Hence, the emergent nature of the patient presentation is not conducive to minimally invasive spinal surgery techniques. However, its application deserves some thought in terms of simplifying surgical spine care in these often multiply injured patients. Stabilization and clearance of the cervical spine are often the number one question to the spine surgeon involved in level I trauma care as other concomitant extremity-, and pelvis fracture, as well as organ injuries, may require open reduction and internal fixation and other surgical care. In this chapter, the authors describe how they employed the spinal endoscope to assist in the posterior reduction of the jumped facet using a case example. Based on their experience with the technique, they will recommend considering this endoscopic facet joint reduction to simplify the surgical treatment of these grave cervical spine injuries.

## AN EXEMPLARY CASE

The authors present their endoscopically assisted cervical facet joint reduction technique using the example of a 50-year-old female. The patient presented to the emergency room with a nine-hour history of severe neck pain and lower extremity paralysis after a high-energy injury to the cervical spine. The patient was accidentally hit into the head by a falling coconut tree while working outdoors. There was a loss of consciousness (LOC) for approximately 10 minutes with a closed head injury resulting in a concussion and cognitive impairment. Upon regaining consciousness, the patient immediately complained of severe neck- and upper extremity pain, and the inability to move her lower extremities.

Moreover, physical examination of the injured revealed neck stiffness, cervical spinous process space, bilateral trapezius muscle tenderness, and no significant sensory loss in both arms. The patient had severely limited cervical spine movement. Motor strength in both arms was limited to 4/5 and 3/5 in the lower extremities, respectively. Both patella tendon reflexes were hyperactive. There was a positive Hoffman's sign bilaterally. The patient had an incomplete spinal cord injury consistent with ASIA Grade D. Advanced imaging examination showed that the C6-7 bilateral cervical facet joints were locked with anterolisthesis of C6 on C7, causing compression of the spinal cord (Fig. **1**). Fracture of the right-sided articular process was best visualized with 3D-rendering of the patient's CT-scan (Fig. **2**).

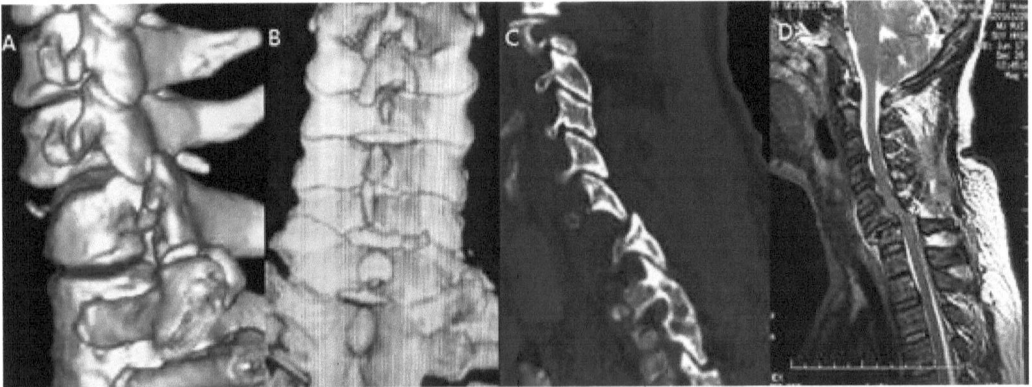

**Fig. (1).** Preoperative three-dimensional computed tomography (CT) scan **(A, B)**, and sagittal CT scan showing the locking of the C6-7 facet joint **(C)** with associated spinal cord compression confirmed on the sagittal T2-weighted magnetic resonance image (MRI) **(D)**.

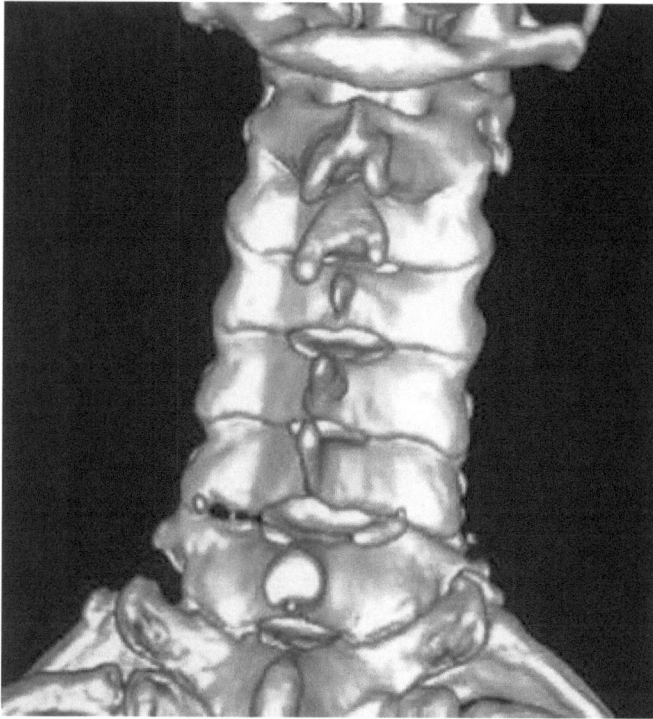

**Fig. (2).** Shown is the preoperative three-dimensional CT-scan confirming fracture of the right-sided articular process. The patient had an incomplete spinal cord lesion with 4/5 motor strength in the upper extremity, and 3/5 in the lower extremities. There was a positive Hoffman's sign. Posterior endoscopic decompression was performed to facilitate the reduction of the "jumped" and locked C6/7 facets.

## ENDOSCOPIC DECOMPRESSION & REDUCTION

The patient was admitted to the hospital and initially placed in skull traction. Repeated attempts to achieve reduction with increasing weights for two weeks failed. The locked un-fractured left-sided articular process prevented the reduction. Therefore, the authors decided to employ the posterior endoscopic approach on the left side before the anterior decompression and fusion to facilitate the reduction (Figs. **3A - 3C**). Under local anesthesia, the upper portion of the left articular process of C7 was drilled down, and the jumped and locked C6/7 facet joint spontaneously reduced under direct endoscopic visualization while manipulating the skull traction.

## DEFINITIVE STABILIZATION

Following the posterior endoscopic decompression, an ACDF was performed employing a cage and an anterior buttress plate (Figs. **3D - 3E**). Successful reduction and anterior column reconstruction was confirmed on postoperative 3D CT scan. This postoperative CT scan also visualized the small portion of the left upper articular process, and the fractured right-sided C7 articular process and an associated right-sided C7 lamina fracture.

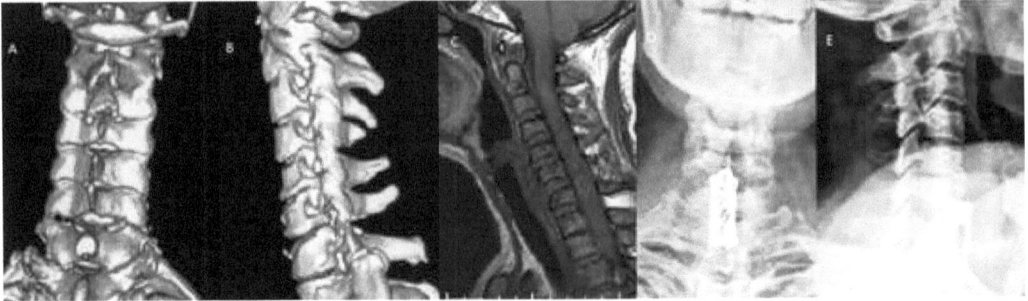

**Fig. (3).** Postoperative three-dimensional computed tomography (CT) scan **(A, B)**, and sagittal MRI scan **(C)** showing the reduction of the locked C6-7 facet joint. The endoscopic resection of the left-sided upper portion of the C7 lateral mass is visualized **(C)**. Postoperative anterior- posterior **(D)**, and lateral **(E)** radiographs confirm stabilization of this unstable cervical spine injury. The patient.

## DISCUSSION

Reduction of jumped cervical facet joints can be difficult at times and may not be accomplished by cervical traction alone. Traditionally, open reduction and stabilization surgery often require anterior and posterior approaches. More recent articles have published on the merits of anterior only techniques to accomplish reduction and stabilization of the injured cervical spinal motion segment. Percutaneous endoscopic decompression of the locked and jumped cervical facet(s) appeared attractive to the authors since it diminishes access trauma and surgery time. Besides, it can be done under local anesthesia without the need for general anesthesia, which in turn makes the subsequent reduction maneuver under skeletal traction safer as the surgeon can communicate with the patient during these dangerous maneuvers. There has been controversy about whether or not a pre-reduction MRI scan is needed in the neurologically intact and injured patient. At least theoretically, the risk of a sudden neurological deficit exists if an extrusion of a large cervical disc herniation occurs during the reduction maneuver. This risk may exist without a preoperative MRI scan. Still, it may be meliorated with the resection of the tip of the jumped articular process, typically piercing the lower facet leading to a high-stress concentration in the injured facet joint. This injury may require large distractive forces during the skeletal traction maneuver aimed at providing enough distraction to reduce the jumped facet. Resecting the tip of the jammed articular process may lessen the distraction forces required to accomplish the reduction significantly.

## CONCLUSIONS

Percutaneous endoscopic release of a locked jumped cervical facet to facilitate spontaneous reduction under skeletal traction is an attractive alternative to open reduction. Decreased approach-related morbidity and lower risk for neurological compromise during the reduction maneuver are apparent advantages. The endoscopic procedure can be done under local anesthesia while releasing the jumped facet under increasing distraction forces. The spontaneous reduction can be observed videoendoscopically under direct visualization simplifying the post-reduction diagnostic algorithm and obviating the need for confirmatory advanced postoperative imaging studies. Staged endoscopic posterior and open anterior procedures are feasible within the same day with lower risk exposure to the patient because diminished blood loss and other associated procedure complications are to be expected. The authors are planning to investigate the merits of the percutaneous endoscopic decompression, release, and reduction in more patients whenever the opportunity arises in their current practice setting. The authors anticipate that their endoscopic technique can be validated in a more extensive patient study and plan to report back once such studies are completed.

## CONSENT FOR PUBLICATION

Not applicable.

## CONFLICT OF INTEREST

The author declares no conflict of interest, financial or otherwise.

## ACKNOWLEDGEMENTS

Declared none.

## REFERENCES

[1]    Panjabi MM, Simpson AK, Ivancic PC, Pearson AM, Tominaga Y, Yue JJ. Cervical facet joint kinematics during bilateral facet dislocation. Eur Spine J 2007; 16(10): 1680-8.
[http://dx.doi.org/10.1007/s00586-007-0410-2] [PMID: 17566792]

[2]    Ivancic PC, Pearson AM, Tominaga Y, Simpson AK, Yue JJ, Panjabi MM. Mechanism of cervical spinal cord injury during bilateral facet dislocation. Spine 2007; 32(22): 2467-73.
[http://dx.doi.org/10.1097/BRS.0b013e3181573b67] [PMID: 18090087]

[3]    Takao T, Kubota K, Maeda T, *et al.* A radiographic evaluation of facet sagittal angle in cervical spinal cord injury without major fracture or dislocation. Spinal Cord 2017; 55(5): 515-7.
[http://dx.doi.org/10.1038/sc.2016.172] [PMID: 27995938]

[4]    Harshfield DL, Jordan R, Grigg K. Radiological case of the month. A facet dislocation (perched or jumped facet) on the right at C4-C5. J Ark Med Soc 1994; 90(8): 403-4.
[PMID: 8175619]

[5]    Ahmed WA, Naidoo A, Belci M. Rapid incremental closed traction reduction of cervical facet fracture

dislocation: the Stoke Mandeville experience. Spinal Cord Ser Cases 2018; 4: 86.
[http://dx.doi.org/10.1038/s41394-018-0109-0] [PMID: 30275978]

[6]    Wimberley DW, Vaccaro AR, Goyal N, *et al.* Acute quadriplegia following closed traction reduction of a cervical facet dislocation in the setting of ossification of the posterior longitudinal ligament: case report. Spine 2005; 30(15): E433-8.
[http://dx.doi.org/10.1097/01.brs.0000172233.05024.8f] [PMID: 16094262]

[7]    Song KJ, Park H, Lee KB. Treatment of irreducible bilateral cervical facet fracture-dislocation with a prolapsed disc using a prefixed polyetheretherketone cage and plate system. Asian Spine J 2013; 7(2): 111-4.
[http://dx.doi.org/10.4184/asj.2013.7.2.111] [PMID: 23741548]

[8]    Li Y, Zhou P, Cui W, *et al.* Immediate anterior open reduction and plate fixation in the management of lower cervical dislocation with facet interlocking. Sci Rep 2019; 9(1): 1286.
[http://dx.doi.org/10.1038/s41598-018-37742-w] [PMID: 30718730]

[9]    Kim SG, Park SJ, Wang HS, Ju CI, Lee SM, Kim SW. Anterior Approach Following Intraoperative Reduction for Cervical Facet Fracture and Dislocation. J Korean Neurosurg Soc 2020; 63(2): 202-9.
[http://dx.doi.org/10.3340/jkns.2019.0139] [PMID: 31805759]

[10]   Miao DC, Qi C, Wang F, Lu K, Shen Y. Management of Severe Lower Cervical Facet Dislocation without Vertebral Body Fracture Using Skull Traction and an Anterior Approach. Med Sci Monit 2018; 24: 1295-302.
[http://dx.doi.org/10.12659/MSM.908515] [PMID: 29500927]

[11]   Shinohara K, Soshi S, Kida Y, Shinohara A, Marumo K. A rare case of spinal injury: bilateral facet dislocation without fracture at the lumbosacral joint. J Orthop Sci 2012; 17(2): 189-93.
[http://dx.doi.org/10.1007/s00776-011-0082-y] [PMID: 21559956]

[12]   Ngo LM, Aizawa T, Hoshikawa T, *et al.* Fracture and contralateral dislocation of the twin facet joints of the lower cervical spine. Eur Spine J 2012; 21(2): 282-8.
[http://dx.doi.org/10.1007/s00586-011-1956-6] [PMID: 21830078]

[13]   Gomes S, Rudkin S, Tsai F, Lotfipour S. Bilateral cervical spine facet fracture-dislocation. West J Emerg Med 2009; 10(1): 19.
[PMID: 19561761]

[14]   Schmidt-Rohlfing B, Nossek M, Knobe M, Das M. Combined approach for a locked unilateral facet fracture-dislocation of the cervicothoracic junction. Acta Orthop Belg 2008; 74(6): 875-80.
[PMID: 19205340]

[15]   Isla A, Alvarez F, Perez-López C, *et al.* Posterior approach for low cervical fractures with unilateral or bilateral facet dislocation. Eur J Orthop Surg Traumatol 2002; 12(3): 123-8.
[http://dx.doi.org/10.1007/s00590-002-0039-0] [PMID: 24573888]

[16]   Hadley MN, Fitzpatrick BC, Sonntag VK, Browner CM. Facet fracture-dislocation injuries of the cervical spine. Neurosurgery 1992; 30(5): 661-6.
[PMID: 1584374]

[17]   Ndoumbé A, Motah M, Mballa Amougou JC, Guifo Marc ML, Takongmo S, Sosso Maurice A. A case of unilateral dislocation of C3 right facet joint treated with lateral mass plating. Neurochirurgie 2011; 57(2): 100-4.
[PMID: 21087778]

[18]   Quarrington RD, Jones CF, Tcherveniakov P, *et al.* Traumatic subaxial cervical facet subluxation and dislocation: epidemiology, radiographic analyses, and risk factors for spinal cord injury. Spine J 2018; 18(3): 387-98.
[http://dx.doi.org/10.1016/j.spinee.2017.07.175] [PMID: 28739474]

[19]   Sun D, Liu P, Cheng J, Ma Z, Liu J, Qin T. Correlation between intervertebral disc degeneration, paraspinal muscle atrophy, and lumbar facet joints degeneration in patients with lumbar disc

herniation. BMC Musculoskelet Disord 2017; 18(1): 167.
[http://dx.doi.org/10.1186/s12891-017-1522-4] [PMID: 28427393]

[20]    Prabhat V, Boruah T, Lal H, Kumar R, Dagar A, Sahu H. Management of post-traumatic neglected cervical facet dislocation. J Clin Orthop Trauma 2017; 8(2): 125-30.
[http://dx.doi.org/10.1016/j.jcot.2016.10.002] [PMID: 28720987]

[21]    Broekema AE, Kuijlen JM, Lesman-Leegte GA, *et al.* FACET study group investigators. Study protocol for a randomised controlled multicentre study: the Foraminotomy ACDF Cost-Effectiveness Trial (FACET) in patients with cervical radiculopathy. BMJ Open 2017; 7(1): e012829.
[http://dx.doi.org/10.1136/bmjopen-2016-012829] [PMID: 28057652]

[22]    Lins CC, Prado DT, Joaquim AF. Surgical treatment of traumatic cervical facet dislocation: anterior, posterior or combined approaches? Arq Neuropsiquiatr 2016; 74(9): 745-9.
[http://dx.doi.org/10.1590/0004-282X20160078] [PMID: 27706424]

[23]    Du W, Wang C, Tan J, Shen B, Ni S, Zheng Y. Management of subaxial cervical facet dislocation through anterior approach monitored by spinal cord evoked potential. Spine 2014; 39(1): 48-52.
[http://dx.doi.org/10.1097/BRS.0000000000000046] [PMID: 24108291]

[24]    Chen Y, Wang X, Chen D, Liu X. Surgical treatment for unilateral cervical facet dislocation in a young child aged 22 months old: a case report and review of the literature. Eur Spine J 2013; 22 (Suppl. 3): S439-42.
[http://dx.doi.org/10.1007/s00586-012-2590-7] [PMID: 23179987]

[25]    Cosar M, Khoo LT, Yeung CA, Yeung AT. A comparison of the degree of lateral recess and foraminal enlargement with facet preservation in the treatment of lumbar stenosis with standard surgical tools *versus* a novel powered filing instrument: a cadaver study. SAS J 2007; 1(4): 135-42.
[http://dx.doi.org/10.1016/S1935-9810(07)70059-2] [PMID: 25802591]

[26]    O'Shaughnessy J, Grenier JM, Stern PJ. A delayed diagnosis of bilateral facet dislocation of the cervical spine: a case report. J Can Chiropr Assoc 2014; 58(1): 45-51.
[PMID: 24587496]

[27]    Mishra A, Agrawal D, Singh PK. Delayed presentation of post-traumatic bilateral cervical facet dislocation: a series of 4 cases. Neurol India 2014; 62(5): 540-2.
[http://dx.doi.org/10.4103/0028-3886.144454] [PMID: 25387625]

[28]    Shimada T, Ohtori S, Inoue G, *et al.* Delayed surgical treatment for a traumatic bilateral cervical facet joint dislocation using a posterior-anterior approach: a case report. J Med Case Reports 2013; 7: 9.
[http://dx.doi.org/10.1186/1752-1947-7-9] [PMID: 23302494]

[29]    Payer M, Tessitore E. Delayed surgical management of a traumatic bilateral cervical facet dislocation by an anterior-posterior-anterior approach. J Clin Neurosci 2007; 14(8): 782-6.
[http://dx.doi.org/10.1016/j.jocn.2006.04.021] [PMID: 17531492]

[30]    Bartels RH, Donk R. Delayed management of traumatic bilateral cervical facet dislocation: surgical strategy. Report of three cases. J Neurosurg 2002; 97(3) (Suppl.): 362-5.
[PMID: 12408394]

[31]    Kahn A, Leggon R, Lindsey RW. Cervical facet dislocation: management following delayed diagnosis. Orthopedics 1998; 21(10): 1089-91.
[http://dx.doi.org/10.3928/0147-7447-19981001-07] [PMID: 9801232]

[32]    Bodman A, Chin L. Bony fusion in a chronic cervical bilateral facet dislocation. Am J Case Rep 2015; 16: 104-8.
[http://dx.doi.org/10.12659/AJCR.892173] [PMID: 25702178]

[33]    Liu K, Zhang Z. A novel anterior-only surgical approach for reduction and fixation of cervical facet dislocation. World Neurosurg 2019; 128: e362-9.
[http://dx.doi.org/10.1016/j.wneu.2019.04.153] [PMID: 31029820]

[34]    Liu K, Zhang Z. Comparison of a novel anterior-only approach and the conventional posterior-anterior

approach for cervical facet dislocation: a retrospective study. Eur Spine J 2019; 28(10): 2380-9.
[http://dx.doi.org/10.1007/s00586-019-06073-3] [PMID: 31332570]

[35]    Kanna RM, Shetty AP, Rajasekaran S. Modified anterior-only reduction and fixation for traumatic cervical facet dislocation (AO type C injuries). Eur Spine J 2018; 27(6): 1447-53.
[http://dx.doi.org/10.1007/s00586-017-5430-y] [PMID: 29279998]

[36]    Raizman NM, Yu WD, Jenkins MV, Wallace MT, O'Brien JR. Traumatic C4-C5 unilateral facet dislocation with posterior disc herniation above a prior anterior fusion. Am J Orthop 2012; 41(6): E85-8.
[PMID: 22837997]

[37]    Feng G, Hong Y, Li L, *et al.* Anterior decompression and nonstructural bone grafting and posterior fixation for cervical facet dislocation with traumatic disc herniation. Spine 2012; 37(25): 2082-8.
[http://dx.doi.org/10.1097/BRS.0b013e31825ee846] [PMID: 22614801]

**CHAPTER 14**

# Endoscopically Assisted Minimally Invasive Laminoplasty in The Treatment of Cervical Spondylotic Myelopathy

**Xifeng Zhang**[1,*], **Li Dongzhe**[1] and **Jiang Hongzhen**[1]

[1] *Department of Orthopedics, First Medical Center, PLA General Hospital, Beijing 100853, China*

**Abstract:** The authors present a case of cervical myelopathy due to degenerative stenosis of the spinal canal. They employed an endoscope to aid in the improved visualization during the release of ligamentous attachments between the cervical dural sac and the ventral aspect of the cervical lamina during laminoplasty. The patient had two paraspinal 2 cm incisions through which a MED tubular retractor was placed, and most of the bony decompression was done using an operating microscope. The lamina was detached from the lateral masses with a high-speed drill. The bony cuts in this lateral groove were completed with Kerrison rongeurs. Silk stitches were passed through the spinous processes to elevate the cervical laminae from the dural sac and create the posterior expansion of the cord's space. This bilateral laminoplasty was then secured with mini-titanium plates. The authors present their utilization of the spinal endoscope in improved visualization of the surgical dissection, which can be problematic even with an operating microscope through the small exposure afforded by the MED tubular retractor system. The illumination and magnification helped safely execute this hybrid operation that employed two different minimally invasive spinal surgery technologies, including the operating microscope and a spinal endoscope. In the authors' opinion, such hybridizations may be the stepping stone towards next-generation advances in the cervical spine's minimally invasive surgery.

**Keywords:** Cervical spondylotic myelopathy, Endoscopy, Laminoplasty.

## INTRODUCTION

Cervical spondylotic myelopathy (CSM) is a common condition affecting patients with advanced degeneration of the cervical spine leading to a significant reduction of the space available for the spinal cord, which results in decreased neurological function [1 - 9]. Common symptoms include tingling or numbness in the arms,

* **Corresponding author Zhang Xifeng:** Department of Orthopedics, First Medical Center, PLA General Hospital, Beijing 100853, China; Tel: 086-010-5325 9627; E-mails: XifengZhangChina@hotmail.com and 656780949@qq.com

**Kai-Uwe Lewandrowski, Jorge Felipe Ramírez León, Anthony Yeung, Hyeun-Sung Kim, Xifeng Zhang, Gun Choi, Stefan Hellinger and Álvaro Dowling (Eds.)**

fingers, or hands, weakness in the arms, shoulders, or hands. Some patients also report trouble grasping and holding on to items. Others describe impairment of their walking ability with the imbalance and other coordination problems, loss of fine motor skills, and pain or stiffness in the neck [10 - 13]. Spinal cord decompression is at the center of surgical treatment. Laminoplasty has been associated with improved clinical outcomes in CSM patients [10, 14 - 19]. Its reported advantages include lower incidence postlaminectomy kyphosis, adjacent segment disease following decompression fusion procedures with lower blood loss, and diminished surgical trauma [12, 18, 20, 21]. The reported disadvantages include axial neck pain and closure of the laminoplasty site with recurrent cervical canal stenosis [8, 22 - 24]. In this chapter, the authors report on their spinal endoscope application during minimally invasive access to the posterior cervical spine during laminoplasty using a MED tubular retractor system. Their hybridized version of the MIS laminoplasty procedure highlights an imminent technology transition in spinal endoscopy from simple uniportal decompression procedures to more complex applications such as reconstructive surgeries of the cervical spine.

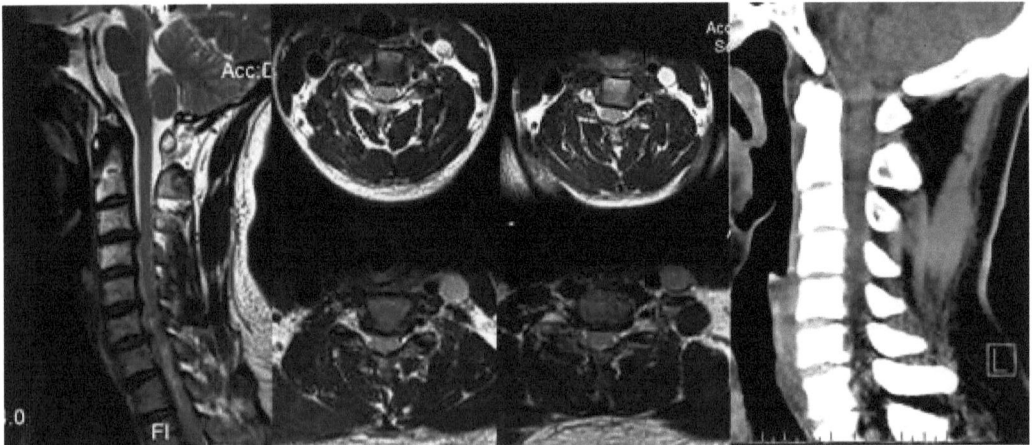

**Fig. (1).** MRI and CT showed multi-segment cervical disc herniation, cervical spinal stenosis, and no obvious posterior longitudinal ligament calcification.

## CASE INTRODUCTION

The patient in a 52-year-old female with a chief complaining of repetitive episodes of the neck- and shoulder pain for more than ten years, which worsened with weakness in the upper- and lower extremities for the last four months before presenting for consultation in our facility. Moreover, the patient reported difficulty holding objects, complained of unstable gait, and limited walking endurance. Physical examination revealed stiffness of the neck muscles and decreased sensation on the radial side of the left forearm and thumb. There was decreased motor strength in the bilateral elbow extensors and flexors 4/5.

Moreover, the grip strength was reduced to 3/5 in both hands. The patient also had a positive Hoffman's sign bilaterally and hyperreflexia in both biceps, triceps, and patella tendon reflexes. The advanced imaging studies showed multi-segment cervical disc herniation and cervical spinal stenosis. Preoperative CT showed a loss of the cervical spine's physiological curvature with straightening without apparent cervical spine instability and calcification of the posterior longitudinal ligament (Fig. **1**).

## INDICATION FOR SURGERY & TECHNIQUE

The patient had apparent cervical spinal cord compression symptoms, and imaging confirmed cervical spinal canal stenosis and compression of the dural sac. Plain film radiographs showed no evident cervical spine instability. The decision was made to offer the patient a cervical laminoplasty under the MED microscope to expand the cervical spinal canal, thereby improving the cervical spinal cord's compression. The adjunctive use of a spinal endoscope was anticipated for the lysis of adhesions and to aid in the dissection of the dural sac's soft tissue just before lifting the posterior lamina to accomplish the posterior spinal canal expansion.

After induction of general anesthesia and intraoperative administration of perioperative antibiotic coverage for 24 hours, the patient is placed in a prone position, a 20mm long and straight incision is made in the posterior median skin positioned at the C3/4 level. Drill holes are drilled on both sides of each spinous process to pass a silk suture thread through the drill hole intended to aid in lifting the lamina upon completion of the bony cuts. After minimal muscle dissection, a MED tubular retractor was inserted just next to the spinous process until it touches the lamina. After exposing the bone surface, the surgeons' preference was to use a curette to determine the transition from the spinous process to the lateral lower edge of the lamina to the facet joint's medial border.

Before the bony cuts, drill holes were placed at the spinous process base, pointing to the opposite side of the lamina to prepare for micro titanium plate fixation. A high-speed drill to score the bone at the lateral lamina's junction with the medial aspect of the lateral mass. The bone cuts are then completed with the use of the cervical Kerrison rongeur. The bone troughs cut are typically 2-3 mm in width. At this junction, the endoscopic hook is used deployed through a spinal endoscope through the MED tube (> 20 mm) to improve visualization of the soft tissue dissection required to free up the posterior lamina to complete the laminoplasty. The authors found this technique very useful in dissecting and cutting the ligamentum flavum and fiber bundles that are typically attached to the dural sac through the grooved window provided by the bone cuts. Once the dura mater is exposed on one side, the whole process is completed on the other side. At this juncture, the previously placed silk thread is pulled posteriorly to mobilize the lamina-spinous process complex of the surgical level(s) and produce the laminoplasty effect by posterior canal expansion approximately 3 mm on each side. This requires some patients and perhaps repeated dissections of the adhesions between the cervical spinal cord's dural sac to accomplish this. Suppose the segment of the posterior bony elements mobilized during the laminoplasty preparation with the bone cuts' placement does not readily displace posteriorly. In that case, repeated use of the spinal endoscope to take a detailed look at the soft tissue preparation and dissection may come in handy. On the medial side, the mini-titanium plates were fixed on the base of the spinous process, and on the lateral side, the same mini-titanium plate was fixed to the lateral mass using the Magerl technique. These surgical steps are carried out on both sides, repositioning the MED tube to the opposite side at the same level. In the authors' opinion, this surgery can be carried out at two to three consecutive levels. After surgery completion, the fascia and skin are sutured, and a wound is drained with an indwelling drain that is typically removed on postoperative day 2 or 3 (Figs. **2** & **3**).

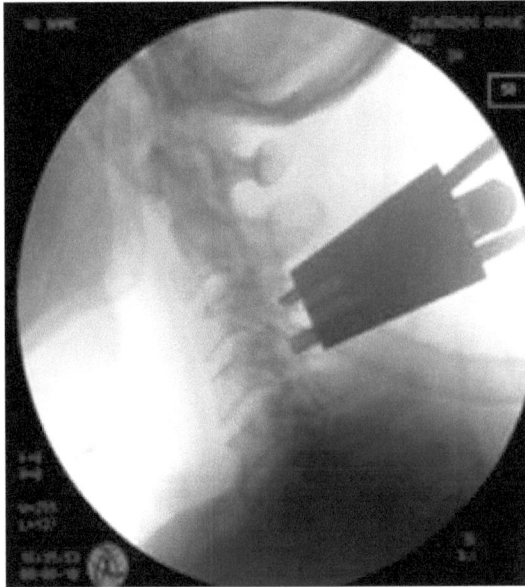

**Fig. (2).** Intraoperative fluoroscopy lateral view of the cervical spine showing the positioning of the MED tubular retractor used during the microsurgical laminoplasty.

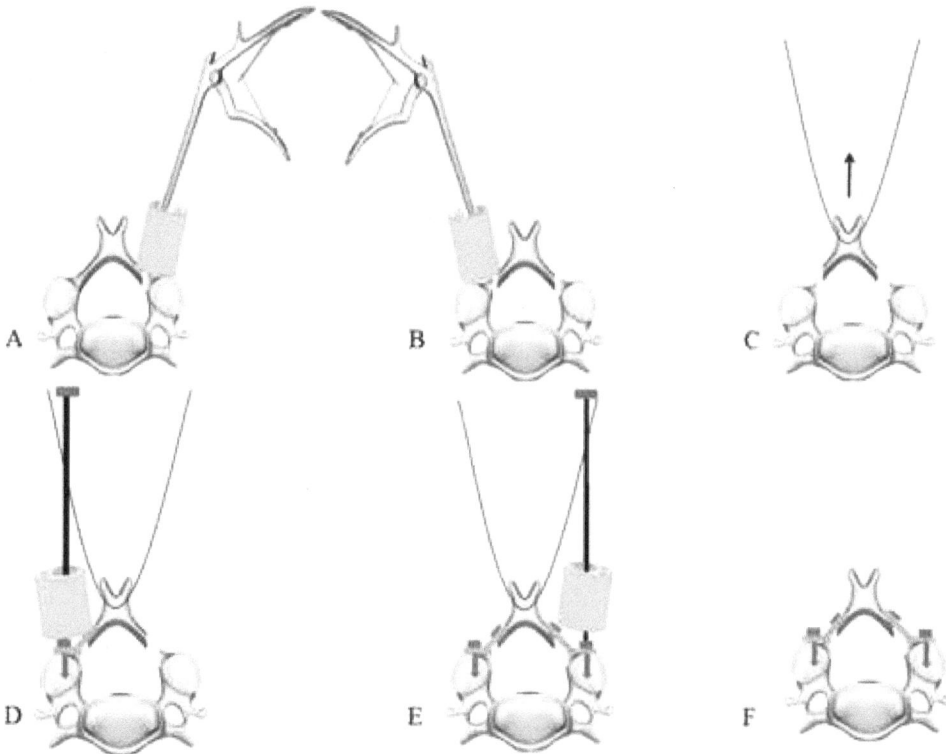

**Fig. (3).** Schematic diagram of the laminoplasty surgery using the MED tubular retractor (**A & B**), the endoscopic hook was used to release soft tissue adhesions between the dura and the posterior laminoplasty bone block formed by spinous process and the remaining lamina (**C-F**).

## CLINICAL COURSE

The patient did well with the minimally invasive laminoplasty surgery. The drain was removed one day after surgery. The patient was encouraged to wear a neck brace and get out of bed for supervised mobilization with the occupational and physical therapist. After the operation, the patient felt that her limbs were relieved of fatigue. Six months after the operation, the patient's upper limb muscle strength recovered to grade 5/5. The patient's cervical JOA score was 8 points before surgery and improved to 13 points one year after surgery. The VAS score for cervical and shoulder pain was 8 points before surgery and reduced to 2 points one year after surgery. A postoperative MRI scan was done 7 days after surgery showed that the cervical spinal canal was significantly enlarged. One year after surgery, X-rays of the cervical spine showed that the titanium plates were in a good position, and there was no loosening. Cross-sectional CT showed bone healing at the lamina notch (Figs. **4** & **5**).

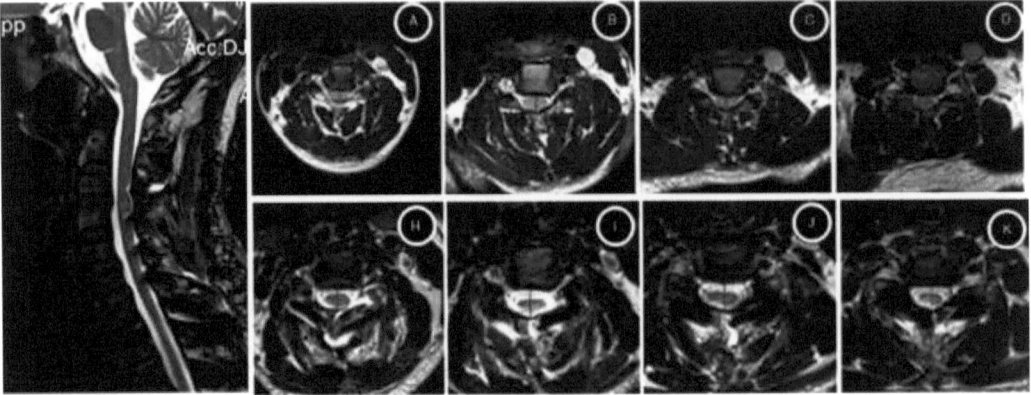

**Fig. (4).** Postoperative sagittal and multiple axial MRI scan images seven days following the hybrid MED-Endoscopy laminoplasty are shown. The spinal endoscope was used to directly visualize the interface between the dura and the posterior laminoplasty block through the 2 to 3 mm wide trough formed between the lateral portion of the lamina and the medial portion the lateral mass created by the bone cuts. The MRI scan showed that the surgical level's cervical spinal canal diameter was significantly enlarged than before the operation (A *vs.* H, B *vs.* I, C *vs.* J, D *vs.* K. The red line indicates the increase in anteroposterior diameter).

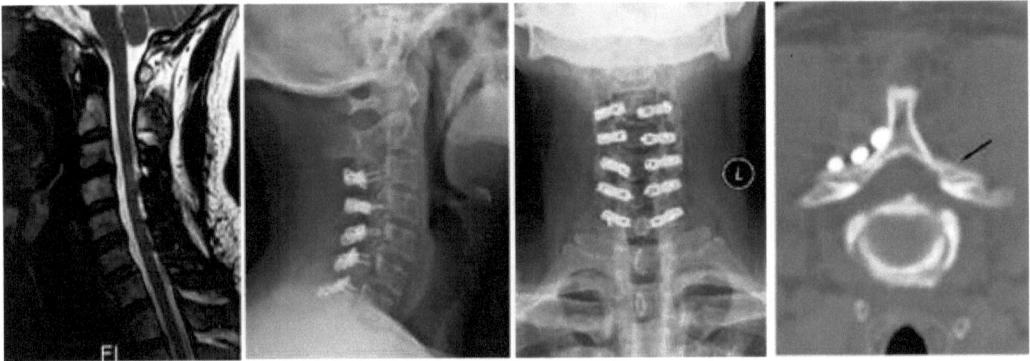

**Fig. (5).** One-year postoperative sagittal MRI scan, lateral and anterior-posterior plain films, and CT scan showed that the spinal canal did not reappear to be stenotic. The x-rays showed that the titanium plates were in a good position, and there was no loosening. The cross-sectional CT showed bone healing of the groove at the laminoplasty cuts.

## DISCUSSION

The treatment of cervical spondylotic myelopathy is still based on various traditional operations, mainly including anterior, posterior, and combined anterior and posterior surgery [6, 12, 25 - 31]. The posterior approach is suitable for the compression of multiple cervical spinal cord segments but does not require particular anterior surgery [28]. The early posterior cervical surgery used extensive laminectomy. It fell out of favor because the postoperative scar tissue can easily cause the spinal cord's recompression, and the long-term outcomes were inferior. Since the single-hinge open-door cervical laminoplasty was first proposed in 1979 [32, 33], various techniques have been popularized and used in clinical practice. The modified anchor single-opening, the cervical spinal "Z"-shaped laminoplasty surgery, and the mini-titanium plate internal fixation are examples of these techniques. Open door, double-door cervical spinal canal enlargement surgery, and others are additional examples. Although these procedures have a relatively positive long-term effect, problems such as C5 nerve root palsy, postoperative re-closure of the laminoplasty with recurrent central cervical canal stenosis, and postoperative kyphosis [8]. Besides, it is reported in the literature that 45%-80% of patients have postoperative axial pain, such as neck- and shoulder pain, soreness, stiffness, muscle spasm, *etc.*, and the duration of symptoms can last up to more than ten years [5, 7, 34]. This may be related to the severe damage of the cervical spine ligamentous complex during the operation or the stripping of the posterior elements' muscles, especially the muscles attachments to C2-C7. Additional factors may include reducing the total range of motion of the cervical spine after the operation, the stimulation of the soft tissue of the cervical spine, and the variable displacement of each laminoplasty segment.

The endoscopically assisted MED cervical laminoplasty completely preserves the spinous process, supraspinous ligament, interspinous ligament, and other essential structures and the attachment of the posterior cervical muscles to the spinous process, which reduces or avoids the destruction of crucial tissue structures in the posterior cervical spine. An endoscope is a useful tool to directly visualize and minimize the necessary dissection necessary to loosen up the posterior laminoplasty bone block formed by the spinous and detached laminae. Thus, the endoscopically assisted MED technique presented by the authors aids in preserving the structural and functional integrity of the posterior cervical muscles, especially the splenius capitus, and the semispinalis capitis muscles C2 cervical spinal muscles, including the obliquus capitis inferior and the rectus capitis posterior major. The detachment should be avoided at all cost. Aiming to achieve sufficient decompression and significant expansion of the spinal canal, the mini-titanium plate rigidly fixes the bony spinal canal and restores its immediate stability. The authors recommend an early postoperative physical therapy and mobilization program to reduce cervical spine lordosis loss and prevent the decline of cervical motion. Postoperative closure of the cervical spinal canal is a common postoperative sequela effectively avoided by the titanium plate fixation. The authors also stipulate that C5 nerve palsy's occurrence should be lower because of the minimal manipulation laminoplasty block.

## CONCLUSIONS

Endoscopic visualization during minimally invasive cervical spinal laminoplasty is only used for cutting the bone groove and during the dissection of soft tissue attachments from the dural sac to facilitate the posterior expansion of the spinal canal when pulling the lamina from the lateral mass *via*the percutaneously place silk stitches. There is minimal traction of the cervical nerve roots. The technique takes some practice but is impossible to master since most surgeons nowadays are familiar with the MED technique. The authors recommend that the prospective surgeon adopt this technique to monitor the amount of deflection of the laminoplasty bone block. It may make the installation of the mini-titanium plates more cumbersome. This part of the operation requires improvement. The authors will continue to research the clinical outcomes with this technique and present their results of more extensive clinical trials in the future. For now, they offer up the method in this case report based on its merits.

## CONSENT FOR PUBLICATION

Not applicable.

## CONFLICT OF INTEREST

The author declares no conflict of interest, financial or otherwise.

## ACKNOWLEDGEMENTS

Declared none.

## REFERENCES

[1]    Yuan H, Zhang X, Zhang LM, Yan YQ, Liu YK, Lewandrowski KU. Comparative study of curative effect of spinal endoscopic surgery and anterior cervical decompression for cervical spondylotic myelopathy. J Spine Surg 2020; 6 (Suppl. 1): S186-96.
       [http://dx.doi.org/10.21037/jss.2019.11.15] [PMID: 32195427]

[2]    Qi Q, Huang S, Ling Z, *et al.* A New Diagnostic Medium for Cervical Spondylotic Myelopathy: Dynamic Somatosensory Evoked Potentials. World Neurosurg 2020; 133: e225-32.
       [http://dx.doi.org/10.1016/j.wneu.2019.08.205] [PMID: 31493599]

[3]    Nouri A, Gondar R, Cheng JS, Kotter MRN, Tessitore E. Degenerative cervical myelopathy and the aging spine: introduction to the special issue. J Clin Med 2020; 9(8): E2535.
       [http://dx.doi.org/10.3390/jcm9082535] [PMID: 32781513]

[4]    Li X, An B, Gao H, *et al.* Surgical results and prognostic factors following percutaneous full endoscopic posterior decompression for thoracic myelopathy caused by ossification of the ligamentum flavum. Sci Rep 2020; 10(1): 1305.
       [http://dx.doi.org/10.1038/s41598-020-58198-x] [PMID: 31992790]

[5]    Li Q, Han X, Wang R, Zhang Y, Liu P, Dong Q. Clinical recovery after 5 level of posterior decompression spine surgeries in patients with cervical spondylotic myelopathy: A retrospective cohort study. Asian J Surg 2020; 43(5): 613-24.
       [http://dx.doi.org/10.1016/j.asjsur.2019.08.003] [PMID: 31481282]

[6]    El-Ghandour NMF, Soliman MAR, Ezzat AAM, Mohsen A, Zein-Elabedin M. The safety and efficacy of anterior *versus* posterior decompression surgery in degenerative cervical myelopathy: a prospective randomized trial. J Neurosurg Spine 2020; 1-9.
       [PMID: 32357329]

[7]     Dobran M, Mancini F, Paracino R, *et al.* Laminectomy *versus* open-door laminoplasty for cervical spondylotic myelopathy: A clinical outcome analysis. Surg Neurol Int 2020; 11: 73.
[http://dx.doi.org/10.25259/SNI_85_2020] [PMID: 32363068]

[8]     Yuan X, Wei C, Xu W, Gan X, Cao S, Luo J. Comparison of laminectomy and fusion *vs* laminoplasty in the treatment of multilevel cervical spondylotic myelopathy: A meta-analysis. Medicine (Baltimore) 2019; 98(13): e14971.
[http://dx.doi.org/10.1097/MD.0000000000014971] [PMID: 30921202]

[9]     Lin Y, Rao S, Li Y, Zhao S, Chen B. Posterior percutaneous full-endoscopic cervical laminectomy and decompression for cervical stenosis with myelopathy: a technical note. World Neurosurg 2019; 8750 (19): 30051-8..
[http://dx.doi.org/10.1016/j.wneu.2018.12.180] [PMID: 30648610]

[10]    Kato S, Oshima Y, Oka H, *et al.* Comparison of the Japanese Orthopaedic Association (JOA) score and modified JOA (mJOA) score for the assessment of cervical myelopathy: a multicenter observational study. PLoS One 2015; 10(4): e0123022.
[http://dx.doi.org/10.1371/journal.pone.0123022] [PMID: 25837285]

[11]    Jho HD. Spinal cord decompression *via* microsurgical anterior foraminotomy for spondylotic cervical myelopathy. Minim Invasive Neurosurg 1997; 40(4): 124-9.
[http://dx.doi.org/10.1055/s-2008-1053432] [PMID: 9477400]

[12]    Law MD Jr, Bernhardt M, White AA III. Cervical spondylotic myelopathy: a review of surgical indications and decision making. Yale J Biol Med 1993; 66(3): 165-77.
[PMID: 8209553]

[13]    Hattori T, Sakakibara R, Yasuda K, Murayama N, Hirayama K. Micturitional disturbance in cervical spondylotic myelopathy. J Spinal Disord 1990; 3(1): 16-8.
[http://dx.doi.org/10.1097/00002517-199003000-00003] [PMID: 2134406]

[14]    Deora H, Kim SH, Behari S, *et al.* World Federation of Neurosurgical Societies (WFNS) Spine Committee. Anterior Surgical Techniques for Cervical Spondylotic Myelopathy: WFNS Spine Committee Recommendations. Neurospine 2019; 16(3): 408-20.
[http://dx.doi.org/10.14245/ns.1938250.125] [PMID: 31607073]

[15]    An B, Li XC, Zhou CP, *et al.* Percutaneous full endoscopic posterior decompression of thoracic myelopathy caused by ossification of the ligamentum flavum. Eur Spine J 2019; 28(3): 492-501.
[http://dx.doi.org/10.1007/s00586-018-05866-2] [PMID: 30656471]

[16]    Minamide A, Yoshida M, Simpson AK, *et al.* Microendoscopic laminotomy *versus* conventional laminoplasty for cervical spondylotic myelopathy: 5-year follow-up study. J Neurosurg Spine 2017; 27(4): 403-9.
[http://dx.doi.org/10.3171/2017.2.SPINE16939] [PMID: 28708041]

[17]    Blizzard DJ, Caputo AM, Sheets CZ, *et al.* Laminoplasty *versus* laminectomy with fusion for the treatment of spondylotic cervical myelopathy: short-term follow-up. Eur Spine J 2017; 26(1): 85-93.
[http://dx.doi.org/10.1007/s00586-016-4746-3] [PMID: 27554354]

[18]    Laiginhas AR, Silva PA, Pereira P, Vaz R. Long-term clinical and radiological follow-up after laminectomy for cervical spondylotic myelopathy. Surg Neurol Int 2015; 6: 162.
[http://dx.doi.org/10.4103/2152-7806.167211] [PMID: 26543671]

[19]    Oshima Y, Takeshita K, Inanami H, *et al.* Cervical microendoscopic interlaminar decompression through a midline approach in patients with cervical myelopathy: a technical note. J Neurol Surg A Cent Eur Neurosurg 2014; 75(6): 474-8.
[http://dx.doi.org/10.1055/s-0034-1373663] [PMID: 24819630]

[20]    Oshima Y, Seichi A, Takeshita K, *et al.* Natural course and prognostic factors in patients with mild cervical spondylotic myelopathy with increased signal intensity on T2-weighted magnetic resonance imaging. Spine 2012; 37(22): 1909-13.

[http://dx.doi.org/10.1097/BRS.0b013e318259a65b] [PMID: 22511231]

[21]  Kato Y, Iwasaki M, Fuji T, Yonenobu K, Ochi T. Long-term follow-up results of laminectomy for cervical myelopathy caused by ossification of the posterior longitudinal ligament. J Neurosurg 1998; 89(2): 217-23.
[http://dx.doi.org/10.3171/jns.1998.89.2.0217] [PMID: 9688116]

[22]  Phan K, Scherman DB, Xu J, Leung V, Virk S, Mobbs RJ. Laminectomy and fusion *vs* laminoplasty for multi-level cervical myelopathy: a systematic review and meta-analysis. Eur Spine J 2017; 26(1): 94-103.
[http://dx.doi.org/10.1007/s00586-016-4671-5] [PMID: 27342611]

[23]  Yabuki S, Kikuchi S. Endoscopic surgery for cervical myelopathy due to calcification of the ligamentum flavum. J Spinal Disord Tech 2008; 21(7): 518-23.
[http://dx.doi.org/10.1097/BSD.0b013e31815a6151] [PMID: 18836365]

[24]  Yabuki S, Kikuchi S. Endoscopic partial laminectomy for cervical myelopathy. J Neurosurg Spine 2005; 2(2): 170-4.
[http://dx.doi.org/10.3171/spi.2005.2.2.0170] [PMID: 15739529]

[25]  Hitchon PW, Woodroffe RW, Noeller JA, Helland L, Hramakova N, Nourski KV. Anterior and posterior approaches for cervical myelopathy: clinical and radiographic outcomes. Spine 2019; 44(9): 615-23.
[http://dx.doi.org/10.1097/BRS.0000000000002912] [PMID: 30724826]

[26]  Yadav YR, Ratre S, Parihar V, Dubey A, Dubey MN. Endoscopic partial corpectomy using anterior decompression for cervical myelopathy. Neurol India 2018; 66(2): 444-51.
[http://dx.doi.org/10.4103/0028-3886.227270] [PMID: 29547169]

[27]  Yadav YR, Parihar V, Ratre S, Kher Y, Bhatele PR. Endoscopic decompression of cervical spondylotic myelopathy using posterior approach. Neurol India 2014; 62(6): 640-5.
[http://dx.doi.org/10.4103/0028-3886.149388] [PMID: 25591677]

[28]  König SA, Spetzger U. Surgical management of cervical spondylotic myelopathy - indications for anterior, posterior or combined procedures for decompression and stabilisation. Acta Neurochir (Wien) 2014; 156(2): 253-8.
[http://dx.doi.org/10.1007/s00701-013-1955-y] [PMID: 24292777]

[29]  Dahdaleh NS, Wong AP, Smith ZA, Wong RH, Lam SK, Fessler RG. Microendoscopic decompression for cervical spondylotic myelopathy. Neurosurg Focus 2013; 35(1): E8.
[http://dx.doi.org/10.3171/2013.3.FOCUS135] [PMID: 23815253]

[30]  Jho HD. Decompression *via* microsurgical anterior foraminotomy for cervical spondylotic myelopathy. Technical note. J Neurosurg 1997; 86(2): 297-302.
[http://dx.doi.org/10.3171/jns.1997.86.2.0297] [PMID: 9010435]

[31]  Hohmann D, Liebig K. Surgical therapy of spondylogenic cervical myelopathy. Indications and techniques. Orthopade 1996; 25(6): 558-66.

[32]  Casella E, Chiappetta F, Dell'Aquila G, Fiume D, Massari A, Scarda G. Surgical treatment of cervical spondylogenic myelopathy (surgical indications and long-term results). Riv Neurobiol 1979; 25(4): 435-48.
[PMID: 262056]

[33]  Hattori S, Saiki K, Kawai S. Diagnosis of the level and severity of cord lesion in cervical spondylotic myelopathy. Spinal evoked potentials. Spine 1979; 4(6): 478-85.
[http://dx.doi.org/10.1097/00007632-197911000-00005] [PMID: 515838]

[34]  Epstein NE. Laminectomy for cervical myelopathy. Spinal Cord 2003; 41(6): 317-27.
[http://dx.doi.org/10.1038/sj.sc.3101477] [PMID: 12746738]

**CHAPTER 15**

# A Case Series Report of Endoscopic Debridement and Placement of an Intralesional Catheter for Chemotherapy of Cervical Tuberculosis

**Xifeng Zhang[1,*], Bu Rongqiang[1], Yuan Heng[1]** and **Jiang Hongzhen[1]**

[1] *Department of Orthopedics, First Medical Center, PLA General Hospital, Beijing 100853, China*

**Abstract:** The authors present a small case series to demonstrate the feasibility of employing the percutaneous approach to treating cervical spine tuberculosis. They placed a puncture needle under CT-guidance into the abscess to drain and debride pre- and paravertebral and retropharyngeal abscesses with endoscopically assisted technique. A pigtail catheter was placed into the abscess cavity for continuous intralesional delivery of antituberculous chemotherapy. Clinical outcomes were favorable. None of the three patients in this case series report experienced neurological function deterioration or needed more aggressive follow-up surgery. In this chapter, the authors set out to demonstrate the utility of the spinal endoscope in other areas of application distinct from decompression commonly required in degenerative spine disease.

**Keywords:** Cervical tuberculosis, Endoscopic debridement, Intralesional chemotherapy.

## INTRODUCTION

Tuberculosis of the cervical spine can be of devastating consequence to the patient if left untreated. Patients frequently complain of neck pain and stiffness. The fifth vertebral body has been reported as the most commonly involved segment [1]. Multi-drug chemotherapy is still the mainstay of treatment, especially for treating the lower subaxial cervical spine [2]. However, surgical debridement contributions to the overall cure of the disease are still debated [2]. Nevertheless, surgical debridement seems preferred by most spine surgeons. A recent review of the literature, including 456 patients, showed that most of them

---
* **Corresponding author Zhang Xifeng:** Department of Orthopedics, First Medical Center, PLA General Hospital, Beijing 100853, China; Tel: 086-010-5325 9627; E-mails: XifengZhangChina@hotmail.com and 656780949@qq.com

(329; 72.1%) underwent surgical debridement. However, the indication for surgery – particularly aggressive debridement – remains controversial. At the same time, surgery has been linked with better recovery of neurologic function.

The additional use of instrumentation maintained better correction of cervical alignment. This chapter's authors stipulated that the high morbidity [3] associated with aggressive surgical debridement of the anterior cervical spine for retropharyngeal abscess and bony destruction could be decreased by minimally invasive endoscopic debridement and decompression of neural elements.

## CASE 1

The patient is a 19-year-old male with a chief complaint of pain in the neck, both arms and dysphagia and bilateral arm pain for the last two months. He was transferred to our hospital from a local healthcare facility where physicians considered an infection of the cervical spine in the differential diagnosis after review of the initial spinal imaging studies and a failed one-month trial of anti-inflammatory and other supportive care measures. The patient was placed in a rigid halo orthosis while undergoing workup. Advanced imaging studies including computed tomography (CT) and magnetic resonance imaging (MRI) showed abnormal signals and destruction of the cervical three to six vertebral bodies and a paravertebral phlegmon (Figs. 1 and 2). In conjunction with additional laboratory studies the patient was diagnosed tuberculosis of the cervical spine with a paravertebral abscess. The cervical four and five vertebral bodies were severely damaged resulting in progressive focal kyphosis in spite of the external halo fixation.

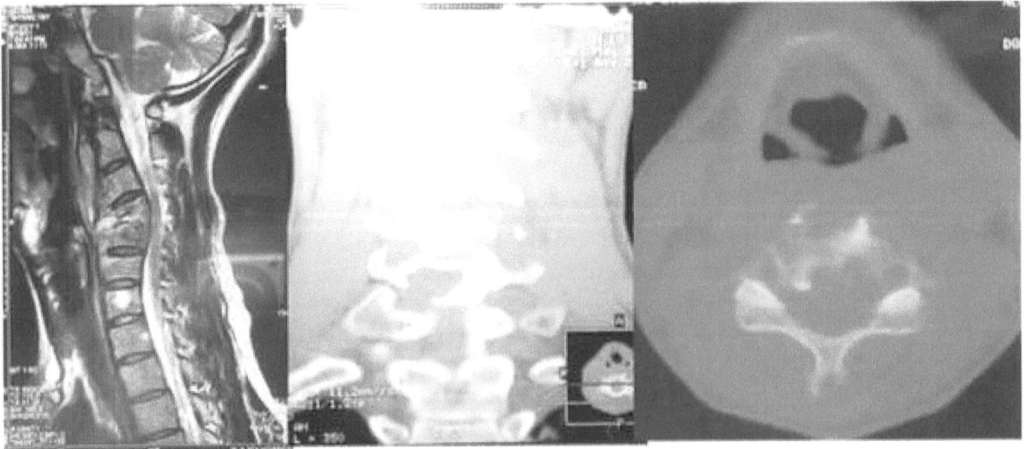

**Fig. (1).** MRI and CT show abnormal signals of C3-6 vertebral body and paravertebral body, and some bone destruction.

The patient underwent anterior minimally invasive endoscopic approach to the infected area in a supine position under general anesthesia. The access was not tricky after initial dissection *via* serial dilation through the tracheoesophageal groove. The abscessed area was lavaged and carefully debrided under direct endoscopic visualization. At the end of the case, a pigtail catheter was placed into the lesion for local intralesional application of antituberculosis chemotherapy. The regional chemotherapy was continued after the operation for three months under the direction of the infectious disease service, who also confirmed the diagnosis. The postoperative MRI scan showed that the retropharyngeal abscess had disappeared after three months of intralesional treatment. Plain films of the cervical spine showed fusion as well. The patient responded favorably to the endoscopic debridement, followed by three-months of intralesional chemotherapy and continued halo immobilization. Postoperative surveillance studies some three-and-a-half years later showed spontaneous fusion of the disease spinal motion segments (Fig. **3**).

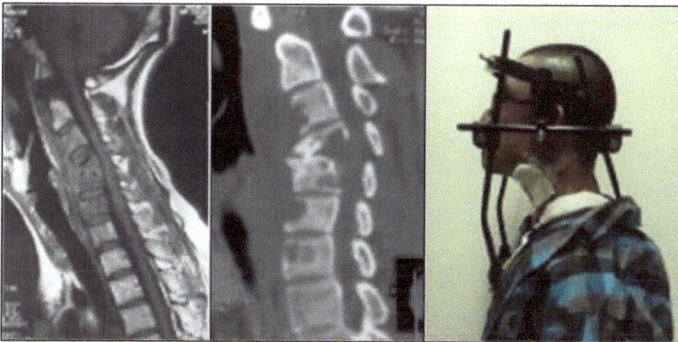

**Fig. (2).** Three months after the operation, MRI showed that the posterior pharynx's abscess disappeared, CT showed that the C4-5 was fused.

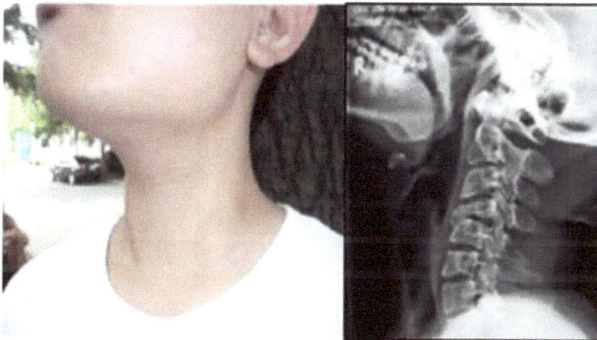

**Fig. (3).** Follow-up examination 3 1/2 years after intervention showed spontaneous fusion with minimal focal kyphosis about the cervical four vertebral body.

## CASE 2

The patient is a 31-year-old male with a chief complaint of neck pain three weeks before admission to our hospital. It worsened significantly in the last week ere admission, during which the patient also had a low-grade fever (38.0°C). Head movements aggravated symptoms. However, there were no paresthesias or motor weakness in any of the extremities. There was no limb numbness and weakness. The patient received supportive conservative care measures at the local hospital, including topical medicine and massage therapy, without relief. After admission to our facility, MRI examination showed cervical 4-5 destruction and a paravertebral abscess (Fig. **4**).

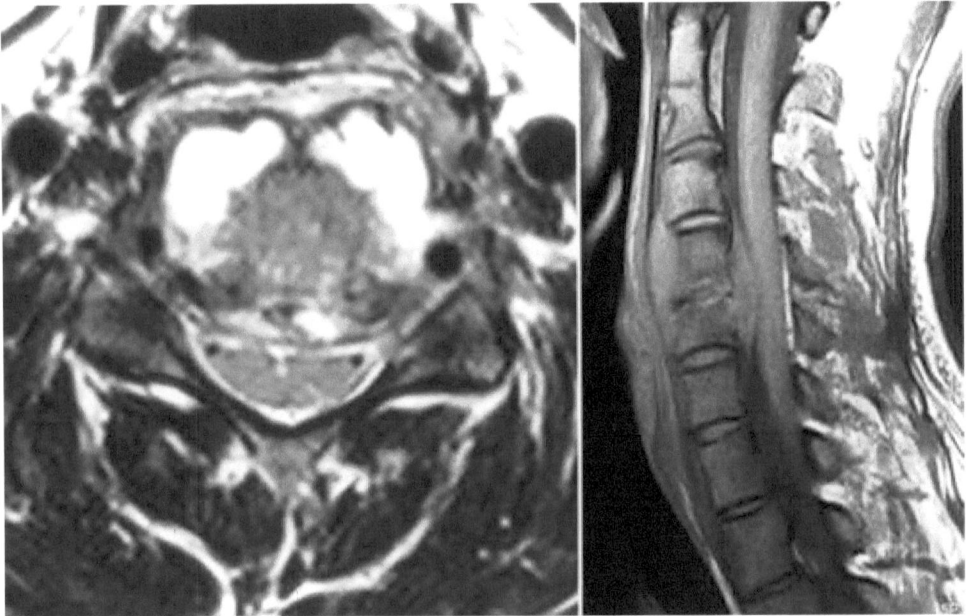

**Fig. (4).** Cervical MRI showed tuberculosis of cervical 4-5 vertebrae with abscess.

The patient had limited neck motion with severe pain provoked by left- and right head rotation and bending. The patient continued to show a normal neurological examination without any upper motor neuron signs. The patient underwent a CT-guided anterior puncture followed by endoscopic debridement and catheterization (Fig. **5**). Although the surgical dissection into the abscess cavity may not be difficult, care should be taken, not injury the content of the carotid sheath or the thyroid. Anti-tuberculous chemotherapy resulted in control of the infection and produced a spontaneous fusion. The pigtail catheter was removed after three months of intralesional treatment, and surveillance MRI suggested cure of the infection (Fig. **6**). At the direction of the infectious disease service, he remained on oral anti-tuberculosis medication for an additional one year after the operation. Two years after the operation, final follow-up films showed resolution of the infection and spontaneous fusion at the C4/5 level (Fig. **7**).

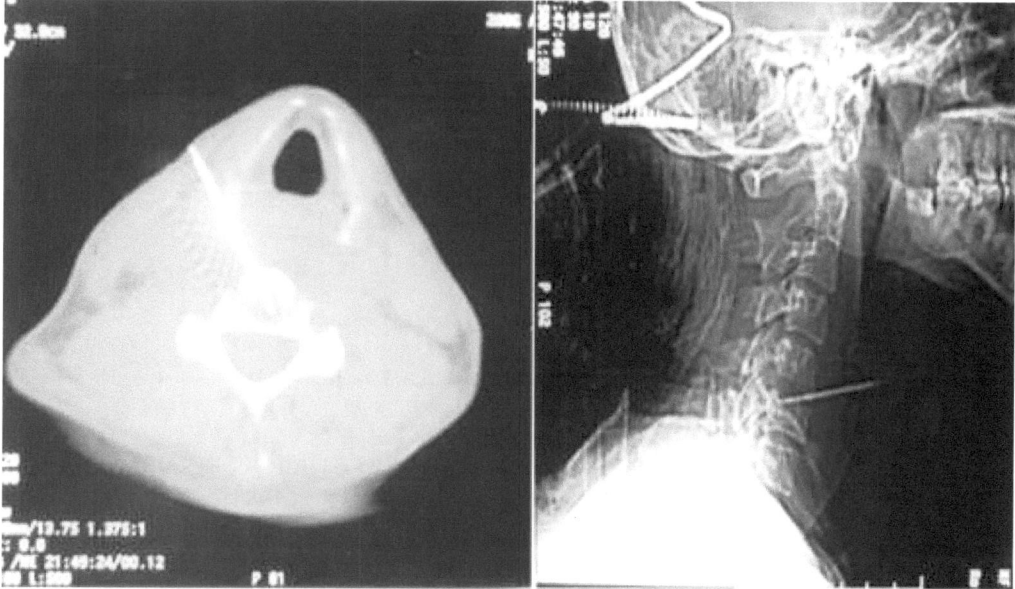

**Fig. (5).** Intraoperative CT positioning phase and horizontal phase puncture to the diseased vertebral body, the puncture position is good.

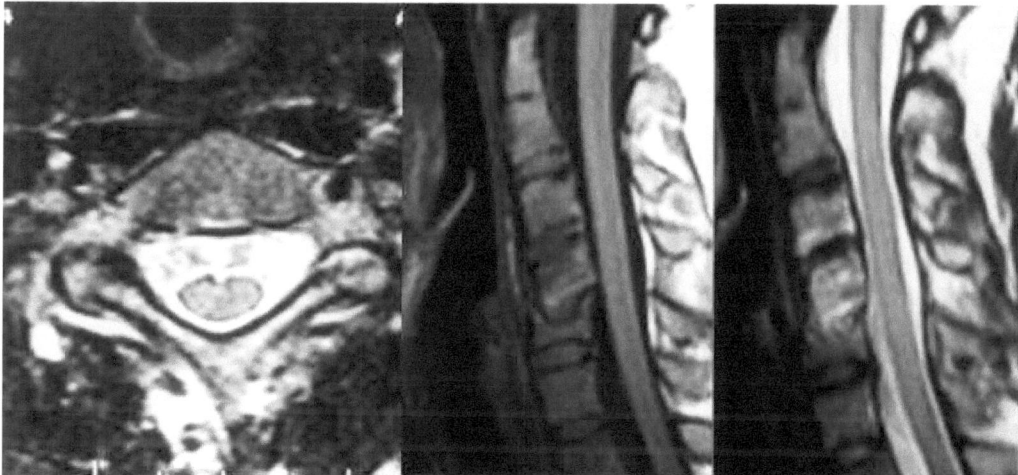

**Fig. (6).** Re-examination of MRI 3 months after surgery showed that the vertebral body was fused at the lesion site and the abscess disappeared.

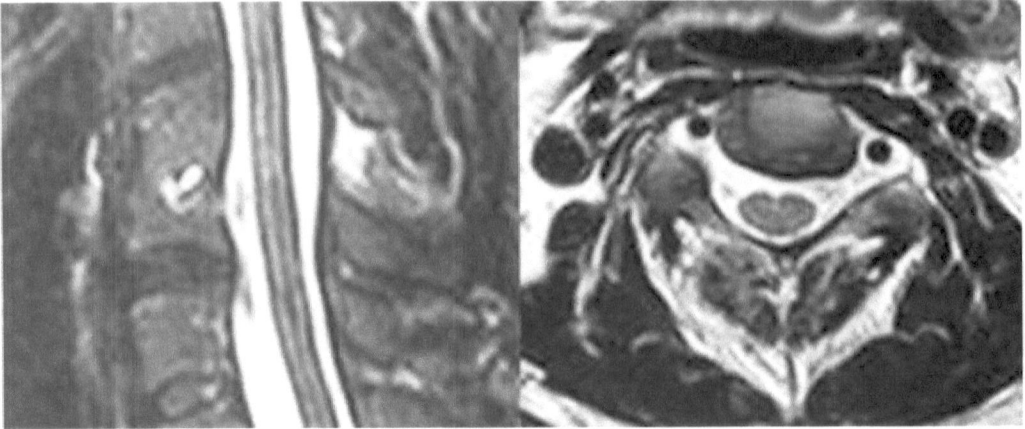

**Fig. (7).** Re-examination of MRI lesions 2 years after operation is stable, and there is no obvious deformity of the cervical spine.

## CASE 3

The patient is a 6-year-old boy with a 3-months chief complaint of neck discomfort and bilateral arm pain. He had slight torticollis to the left when standing. He was treated at a local hospital with anti-rheumatic and calcium supplementation treatments without success. CT and MRI scan of the cervical spine and adjunctive laboratory examinations were suggestive tuberculosis of the C6/7 vertebral level with an associated paravertebral abscess. The MRI scan also demonstrated a substantial prevertebral abscess with a large intracanal component compressing the anterior dural sac (Fig. **8**).

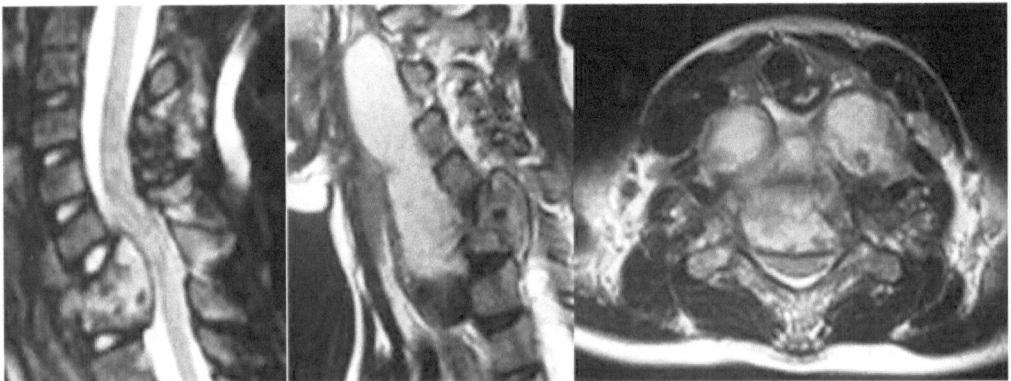

**Fig. (8).** Sagittal and axial MRI scans showed abnormal signals of the cervical vertebral body and paravertebral body, and the C6-7 vertebral body was seriously damaged.

The plain film radiographs showed destruction of the C6 and C7 vertebral body (Fig. **9**). On examination, the boy limited neck movement and severe pain. His neurological examination did not show any paresthesias, normal muscle strength in all four extremities. There were no upper motor neuron signs.

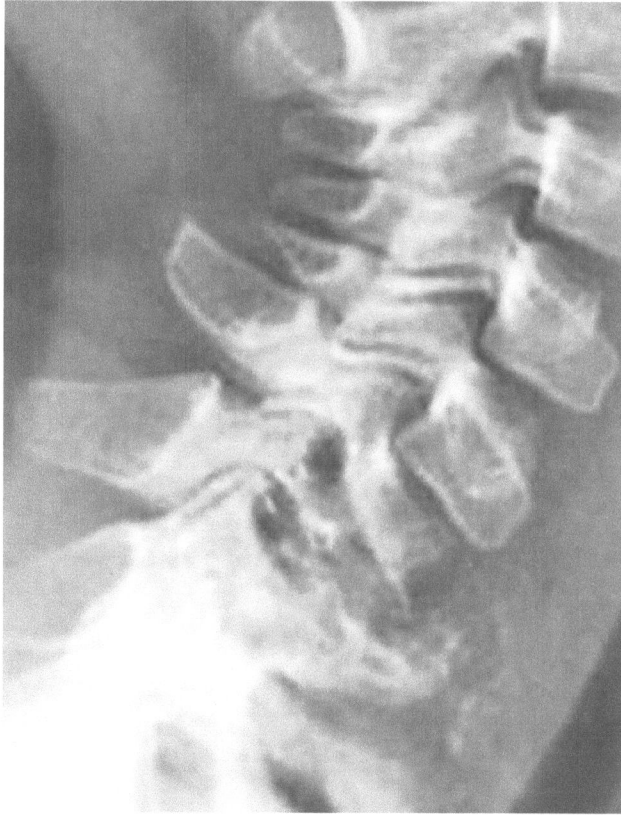

**Fig. (9).** The X-ray shows that C6-7 is severely damaged, the cervical 7 vertebrae almost disappeared, the chest 1 is involved, and the prevertebral space is significantly widened.

The patient was considered minimally invasive drainage and lavage, similar to the methods presented in cases 1 and 2. The treating surgeon feared that the deformity would progress if left untreated, and the patient's neurological function could deteriorate and render him possibly quadriplegic. The initial puncture needle was placed under CT guidance, and the patient underwent endoscopic lavage and drainage to follow. As in the other two patients, the boy was treated with anti-tuberculosis chemotherapy under the direction of the infectious disease service (Fig. **10**). The destruction of the C6 and C7 vertebral body was visualized, and the patient was braced for the next three months to prevent kyphosis and neurological deterioration. Interestingly, the bone loss in the C6 and C7 vertebral body was reconstituted over time. Long-term follow-up imaging studies showed a nearly average growth of the cervical spine without kyphosis some eight years later (Fig.

11).

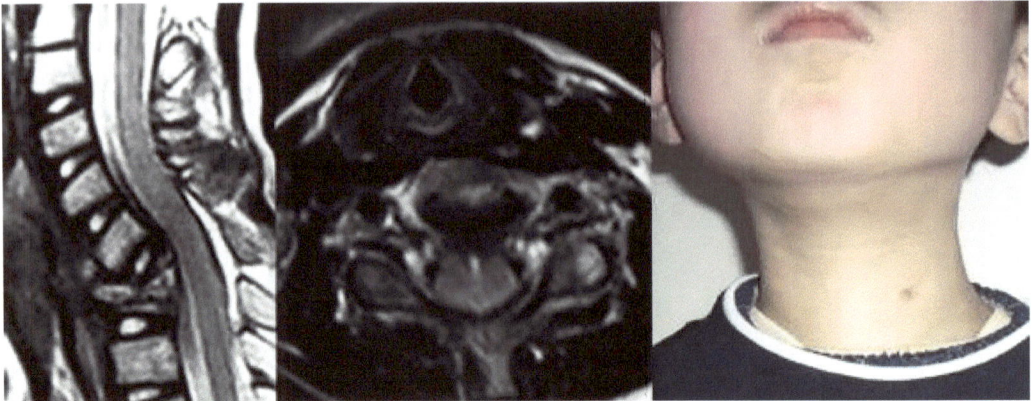

**Fig. (10).** The 1-year follow-up X-ray film showed that the damaged part of the vertebral body was stable and the wound healed well.

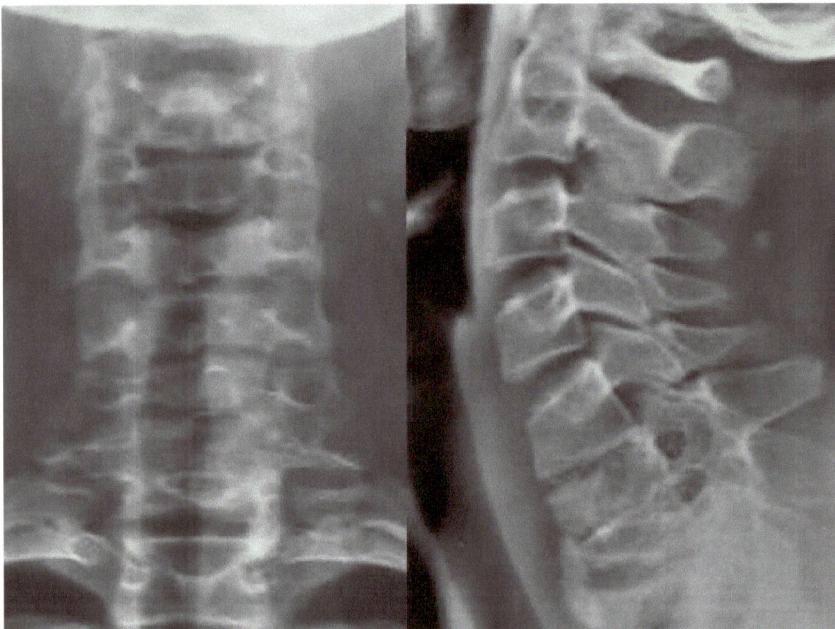

**Fig. (11).** Eight years after the operation, X-rays showed no excessive focal kyphotic deformity. The cervical 7 vertebra appears well healed.

## DISCUSSION

The prior literature indicates that tuberculosis (TB) of the subaxial cervical spine is less common, but it may lead to severe neurological complications if ignored and left untreated. A recent study compared the characteristics of patients with TB of the cervical spine to those of patients TB in other spinal areas [4]. The record review performed by these authors in a tertiary hospital setting provided 51 TB cases of the spine, of which 14 affected the cervical spine. The demographic and clinical data analysis showed that the median age of affected patients was 39 years of age. Multifocal lesions were statistically significantly more common in the cervical spine than in other areas of the spine. Two-thirds of patients eventually required surgery. Clinical outcomes at the final follow-up of 20 months were similar between TB patients with cervical spine involvement *versus* other areas of the spine. However, the authors found that the incidence of disability from deterioration of neurological function was more common in cervical spine TB patients.

All of our patients were treated with the anterior approach to the cervical spine. Its effectiveness has been recently investigated in the treatment of TB affecting the lower cervical spine for cervicothoracic junction [5]. These authors performed lesion removal, bone grafting and internal fixation. Their statistical analysis of clinical outcomes was based on the kyphotic Cobb angle, visual analog scale (VAS), Frankel grade, erythrocyte sedimentation rate (ESR), and C-reactive protein (CRP). In comparison to our minimally invasive approach, these authors performed an open debridement and irrigation at a mean operation time was 145 minutes, and a mean intraoperative blood loss was 425 ml. The time to bony fusion time averaged 7.4 months. In comparison, our patients achieved bony fusion typically within 3 months following a simplified and much shorter endoscopically assisted percutaneous debridement and irrigation. While our case series report is obviously limited by a small number of cases and was merely intended to demonstrate feasibility of the endoscopic technique to offer patients a simplified treatment of a disease that can take on a complicated course with potential for spinal deformity, neurological deficits, and complications if intervention is instituted. For example, the complication rate in the study provided by Li *et al.* [5] was 25% within the first three postoperative months. While there is no doubt that the anterior approach to treat TB of the cervical spine is the most effective approach since the disease process plays out predominantly in the anterior column, the endoscopic debridement with placement of a pigtail cather allowing continuous irrigation may be an attractive alternative to open treatment. It should be considered at least in the initial treatment of cervical spine TB to control the disease. The authors of this chapter recommend to consider aggressive treatments if the initial endoscopically assisted debridement fails.

The successful treatment in our three cases shows that local catheterization and irrigation and local intralesional chemotherapy have apparent advantages in treating cervical tuberculosis. Minimally invasive and endoscopic surgery with continuous perfusion and drainage reduces tuberculosis lesions. It drains the paravertebral abscesses and the posterior pharynx, reduces the abscess on the spinal cord and throat, and relieves the symptoms of numbness and dysphagia in the upper extremities. Continuous local chemotherapy can cure Mycobacterium tuberculosis, inhibit the pathogenic factors that form the sinus. Compared with traditional open surgery, patients with cervical spine tuberculosis who underwent minimally invasive surgery may be successfully treated with just a cervical collar and can be mobilized early. Only one of our three patients was treated in a halo-vest as this treatment was started in a local hospital before the referral to our institution. None of our patients underwent additional radical surgery, thus, avoiding the complications common to radical surgery. Other advantages are less pain, shorter hospitalization time, and faster treatment course. The authors emphasize that aggressive removal of dead bone should be avoided during the initial endoscopic debridement since it was intended to serve as a bone graft incorporated into the anterior column fusion.

## CONCLUSIONS

The tuberculosis of the cervical spine is by far less common than in the thoracolumbar spine. Approximately one-quarter of all spinal tuberculosis cases affect the cervical spine. If left untreated, the disease process can be aggressive and preferentially destroy the anterior column, leading to kyphosis with a deterioration of neurological function. The anterior approach affords the surgeon the ability to debride, irrigate, and reconstruct the cervical spine. Nearly one-quarter of patients undergoing open anterior approach in the surgical treatment of cervical spine TB may experience complications within the first three postoperative months. Therefore, the authors recommend considering percutaneous endoscopically assisted debridement of the TB lesions and any associated paraspinal or retropharyngeal abscesses with a pigtail catheter's intralesional placement continuous delivery of anti-tuberculous chemotherapy as an alternative to open approaches. Although our case series is small, none of the patients required reconstruction of the anterior column with bone graft and instrumentation. Therefore, the authors will continue to investigate our technique's feasibility as an initial treatment with the intent of reserving open surgery only for those patients in whom the initial endoscopic treatment failed.

## CONSENT FOR PUBLICATION

Not applicable.

## CONFLICT OF INTEREST

The author declares no conflict of interest, financial or otherwise.

## ACKNOWLEDGEMENTS

Declared none.

## REFERENCES

[1]    Yin XH, He BR, Liu ZK, Hao DJ. The clinical outcomes and surgical strategy for cervical spine tuberculosis: A retrospective study in 78 cases. Medicine (Baltimore) 2018; 97(27): e11401.
[http://dx.doi.org/10.1097/MD.0000000000011401] [PMID: 29979434]

[2]    Wu W, Li Z, Lin R, Zhang H, Lin J. Anterior debridement, decompression, fusion and instrumentation for lower cervical spine tuberculosis. J Orthop Sci 2020; 25(3): 400-4.
[http://dx.doi.org/10.1016/j.jos.2019.06.008] [PMID: 31262450]

[3]    Srivastava S, Raj A, Bhosale S, Purohit S, Marathe N, Shah S. Does kyphosis in healed subaxial cervical spine tuberculosis equate to a poor functional outcome? J Craniovertebr Junction Spine 2020; 11(2): 86-92.
[http://dx.doi.org/10.4103/jcvjs.JCVJS_53_20] [PMID: 32904986]

[4]    Pourbaix A, Zarrouk V, Allaham W, *et al.* More complications in cervical than in non-cervical spine tuberculosis. Infect Dis (Lond) 2020; 52(3): 170-6.
[http://dx.doi.org/10.1080/23744235.2019.1690675] [PMID: 31718363]

[5]    Li Z, Li K, Tang B, *et al.* Analysis of the curative effect of the anterior approach to the lower cervical spine for cervicothoracic spinal tuberculosis. J Craniofac Surg 2020; 31(2): 480-3.
[http://dx.doi.org/10.1097/SCS.0000000000006097] [PMID: 31895841]

# CHAPTER 16

# Cervical Endoscopic Spinal Surgery: Sequela, Failure to Cure, Complications and Their Management

**Kai-Uwe Lewandrowski[1,2,3,*], Xi Jiancheng, Zheng Zeze[4], Wang Yipeng[4], Li Jinlong[4], Jiang Hongzhen[4], Stefan Hellinger[5] and Hyeun Sung Kim[6,7,8,9,10]**

[1] *Center for Advanced Spine Care of Southern Arizona and Surgical Institute of Tucson, Tucson, AZ, USA*

[2] *Department of Orthopaedic Surgery, UNIRIO, Rio de Janeiro, Brazil*

[3] *Department of Orthoapedic Surgery, Fundación Universitaria Sanitas, Bogotá, D.C., Colombia, USA*

[4] *Department of Orthopedics, The Eighth Medical Center, PLA General Hospital, 100091 Beijing, China;*

[5] *Department of Orthopedic and Spine Surgery, Arabellaklinik, Munich, Germany*

[6] *Department of Neurosurgery, Nanoori Gangnam Hospital, Seoul, Republic of Korea*

[7] *A President of the Korean Research Society of the Endoscopic Spine Surgery (KOSESS), South Korea*

[8] *A Faculty of the KOrean Minimally Invasive Spine Surgery Society (KOMISS), South Korea*

[9] *A Chairman of the Nanoori Hospital Group Scientific Team, South Korea*

[10] *An Adjunct Professor of the Medical College of the Chosun University, Gwangju, South Korea*

**Abstract:** Sequelae and complications following endoscopic surgery of the cervical spine are rare. They may range from neuropraxia, temporary and self-limiting loss of sensation, motor strength, loss of the voice due to recurrent laryngeal nerve injury, vascular and dural leaks to full-blown spinal cord injury with tetraplegia in the worst cases. In this chapter, the authors systematically review the most concerning problems the endoscopic spine surgeon may run into and discuss their management in the context of the most up-to-date peer-reviewed literature. Surgeon training and high skill level are of the utmost importance in minimizing potentially grave outcomes from the cervical spine's endoscopic spine surgery.

* **Corresponding author Kai-Uwe Lewandrowski:** Center for Advanced Spine Care of Southern Arizona and Surgical Institute of Tucson, Tucson, AZ, USA, Department of Orthopaedic Surgery, UNIRIO, Rio de Janeiro, Brazil and Department of Orthoapedic Surgery, Fundación Universitaria Sanitas, Bogotá, D.C., Colombia, USA; Tel: +1 520 204-1495; Fax: +1 623 218-1215; E-mail: business@tucsonspine.com

**Keywords:** Cervical endoscopy, Complications, Failure to cure, Sequela.

## INTROCUTION

The authors trust that the readers of Contemporary Spinal Endoscopy: Cervical Spine Vol. 1 would not consider their text complete unless there was some discussion of sequela, failure-to-cure scenarios, and complications that could occur during anterior and posterior cervical endoscopy. The endoscopic spine surgeon could encounter any of those in routine clinical practice. Therefore, the authors deem it necessary to discuss some of the pitfalls one should understand and be prepared to manage. They range from incomplete decompression with failure to cure, sequelae defined as unavoidable side effects from an expertly executed surgery, such as neuropraxia or dysesthesia, to outright complications including vascular injury to the carotid sheath or its tributaries, vagal nerve damage, loss of voice, cervical dural tears, and nerve root injuries, and last but not least damage to injury of the cervical spinal cord with grave neurological deficit. While arterial injury can quickly deteriorate into a life-threatening situation that calls for rapid and prompt exploration and intervention with surgical repair, spinal cord injury is undoubtedly the most devastating complication one could encounter as a result of an elective palliative procedure intended to diminish pain. These most severe complications are uncommon to the point where not every one of this chapter's authors has had a case. Therefore, they will present problematic cases that they did have and discuss other problems at least from a theoretical point of view by reviewing the published peer-reviewed literature. Therefore, this chapter is intended to discuss the anatomical basis for peri- and postoperative problems and suggest management protocols the endoscopic spine surgeon should have implemented before embarking on a routine cervical spine endoscopic surgery program.

## THE REFERENCES STANDARDS

Using anterior cervical discectomy and fusion as a standard for comparison with anterior cervical endoscopy, the overall morbidity rates for ACDF has neem published to be in the range from 13.2% to 19.3% [1]. In descending order, common problems with the ACDF surgery are dysphagia (1.7%-9.5%), postoperative hematoma requiring additional surgery (2.4% of 5.6%), epidural hematoma (0.9%), exacerbation of myelopathy (0.2%-3.3%), symptomatic recurrent laryngeal nerve palsy (0.9%-3.1%), cerebrospinal fluid (CSF) leak (0.5%-1.7%), wound infection (0.1-0.9%-1.6%), increased radiculopathy (1.3%), Horner's syndrome (0.06%-1.1%), respiratory insufficiency (1.1%), esophageal perforation (0.3%-0.9%, with a mortality rate of 0.1%), and instrument failure (0.1%-0.9%) [1]. Internal jugular vein occlusion and a phrenic nerve injury were only reported in case reports. Pseudarthrosis with ACDF reportedly is dependent on the number of levels fused and may range between 0 to 4.3% (1-level), 24% (2-level), 42% (3 levels) to 56% (4 levels). The reported reoperation rate for symptomatic pseudarthrosis is 11.1%. Readmission rates for ACDF may range from 5.1% (30 days) to 7.7% (90 days postoperatively).

The comparison numbers for posterior cervical foraminotomy have been studied by Skovrij *et al.* who reported the overall complication rates with the minimally invasive version of the posterior foraminotomy as 4.3% [2]. Their study of 70 patients reported 3 patients with complications – 1 patient with a cerebrospinal fluid leak, 1 patient with a postoperative wound hematoma, and another patient with radiculitis. The reoperation rate with ACDF for failure to cure was 7.14% (5/70 patients). Platt *et al.* performed a comparison of outcomes following minimally invasive and open posterior cervical foraminotomy in a systematic review of the literature describing minimally invasive techniques [3]. Employing the Preferred Reporting Items for Systematic Reviews and Meta-Analysis (PRISMA) guidelines the authors searched the PubMed, Cochrane Library, and Scopus libraries for clinical studies comparing minimally invasive posterior cervical foraminotomy (MIS-PCF) to open posterior cervical foraminotomy or percutaneous endoscopic (full-endoscopic) posterior cervical foraminotomy (FE-PCF). A total of 178 abstracts were identified of which 79 full text articles were evaluated. Articles describing laser decompressions or anterior endoscopic techniques were excluded. Platt *et al.* were able to identify 6 eligible studies comparing open to MIS-PCF, including one randomized controlled trial [4 - 9]. Two studies were included in their analysis that compared minimally invasive tubular retractor based posterior cervical foraminotomy to full endoscopic cervical foraminotomy and discectomy [5, 7]. Fessler *et al.* reported no reoperations and three cerebrospinal fluid (CSF) leaks as the only complication in the minimally invasive group including two CSF leaks and one partial thickness dural violation *versus* no complications in the open group [5]. Kim *et al.* (in 2009) had no complications in either group [7]. The complication rates were not statistically different between MIS and open in Winder's *et al.* study [9]. However, reoperations were not specified in three of five studies did not include reoperations [7 - 9]. Another meta-analysis by Fang *et al.* employing the same PRISMA criteria [10, 11] and the Newcastle-Ottawa Scale (NOS) criteria [12] of quality assessment of non-randomized comparative studies [13]. Fang *et al.* found 506 relevant studies, excluded 320 duplicate and 277 irrelevant studies were excluded arriving at 15 studies including 54107 cases which met the the authors predefined inclusion criteria. Three of them were randomized controlled trials [14 - 16], and the other 12 studies were non-randomized comparative studies [17 - 28]. The portion of Fang's meta-analysis relevant for this review of complications with anterior and posterior cervical approaches for cervical radiculopathy revealed

11 studies [15, 17, 19 - 21, 23, 25 - 28]. There was no statistically significant difference in the complication rate between the two groups (P = 0.60, OR 1.15, 95%CI 0.68 to 1.94). The included studies' total complication rate was 4.23% in the ACDF group and 4.55% in the PCF group. Unfortunately, the breakdown of complication- and reoperation rates with PCF is not as detailed in the available literature as with ACDF. However, a brief review of the available data gives the reader of this chapter somewhat of an understanding of the reported rates of some negative fallout with commonly performed surgeries in the treatment of cervical radiculopathy regardless of whether considering sequelae, complication, or failure to cure. It intended to help the endoscopic spine surgeons position the clinical outcomes with their cervical endoscopic spinal surgery program by comparing it to these reported benchmarks.

## ACCESS & WOUND PROBLEMS

Wound problems by the very nature of the ultra-minimally invasive anterior and posterior endoscopic spinal surgery are uncommon—most studies on cervical endoscopy report that their authors did not encounter superficial wound or incisional complications. Infections are unheard of. This chapter's authors could only find one case report where wound infection was mentioned as a possible complication associated with traditional open surgery but not with anterior endoscopic cervical spine decompression [29]. A larger series of 103 endoscopic cervical spine surgery patients reported by Papavero *et al.* indicated one patient with a posterior cervical wound infection [30]. Hematomas are more likely to occur as they have been reported with the transcorporal anterior discectomy [31, 32]. As a result, proponents of this surgical technique suggested applying bone wax to the bony transcorporal drill channel for hemostasis [33]. Posterior endoscopic is also rarely associated with a wound hematoma, but the Papavero study also reports one patient in whom this postoperative complication had occurred [30].

## SEQUALAE

A sequala is considered an unavoidable side-effect or postoperative problem that may occur despite an expertly executed operation. While sequelae such as dysesthesia with increased pain and neuropraxia with postoperative muscle weakness may occur as a result of any operation in the cervical spine aimed at alleviating compression on the symptomatic neural elements, the occurrence and management should be discussed with the patients preoperatively so they are not caught off guard when such problems should arise after surgery. The aforementioned comparative study by Xiao *et al.* on a total of 84 patients – 40 of which had a standard posterior full endoscopic decompression and 44 patients underwent partial pediculectomy during the posterior full endoscopic cervical discectomy (PECD) – determined that the complication rate is substantially lower with the pediculectomy (4.55%) *versus* the standard full endoscopic posterior discectomy surgery (10.0%) [34]. Patients of that study experienced a postoperative increase of numbness (2 patients), pain (1 patient), and weakness (1 patient) with the conventional PECD. The two patients who underwent PECD with partial pediculectomy had a postoperative increase in pain and numbness. Their symptoms were resolved with supportive care measures within three days *versus* seven days in the conventional PECD group. The one patient with motor weakness recovered within six months. This patient underwent conventional PECD. Choi conceptualized that the C5 nerve root is most sensitive to motor palsy after PECD since it typically covers the entire disc space and therefore needs sustained retraction than any other of the cervical nerve roots [35]. Youn *et al.* (11) stipulated that removal of an extruded disc or bony spur requires excessive retraction, thus, setting the stage for motor palsy [36]. These authors concluded that the risk of transient root injury may be increased due to root retraction without discectomy. Lee *et al.* also reported on transient motor weakness and transient sensory changes after posterior cervical foraminotomy and attributed it to excessive traction, mechanical injury during drilling, or possibly thermal injury during PECD [37]. The drilling of the caudal pedicle's superomedial quadrant improves access to the ventral pathology, thus minimizing traction injury-related neuropraxia. The irrigation fluid used during cervical endoscopy may also contribute to improved clarity of the magnified and directly visualized operative field and degrease infection, and enhanced hemostasis because of positive hydraulic pressure of the water column in the semi-open endoscopic spine system. Compared to the static visual field often employed during microendoscopy or microsurgical decompression with the operative microscope, the PECD with cervical endoscopes with off-center viewing angles allows the surgeon to adjust the visualized operative field easily. Thus, surgical trauma to the nerve root may be further minimized with the endoscopy, particularly in conjunction with the partial pediculolectomy procedure. The endoscope may not retract the root as much and is not placed continuously in the same position for prolonged periods. The authors of this chapter advocate employing the partial pediculectomy (described in a different chapter of this textbook) as it could provide enough space for the endoscope to be inserted more, reducing the manipulation of the nerve root required to expose the cervical intervertebral disc and making the procedure safer.

## RECURRENT LARYNGEAL NERVE

Although injury to the recurrent laryngeal nerve (RLN) could be considered a sequela rather than a complication since it is mostly related to sometimes unavoidable prolonged pressure or overstretching [38], most surgeons would categorize it as a complication since the it at least on a theoretical level is perhaps avoidable by employing careful dissection techniques and minimizing retraction of the surgical field [1]. However, during endoscopy and in particular during the initial dissection with serial dilation injury to the RLN could occur. Anatomically the RLN branches of the vagus nerve (CN X) carrying sensory, motor, and parasympathetic fibers into the larynx as the main motor nerve to all of the intrinsic laryngeal muscles with the exception of the cricothyroid, which is innervated by the external laryngeal nerve [39]. With RLN injury being the most common iatrogenic complications associated with any neck surgery [40], the clinical fallout may be temporary or permanent with recovery of symptoms being quite variable depending on the severity of the nerve injury. Bilateral RLN damage produces more significant loss of function including hypophonation, and in rare cases, dyspnea by paralyzing the muscles of the larynx [40]. Unilateral vocal cord paralysis due to RLN injury may be clinically silent and therefore be underdiagnosed. However, it may also present as hypophonia, dysphonia, or dysphagia and aspiration [41]. Many patients undergo multiple anterior cervical surgeries over the years. The endoscopic spine surgeon should consider oropharyngeal visualization of the vocal cords by an ear nose and throat (ENT) specialist should there be any concern about the patient's vocal cord function. This ENT consultation should be considered in any patient with any previous surgery or radiation in the head-and-neck region for cancerous tumors. Such a protocol may not only improve patient care by providing proper preoperative counseling and education, but it may also lower the medicolegal exposure the endoscopic spine surgeon may incur as a result of RLN injury.

There has been a great deal of discussion on the relevancy of the anatomical variations of the RLN in the tracheoesophageal groove as because the left RLN has a longer run into the thoracic region as it loops around the arch of the aorta below the ligamentum arteriosum *versus* on the right side around the subclavian artery before looping back up into the larynx to the inferior pharyngeal constrictor muscle [39, 42]. These anatomical variations have been explained with their different embryonic origin [39] the right RLN taking a more anterior and lateral course than on the left. Initial studies seem to suggest lower RLN injury rates on the left side during ACDF procedures which have subsequently been debunked [43 - 45].

The RLN may be at risk during the anterior endoscopic cervical surgeries and safely avoiding it may prove difficult because of its anatomical variations which may also play out bilaterally in one and the same patient [44]. Moreover, the RLN was shown to be more like a plexus rather than a solitary nerve making it potentially even more vulnerable during the endoscopic cervical surgery [43 - 45].

The stipulation that risk of injury to the RLN should be minimized by properly identifying it seems obvious and may work for open- or other forms of cervical spine surgery but proves impractical for the anterior endoscopic access to the cervical spine. Thomas *et al.* published a cadaver-based study to better understand the relationship between the RLN and other anatomical structures in order to improve the safety of neck surgeries [46]. Their cadaveric studies' findings demonstrated that there is a significant amount of variation in the course and branching pattern of the RLN. The authors found 89% of right RLNs and 74.6% of left RLNs demonstrated 2–5 extra-laryngeal branches [46] – an observation that may be relevant to patients considering anterior endoscopic spine surgery. It suggests that phonation problems due to RLN injury following endoscopic surgery in the anterior cervical spine may occur at lower incidence due to the small tissue dissection and surgical trauma but may also have a better prognosis since multiple "back-up" systems exist that may not be affected by the minimal endoscopic surgical dissection. However, this chapter's authors could not find any peer-reviewed publication that studied the incidence of RLN injury specifically during anterior endoscopic cervical spine surgery.

The gold standard anterior cervical operation – the Anterior cervical discectomy and fusion (ACDF) – is associated with a reported incidence of RLN injury ranging from 0.2–16.7% [47]. A recent meta-analysis by Oh *et al.* included 5 studies [48 - 52] totaling 3,514 patients which they chose from a total of 319 studies found that 41 of these 3,514 patients (1.2%) experienced postoperative symptoms due to RLN injury. Broken down by number of levels operated, two-level ACDF patients (1,162/3,514) RLN palsy was present in 18 (1.55%) cases. Of the single-level procedures (2,144/3,514), 23 patients (1.07%) had a RLN palsy. Employing fixed effect modelling the authors did not find a statistically significant difference between RLN palsy rates for two- or single-level ACDF (OR 1.36; 95% CI: 0.73–2.55; P=0.331; I2=0%). The multiple-level ACDF RLN injury rate was not statistically different to the single-level ACDF rate (OR 1.04; 95% CI: 0.56–1.95; P=0.891, I2=0%) [47]. These benchmark numbers should be used as a gold reference standard for the anterior endoscopic cervical surgery where RLN injury rates should if anything be lower and not higher than with ACDF.

**DURAL LEAK**

Dural injury from either the anterior or the posterior endoscopic approach is undoubtedly a practical consideration. Every spine surgeon attempting to decompress cervical spinal pathology should be prepared to deal with an accidental CSF leak. Reports in the published peer-reviewed literature suggest that this complication is relatively rare. In the same series of 103 patients in whom

Papavera *et al.* had performed a posterior endoscopic cervical decompression, the authors had encountered an incidental durotomy thankfully only in one patient [30]. In 2018, Ruetten *et al.* also described an incidental durotomy encountered during uniportal full-endoscopic posterior cervical foraminotomy and discectomy in their series of 7 patients. Some authors perform an epidurogram during the endoscopic procedure, which at least theoretically carries the risk of a dural injury and CSF leak [53]. Another study by Xiao *et al.* employing a modified posterior endoscopic keyhole technique recommended a partial pediculolectomy to take the endoscopic decompression instruments further lateral and way from the spinal cord. This modified technique resulted in none of the 84 patients suffering from an incidental dural leak [34]. There is no uniform strategy to manage dural tears encountered during the full endoscopic cervical spine surgery in part due to their low incidence. Depending on the location and the durotomy's size and the severity of the associated leakage of cerebrospinal fluid (CSF), rootlet- or cord herniation through the durotomy site, aggressive management may not be required. Proposed management strategies range from observation, placement of Duragen™ or Gelfoam™ patches to simply cover the defect, to conversion to open repair should neurological function deteriorate, spinal headaches or any associated CSF leakage through the wound be unmanageable with conservative care measures. It is evident that this aspect of full endoscopic surgery of the cervical spine will likely get more attention and will require more research to determine the appropriate course of action as more such cases are performed.

## INCOMPLETE DECOMPRESSION & FAILURE TO CURE

Both the anterior and posterior surgical access corridors have anatomical restrictions that may limit the surgeons' ability to completely decompress the offending pathology causing radicular neck, shoulder- and arm pain or myelopathy symptoms due to spinal cord compression and its subsequent dysfunction syndromes. The anterior endoscopic approach to the cervical spine exploits the tracheoesophageal groove to leave the carotid sheath's content laterally safely, and the esophagus and trachea medially. The sternocleidoid muscle may pose additional approach-related restrictions if it is contracted. The transdiscal anterior cervical endoscopic discectomy traverses the cervical disc space, narrowing to the advanced degenerative process resulting in vertical collapse. Hence, maneuvering the endoscope inside the disc space medial-to-lateral or superior-to-inferior in relation to the compressive pathology may be limited. Typically, the compressive lesion is approached from the opposite side to minimize these problems. For example, a left-sided C5/6 uncovertebral osteophyte causing axillary nerve root compression of the exiting C6 nerve root may be best approached from the right side. A right-sided problem should be approached from the right side *etc.* By comparison, the limitations of the posterior approach appear less restrictive. However, extensive bony hypertrophy of the surgical cervical facet joint complex may overwhelm the endoscopic systems' ability to adequately decompress the compressive pathology that is causing a shoulder-type nerve root compression syndrome of the exiting nerve root.

It is clear that all of these considerations may impede the surgeons' ability to carry out an adequate decompression and that incomplete decompression may result, thus, setting the stay for incomplete or delayed recovery or reoperations. This was demonstrated in a retrospective study by Ahn *et al.*, who reported on their clinical outcomes and radiographic changes, including the disc height, the sagittal cervical alignment, and the segmental range of motion after percutaneous endoscopic cervical discectomy (PECD) with high-resolution full endoscopy performed on 36 consecutive patients for herniated discs [54]. The mean follow-up period in Ahn's study was 28.6 months. Employing the Prolo Scale criteria, excellent outcomes were achieved in 52.8% (19 of 36 patients), good outcomes in 33.3% (12 of 26), fair outcomes in 8.3% (3 of 36 patients), and poor outcomes in 5.6% (2 of 26 patients). The authors found that the disc height significantly decreased by 11.2% of the original height (p < 0.001). The authors found that the overall and focal sagittal alignments remained well maintained without postoperative development segmental instability or spontaneous fusion. However, in one patient, an open revision surgery had to be performed as the decompression achieved during the endoscopic index surgery was incomplete. An illustrative case by one of the co-authors of this chapter is shown in Fig. (**1**).

Given the paucity of literature on incomplete decompression with the cervical endoscopy one can only estimate the across-the-board relevancy of this problem. The authors of this chapter could not find any literature regarding incomplete decompression with the cervical endoscopy. As this ultra-minimally spinal surgery technique gains more traction with younger generation surgeons and its patient-self-reported and clinical outcome data become more available it will likely become clearer as to how dependent cervical endoscopy is on surgeon skill level or by the complexity of the underlying cervical pathology to be tackled with *via* one of the two endoscopic approaches. Certainly, there is a learning curve and surgeons should be prepared for having to revise some of their patients with alternative decompression techniques early on until they master the procedure and learn how to overcome difficulty and achieve consistent clinical improvements with the procedure.

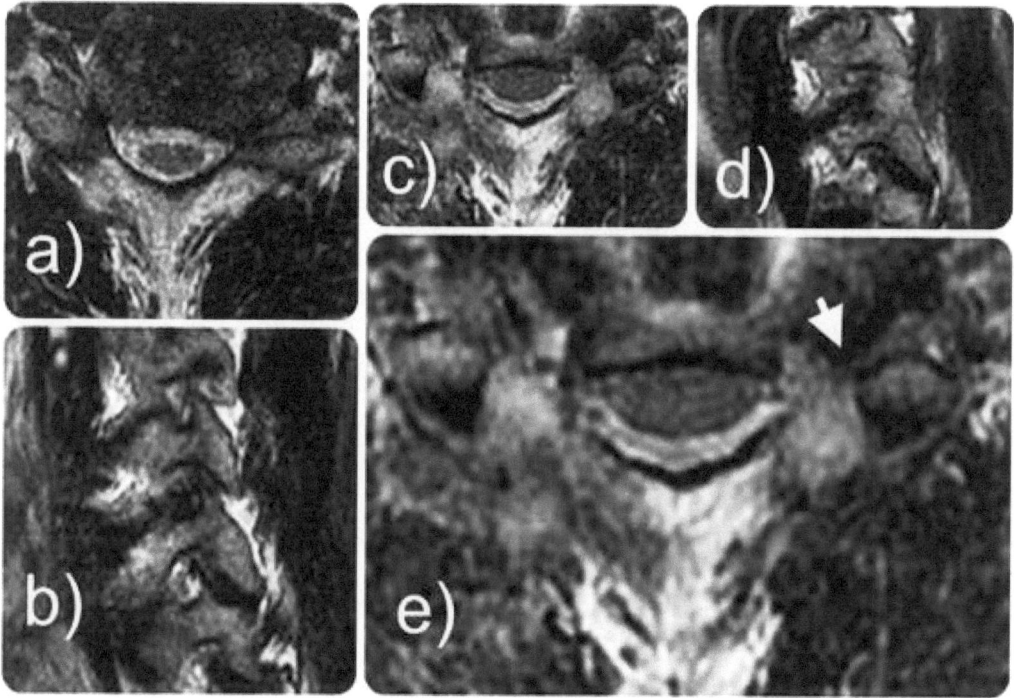

**Fig. (1).** Shown is an illustrative case example of incomplete endoscopic decompression with posterior endoscopic cervical discectomy (PECD) in a 45-year male patient. The preoperative axial **(a)** and sagittal **(b)** MRI scan were compared to postoperative axial **(c)** and sagittal **(d)** scans since the patient did not improve. These postoperative scans showed residual compressive pathology **(c-d)** more lateral in the surgical neuroforamen. The patient underwent an additional posterior cervical decompression employing a tubular retractor system **e**.

## VASCULAR INJURY

The anterior endoscopic approach requires to traverse the content of the tracheoesophageal groove requires and places the content of the carotid sheath, the trachea and the esophagus at risk for injury during serial dilation and final placement of the endoscopic working cannula. Dilators should be tapered to avoid accidental trapping and subsequent cutting of vital structure between the various dilation tubes. The beveled tip of the endoscopic working cannula may act as a cutting blade and cause injury to vital structures as in our case and should be inserted very carefully and slowly to make sure no soft tissue is accidentally entrapped or cut. The authors recommend performing the anterior endoscopic surgery only on one surgical level. Multilevel endoscopic decompressions are conceivably possible but increase the probability of injuring a branch of the carotid artery or jugular vein system that horizontally crosses the surgical field. Moreover, the authors recommend endoscopic discectomy only for soft herniations and advise surgeons to apply extra caution in case of multilevel decompressions. Patients should be scrutinized preoperatively in the office to ensure their carotid pulse can be palpated, particularly in patients with a short stubby neck. Each surgeon should use the best judgment to select patients for the anterior endoscopic discectomy. Considering the potential for life-threatening injury and grave outcome, patients should be considered for alternative decompression surgeries should there be any doubt that the anterior endoscopic discectomy surgery cannot be safely carried out or would be plagued by any additional risk factors that cannot be easily controlled during surgery.

Two of the authors (XiJ & SH) of this chapter had to manage a vascular injury in their cervical endoscopic spinal surgery practice. An illustrative case of a 47-yea--old female who complained of pain and discomfort in the neck, shoulder, and left upper extremity for the past one year and worsening symptoms for the last one month before admission to the hospital department with cervical spondylopathy. Physical examination on admission showed straightening of the cervical spine without pronounced kyphosis, scoliosis, torticollis, or any other deformity about the cervical spine without atrophy of the limbs. She complained of slight tenderness in the neck, shoulder, and back of the neck on bilaterally. Left lateral bending and rotation provoked increasing numbness and dysesthesias in the left arm radiating into the radial forearm, the thumb, the index finger, and the middle finger. There was pronounced left-sided biceps reflex weakness. The left brachial plexus traction test, left intervertebral foramina compression test, intervertebral foraminal separation test, and axial compression test were all positive. Bilateral Babinski's signs were negative. Other upper motor neuron signs, including Hoffmann sign, sustained ankle- and patella clonus, were also negative.

A radiographic cervical spine series showed a loss of the cervical spine's physiological curvature with straightening. Anterior and posterior osteophytes changed the cervical 5 and 6 vertebrae (Fig. **2**). There was a narrowing of the intervertebral space. The cervical spine MRI showed reduced signal intensity in multiple intervertebral discs on the T2-weighted sequence images (Fig. **3**). The C4-5 and C6-7 intervertebral discs were mildly herniated. However, there was a large C5-6 intervertebral disc herniation causing compression of the anterior dural sac. The duration of the symptoms was one year. However, the recent functional downturn and the aggravation of symptoms over the last month prompted the surgical consultation. Based on the physical examination and advanced imaging study findings, the treating surgeon concluded that the anterior spinal cord compression at the C5/6 level needed decompression. An anterior endoscopic C5/6 surgery was planned.

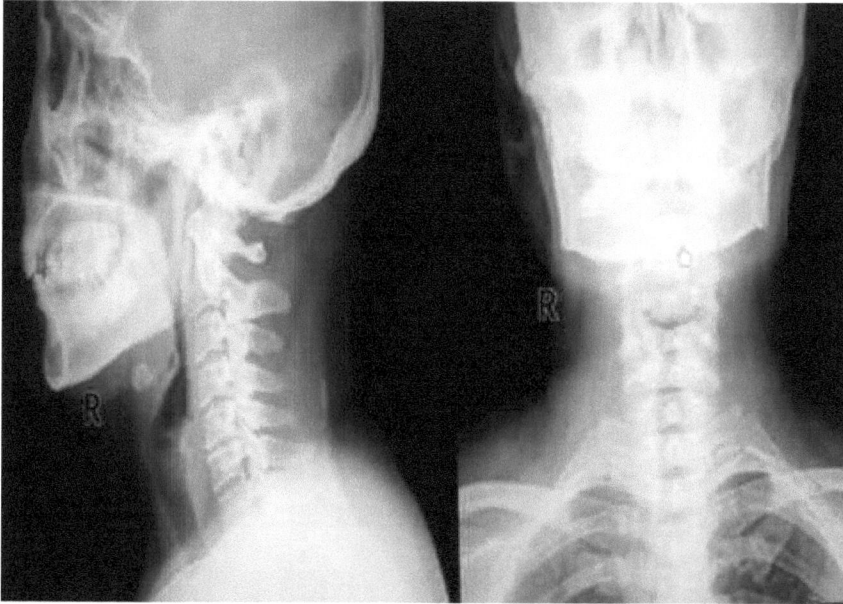

**Fig. (2).** Cervical spine series radiographs showed straightening of the cervical spine and loss of the physiological curvature. There were advanced degenerative changes at the C5/C6 level with anterior osteophytosis.

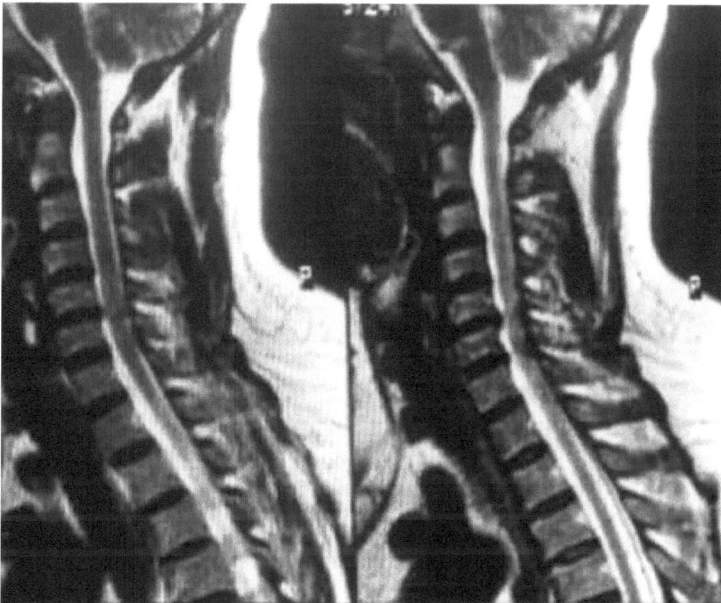

**Fig. (3).** Sagittal T2-weighted MRI scans confirm the loss of the physiological curvature of the cervical spine. There are smaller disc herniations at the C4-5 and C6-7 intervertebral disc levels. The larger C5-6 intervertebral discs herniation causes indentation of the anterior dural sac.

For the C5-6 anterior cervical endoscopic discectomy, the patient was positioned supine. The spinal needle was inserted 2.5 cm lateral of the midline along the horizontal line drawn across the C5-6 level employing the anterior-posterior fluoroscopic view. The right-sided approach was chosen. The tracheoesophageal groove was exploited by digital distraction. The puncture positioning needle was 30 degrees from the trunk's sagittal plane and 10 degrees from the horizontal position, and the carotid artery is pulled laterally. The needle was slowly inserted into the intervertebral disc. A small 4-mm skin incision was made, and the plane between the sternocleidoid muscle laterally and the trachea medially was bluntly dissected until the anterior cervical spine is reached. After a surgical corridor was established, the endoscopic working cannula was inserted over serial dilators into the nucleus pulposus (Fig. **4**). Then, the mechanical removal of the herniated disc, nerve lysis, and low-temperature plasma radiofrequency ablation was performed under direct visualization. The postoperative outcome was satisfactory to the patient with near-complete resolution of symptoms.

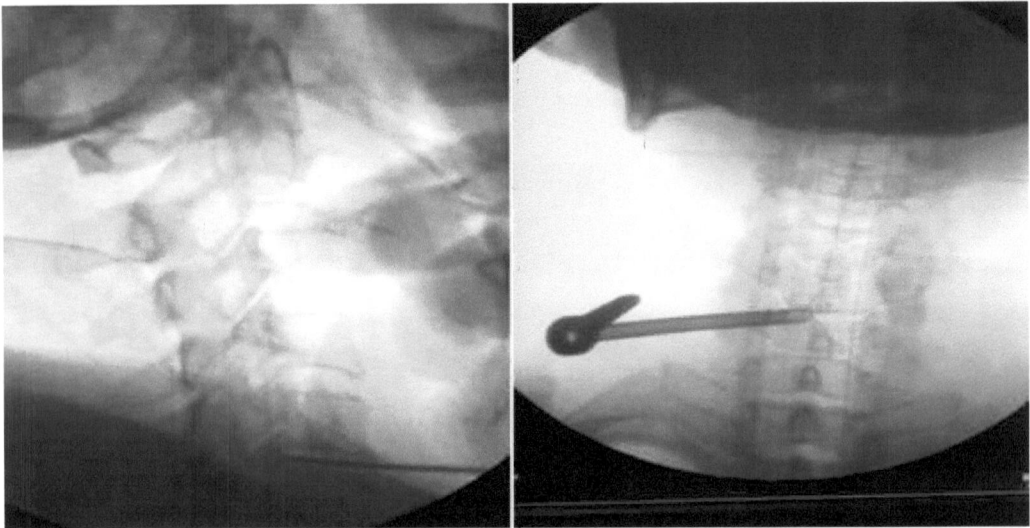

**Fig. (4).** Intraoperative positioning of the endoscopic working cannula during C5-6 anterior cervical endoscopic discectomy.

Immediately, upon removal of the working cannula bright red blood spurted from the surgical incision. The bleeding was gradually controlled by compression. However, the patient experienced severe breathing difficulties and became tachycardic and went into sudden cardiac arrest. The patient was promptly intubated and resuscitated with positive pressure mechanical ventilation as a compressive hematoma accumulated in the anterior neck obstructing the trachea. The patient coded and chest compressions were instituted. The patient was placed on the ventilation until sufficient recovery of cardiopulmonary function and reduction of facial swelling had occurred. Once medically stable, a vascular computed tomography angiogram (CTA) examination (Fig. **5**) suggested an injury to the right carotid artery. Also, there was blood accumulation in the posterior mediastinum and right thoracic cavity. An immediate exploratory surgery, and vascular repair was carried out. The common carotid blood vessel of this patient was found to be injured at the takeoff of the superior thyroid artery. There was a small 2 mm punch hole in the common carotid artery which was repaired by the vascular team.

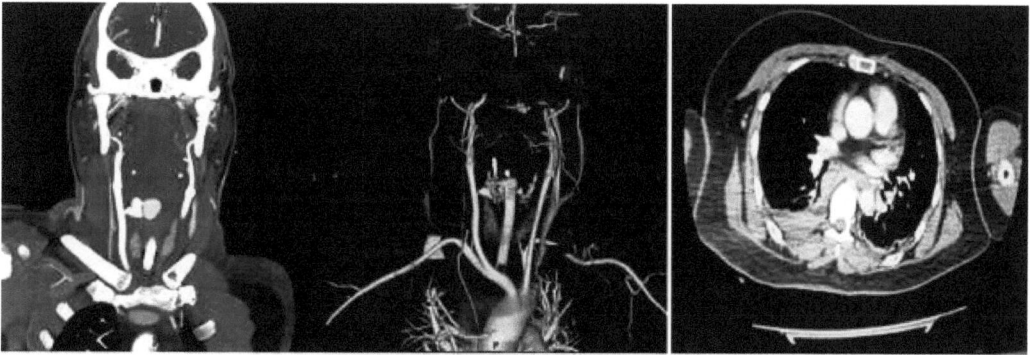

**Fig. (5).** Postoperative cervical vascular CTA and chest CT examination showing hematoma in the posterior mediastinum and right-sided thoracic cavity.

Reports in the literature on significant vascular injury in the anterior neck resulting from cervical endoscopy are currently unavailable. Hence, a discussion of how to manage such a potentially devastating complication is also scant. Based on the observations and discussion of management of the carotid injury observed by one participating author of this chapter (XiJ), several key recommendations should be made. The puncture positioning's intraoperative assessment should be verified several times before introducing the serial dilators or trephines as it may be inaccurate. The neck blood vessels can be easily damaged during the puncture. Serial dilation over a guidewire and placement of the beveled working cannular may also contribute to the carotid injury, particularly if the cannula is placed above the common carotid's bifurcation. The bevel tip may act as a cutting edge similar to a round gauge. The carotid artery's injury very likely occurred with the advancement of the beveled tip of the endoscopic working cannula onto the anterior aspect of the cervical spine. The endoscopic working cannula likely also was occluding the punch hole injury in the common carotid, which instantly started bleeding when upon its removal at the end of the surgery. Therefore, the authors recommend that the surgeon's middle finger be medial to the carotid sheath, and its pulse should still be palpable after placement of the access puncture needle. However, the carotid's palpation above its bifurcation may prove challenging even for experienced surgeons and should be verified during the careful serial dilation process. In the case presented herein, the injury to the common carotid artery at the takeoff of the superior thyroid artery was located and repaired during the open exploration of the anterior neck area. The more considerable distance between the skin and the carotid sheath in obese patients with a short and thick neck may be a relative contraindication to anterior cervical endoscopic discectomy.

## SPINAL CORD INJURY

Neurologic deficit due to irritation or injury of the cervical spinal cord after anterior or posterior endoscopic decompression is a devastating complication. Reports in the literature associated with cervical endoscopy are non-existent. Many of the newest spinal endoscopy publications indicate that no such injury [55 - 57]. However, the risk of spinal cord injury has been reported with other common cervical spine surgeries. One has to assume that eventually, such reports will emerge with endoscopic spinal surgery due to higher surgery rates for common painful degenerative conditions of the cervical spine. The senior author of this chapter has had neurological deterioration after anterior endoscopic cervical discectomy (Fig. 6). Fortunately, that patient experienced near-complete recovery of her finger- and grip weakness. Does the question arise which factors may contribute to such postoperative neurological deterioration, and are there any preoperative prognosticators that may help reduce its incidence? First and foremost, one needs to consider the severity of the underlying disease process. Patients with advanced cervical myelopathy have been shown to have neurological deficits following anterior cervical discectomy and fusion at a higher rate than patients with less advanced disease stages [58]. The white cord syndrome has been widely described in the literature as a rare but disastrous complication presumably related to ischemia and reperfusion injury with early or delayed onset [59 - 70]. It is possible that this occurred in our illustrative case example. Other factors related to the endoscopic technique – specifically the use of irrigation fluid, and small instruments being advanced through small endoscopic access corridors – may be relevant as well. Thermal injury may occur when lasers are used [71]. While it has somewhat fallen out of favor now and is only used in conjunction with modern cervical endoscopy equipment [72, 73], laser discectomy was the starting point of endoscopic cervical discectomy and complications related to laser use in the cervical spine nowadays are unheard of [74, 75].

The management of neurological deficit following cervical endoscopy is potentially as controversial as the complication itself and depends on the clinical presentation with either complete or incomplete loss of neurological function. No validated clinical protocols specific to endoscopy of the cervical spine exist. Whether or not it is appropriate to apply the same principles to postoperative loss of neurological function following cervical endoscopic surgery as in traumatic spinal cord injury by employing the American Spinal Injury Association (ASIA) grading and its associated clinical treatment guidelines remains to be seen and needs to be subject to future clinical research. However, there are a few recommendations the authors of this chapter are making should the endoscopic spine surgeon encounter this unpleasant problem following cervical spine endoscopy.

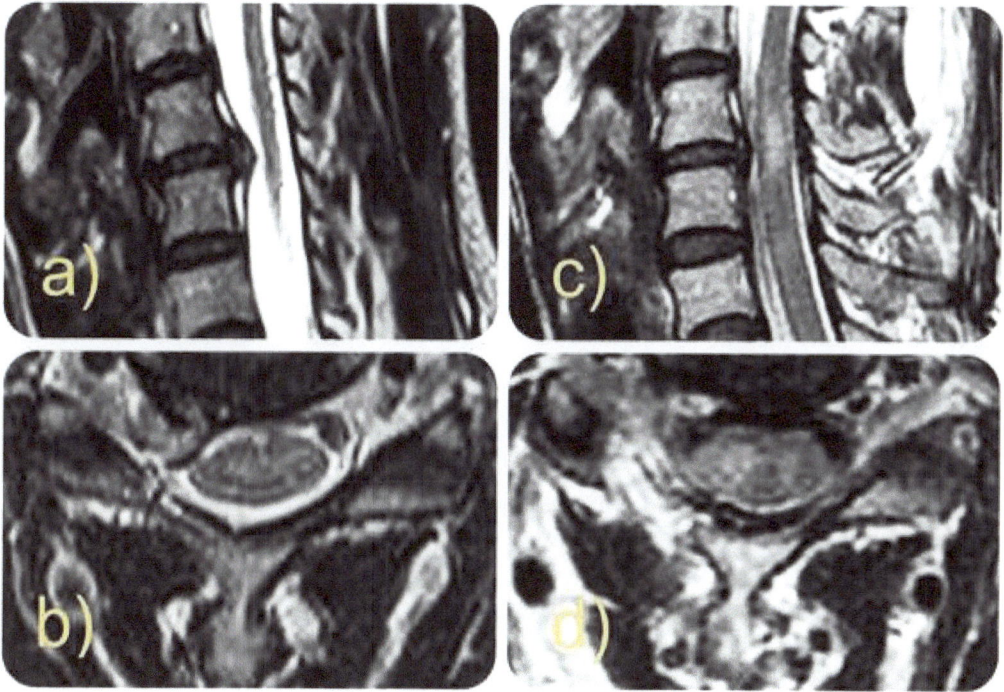

**Fig. (6).** Shown is an illustrative case example of incomplete endoscopic decompression with posterior endoscopic cervical discectomy (PECD) in a 45-year female patient. The preoperative and postoperative axial (**a** and **b**) and sagittal (**c** and **d**) MRI scan were compared to postoperative axial (**c**) and sagittal (**d**) show edema within the spinal cord at the surgical level. The patient underwent anterior endoscopic cervical discectomy for right neck, shoulder, and arm pain. Postoperatively, the patients 2/5 motor weakness in finger extension and grasp in the right hand improved to nearly completely at three months postoperatively.

First, a complete and thorough clinical examination is needed to fully document and understand the extent of the neurological deficit – it is complete with tetraplegia or incomplete with weakness in the motor groups directly related to the surgical level or more distant levels suggesting an expansion of the underlying process. Second, the endoscopic spine surgeon should be highly vigilant and have a low threshold to initiate a rapid transfer of a patient with severe neurological deficits (ASIA grade A through D) to a higher level of care institution where an intensive care unit (ICU) is available if the endoscopy was performed in an outpatient surgery center. Third, postoperative advanced imaging studies, including gadolinium enhanced MRI, are mandatory to demonstrate the spinal cord reaction to the surgical insult visually. Fourth, the treating surgeon should quickly assemble a multidisciplinary care team if the patient is diagnosed with white cord syndrome. This syndrome may take an entirely unpredictable postoperative course where rapid deterioration with multiorgan failure, brady-arrhythmias with hypotension possibly culminating in cardiopulmonary arrest are unfortunately possible [64]. Finally, a high-dose steroid regimen with methylprednisolone and aggressive postoperative rehabilitation programs should be instituted quickly as advocated by many authors [62 - 65]. However, a standardized, validated protocol outlining the dosing or timing of steroid therapy similar to those applied to spinal cord injury patients, where treatment initiation eight hours after injury contrary to former National Acute Spinal Cord Injury Study (NASCIS) standards [76] is no longer recommended, does not exist [77 - 80]. Hence, the authors of this chapter suggest that the endoscopic spine surgeon, who unfortunately may have to manage a patient with neurological deficits following the cervical decompression, employ the spinal cord injury protocols accepted in her or his community by applying the local standards of care regarding steroid treatment endorsed by their leading spine societies and professional physician organizations.

In any patient with neurological deficits following cervical endoscopy, the surgeon should quickly try to understand whether there is an underlying problem responsible for the neurological deterioration and whether it can be rapidly addressed to reverse the loss of function. For example, a hematoma within the spinal canal or the retropharyngeal space may contribute to neurological deficits warranting rapid revision decompression. A CSF leak due to dural tears and associated rootlet- or spinal cord herniation may also be amenable to early postoperative repair as well [65]. Hemiparesis or partial loss of function has also been reported in patients with advanced myelopathy who may be more appropriately considered for an alternative decompression technique without knowing whether that actually would lower the risk with surgery in general [59]. Additional logistical factors may go into the preoperative decision algorithm, particularly if the patient is scheduled for treatment in an ambulatory surgery center setting and to be discharged home within hours following the operation. The lack of resources to deal with potential complications may be the leading reason to consider alternative operations in other clinical settings.

# CONCLUSIONS

After endoscopic decompression surgery of the cervical spine, complications for common painful degenerative conditions are rare. Sequelae are by far more prevalent and typically have a benign postoperative course with a favorable long-term outlook on recovering function related to neuropraxia with early supportive care measures and aggressive rehabilitation. Failure to cure may occur in cases of incomplete decompression. These under treatment scenarios are typically well managed with additional staged and perhaps alternative decompression surgeries. Any vascular injury needs to be repaired quickly as soon as it is recognized and, if necessary, during the same endoscopic operation. Delays for additional diagnostic or imaging studies may pose the patient at undue risk for hemodynamic demise. Unfortunately, there is no validated algorithm in assessing the perioperative risks for complications with endoscopic surgery of the cervical spine concerning spinal cord injury and rapid deterioration of neurological function. In the worst cases, tetraplegia or medical demise of patients with white cord syndrome may occur due to cardiopulmonary collapse or hypoxic brain ischemia. Last but not least, there is the surgeon factor. The surgeon skill level may widely vary, and the need for formalized and accredited postgraduate training programs is evident. Only those surgeons with adequate training and clinical experience and the ability to manage postoperative problems should attempt endoscopic surgery of the cervical spine.

## CONSENT FOR PUBLICATION

Not applicable.

## CONFLICT OF INTEREST

The author declares no conflict of interest, financial or otherwise.

## ACKNOWLEDGEMENTS

Declared none.

## REFERENCES

[1]     Epstein NE. A Review of Complication Rates for Anterior Cervical Diskectomy and Fusion (ACDF). Surg Neurol Int 2019; 10: 100.
[http://dx.doi.org/10.25259/SNI-191-2019] [PMID: 31528438]

[2]     Skovrlj B, Gologorsky Y, Haque R, Fessler RG, Qureshi SA. Complications, outcomes, and need for fusion after minimally invasive posterior cervical foraminotomy and microdiscectomy. Spine J 2014; 14(10): 2405-11.
[http://dx.doi.org/10.1016/j.spinee.2014.01.048] [PMID: 24486472]

[3]     Platt A, Gerard CS, O'Toole JE. Comparison of outcomes following minimally invasive and open posterior cervical foraminotomy: description of minimally invasive technique and review of literature.

J Spine Surg 2020; 6(1): 243-51.
[http://dx.doi.org/10.21037/jss.2020.01.08] [PMID: 32309662]

[4]  Eicker SO, Steiger HJ, El-Kathib M. A Transtubular Microsurgical Approach to Treat Lateral Cervical Disc Herniation. World Neurosurg 2016; 88: 503-9.
[http://dx.doi.org/10.1016/j.wneu.2015.10.037] [PMID: 26525426]

[5]  Fessler RG, Khoo LT. Minimally invasive cervical microendoscopic foraminotomy: an initial clinical experience. Neurosurgery 2002; 51(5) (Suppl.): S37-45.
[http://dx.doi.org/10.1097/00006123-200211002-00006] [PMID: 12234428]

[6]  Kim CH, Kim KT, Chung CK, *et al.* Minimally invasive cervical foraminotomy and diskectomy for laterally located soft disk herniation. Eur Spine J 2015; 24(12): 3005-12.
[http://dx.doi.org/10.1007/s00586-015-4198-1] [PMID: 26298479]

[7]  Kim KT, Kim YB. Comparison between open procedure and tubular retractor assisted procedure for cervical radiculopathy: results of a randomized controlled study. J Korean Med Sci 2009; 24(4): 649-53.
[http://dx.doi.org/10.3346/jkms.2009.24.4.649] [PMID: 19654947]

[8]  Uehara M, Takahashi J, Kuraishi S, *et al.* Mini Open Foraminotomy for Cervical Radiculopathy: A Comparison of Large Tubular and TrimLine Retractors. Asian Spine J 2015; 9(4): 548-52.
[http://dx.doi.org/10.4184/asj.2015.9.4.548] [PMID: 26240713]

[9]  Winder MJ, Thomas KC. Minimally invasive *versus* open approach for cervical laminoforaminotomy. Can J Neurol Sci 2011; 38(2): 262-7.
[http://dx.doi.org/10.1017/S0317167100011446] [PMID: 21320831]

[10]  Hutton B, Salanti G, Caldwell DM, *et al.* The PRISMA extension statement for reporting of systematic reviews incorporating network meta-analyses of health care interventions: checklist and explanations. Ann Intern Med 2015; 162(11): 777-84.
[http://dx.doi.org/10.7326/M14-2385] [PMID: 26030634]

[11]  Poveda-Montoyo I, Belinchón-Romero I, Romero-Pérez D, Ramos-Rincón JM. Topics and PRISMA Checklist Compliance for Meta-analyses in Dermatology: Journal Case Study. Acta Dermatovenerol Croat 2019; 27(4): 275-7.
[PMID: 31969243]

[12]  Cook DA, Reed DA. Appraising the quality of medical education research methods: the Medical Education Research Study Quality Instrument and the Newcastle-Ottawa Scale-Education. Acad Med 2015; 90(8): 1067-76.
[http://dx.doi.org/10.1097/ACM.0000000000000786] [PMID: 26107881]

[13]  Fang W, Huang L, Feng F, *et al.* Anterior cervical discectomy and fusion *versus* posterior cervical foraminotomy for the treatment of single-level unilateral cervical radiculopathy: a meta-analysis. J Orthop Surg Res 2020; 15(1): 202.
[http://dx.doi.org/10.1186/s13018-020-01723-5] [PMID: 32487109]

[14]  Herkowitz HN, Kurz LT, Overholt DP. Surgical management of cervical soft disc herniation. A comparison between the anterior and posterior approach. Spine 1990; 15(10): 1026-30.
[http://dx.doi.org/10.1097/00007632-199010000-00009] [PMID: 2263967]

[15]  Ruetten S, Komp M, Merk H, Godolias G. Full-endoscopic cervical posterior foraminotomy for the operation of lateral disc herniations using 5.9-mm endoscopes: a prospective, randomized, controlled study. Spine 2008; 33(9): 940-8.
[http://dx.doi.org/10.1097/BRS.0b013e31816c8b67] [PMID: 18427313]

[16]  Wirth FP, Dowd GC, Sanders HF, Wirth C. Cervical discectomy. A prospective analysis of three operative techniques. Surg Neurol 2000; 53(4): 340-6.
[http://dx.doi.org/10.1016/S0090-3019(00)00201-9] [PMID: 10825519]

[17]  Alvin MD, Lubelski D, Abdullah KG, Whitmore RG, Benzel EC, Mroz TE. Cost-utility analysis of

Anterior Cervical Discectomy and Fusion With Plating (ACDFP) *versus* Posterior Cervical Foraminotomy (PCF) for patients with single-level cervical radiculopathy at 1-year follow-up. Clin Spine Surg 2016; 29(2): E67-72.
[http://dx.doi.org/10.1097/BSD.0000000000000099] [PMID: 26889994]

[18]  Cho TG, Kim YB, Park SW. Long term effect on adjacent segment motion after posterior cervical foraminotomy. Korean J Spine 2014; 11(1): 1-6.
[http://dx.doi.org/10.14245/kjs.2014.11.1.1] [PMID: 24891864]

[19]  Dunn C, Moore J, Sahai N, *et al.* Minimally invasive posterior cervical foraminotomy with tubes to prevent undesired fusion: a long-term follow-up study. J Neurosurg Spine 2018; 29(4): 358-64.
[http://dx.doi.org/10.3171/2018.2.SPINE171003] [PMID: 29957145]

[20]  Foster MT, Carleton-Bland NP, Lee MK, Jackson R, Clark SR, Wilby MJ. Comparison of clinical outcomes in anterior cervical discectomy *versus* foraminotomy for brachialgia. Br J Neurosurg 2019; 33(1): 3-7.
[http://dx.doi.org/10.1080/02688697.2018.1527013] [PMID: 30450995]

[21]  Korinth MC, Krüger A, Oertel MF, Gilsbach JM. Posterior foraminotomy or anterior discectomy with polymethyl methacrylate interbody stabilization for cervical soft disc disease: results in 292 patients with monoradiculopathy. Spine 2006; 31(11): 1207-14.
[http://dx.doi.org/10.1097/01.brs.0000217604.02663.59] [PMID: 16688033]

[22]  Lin GX, Rui G, Sharma S, Kotheeranurak V, Suen TK, Kim JS. Does the neck pain, function, or range of motion differ after anterior cervical fusion, cervical disc replacement, and posterior cervical foraminotomy? World Neurosurg 2019; 129: e485-93.
[http://dx.doi.org/10.1016/j.wneu.2019.05.188] [PMID: 31150858]

[23]  Mansfield HE, Canar WJ, Gerard CS, O'Toole JE. Single-level anterior cervical discectomy and fusion *versus* minimally invasive posterior cervical foraminotomy for patients with cervical radiculopathy: a cost analysis. Neurosurg Focus 2014; 37(5): E9.
[http://dx.doi.org/10.3171/2014.8.FOCUS14373] [PMID: 25491887]

[24]  Mok JK, Sheha ED, Samuel AM, *et al.* Evaluation of current trends in treatment of single-level cervical radiculopathy. Clin Spine Surg 2019; 32(5): E241-5.
[http://dx.doi.org/10.1097/BSD.0000000000000796] [PMID: 30762836]

[25]  Scholz T, Geiger MF, Mainz V, *et al.* Anterior cervical decompression and fusion or posterior foraminotomy for cervical radiculopathy: results of a single-center series. J Neurol Surg A Cent Eur Neurosurg 2018; 79(3): 211-7.
[http://dx.doi.org/10.1055/s-0037-1607225] [PMID: 29132169]

[26]  Selvanathan SK, Beagrie C, Thomson S, *et al.* Anterior cervical discectomy and fusion *versus* posterior cervical foraminotomy in the treatment of brachialgia: the Leeds spinal unit experience (2008-2013). Acta Neurochir (Wien) 2015; 157(9): 1595-600.
[http://dx.doi.org/10.1007/s00701-015-2491-8] [PMID: 26144567]

[27]  Tumialán LM, Ponton RP, Gluf WM. Management of unilateral cervical radiculopathy in the military: the cost effectiveness of posterior cervical foraminotomy compared with anterior cervical discectomy and fusion. Neurosurg Focus 2010; 28(5): E17.
[http://dx.doi.org/10.3171/2010.1.FOCUS09305] [PMID: 20568933]

[28]  Witiw CD, Smieliauskas F, O'Toole JE, Fehlings MG, Fessler RG. Comparison of anterior cervical discectomy and fusion to posterior cervical foraminotomy for cervical radiculopathy: utilization, costs, and adverse events 2003 to 2014. Neurosurgery 2019; 84(2): 413-20.
[http://dx.doi.org/10.1093/neuros/nyy051] [PMID: 29548034]

[29]  Lin Y, Rao S, Li Y, Zhao S, Chen B. Posterior percutaneous full-endoscopic cervical laminectomy and decompression for cervical stenosis with myelopathy: a technical note. World Neurosurg 2019; S1878-8750 (19): 30051-8.
[http://dx.doi.org/10.1016/j.wneu.2018.12.180] [PMID: 30648610]

[30]　Papavero L, Kothe R. Minimally invasive posterior cervical foraminotomy for treatment of radiculopathy : An effective, time-tested, and cost-efficient motion-preservation technique. Oper Orthop Traumatol 2018; 30(1): 36-45.
[http://dx.doi.org/10.1007/s00064-017-0516-6] [PMID: 28929274]

[31]　Deng ZL, Chu L, Chen L, Yang JS. Anterior transcorporeal approach of percutaneous endoscopic cervical discectomy for disc herniation at the C4-C5 levels: a technical note. Spine J 2016; 16(5): 659-66.
[http://dx.doi.org/10.1016/j.spinee.2016.01.187] [PMID: 26850173]

[32]　Yang J, Chu L, Deng Z, *et al.* Clinical study of single-level cervical disc herniation treated by full-endoscopic decompression *via* anterior transcorporeal approach. Zhongguo Xiu Fu Chong Jian Wai Ke Za Zhi 2020; 34(5): 543-9.
[PMID: 32410418]

[33]　Chu L, Yang JS, Yu KX, Chen CM, Hao DJ, Deng ZL. Usage of bone wax to facilitate percutaneous endoscopic cervical discectomy *via* anterior transcorporeal approach for cervical intervertebral disc herniation. World Neurosurg 2018; 118: 102-8.
[http://dx.doi.org/10.1016/j.wneu.2018.07.070] [PMID: 30026139]

[34]　Xiao CM, Yu KX, Deng R, *et al.* Modified K-hole percutaneous endoscopic surgery for cervical foraminal stenosis: partial pediculectomy approach. Pain Physician 2019; 22(5): E407-16.
[PMID: 31561650]

[35]　Choi KC, Ahn Y, Kang BU, Ahn ST, Lee SH. Motor palsy after posterior cervical foraminotomy: anatomical consideration 2013.
[http://dx.doi.org/10.1016/j.wneu.2011.03.043]

[36]　Youn MS, Shon MH, Seong YJ, Shin JK, Goh TS, Lee JS. Clinical and radiological outcomes of two-level endoscopic posterior cervical foraminotomy. Eur Spine J 2017; 26(9): 2450-8.
[http://dx.doi.org/10.1007/s00586-017-5017-7] [PMID: 28337706]

[37]　Lee U, Kim CH, Chung CK, *et al.* The recovery of motor strength after posterior percutaneous endoscopic cervical foraminotomy and discectomy. World Neurosurg 2018; 115: e532-8.
[http://dx.doi.org/10.1016/j.wneu.2018.04.090] [PMID: 29689395]

[38]　Dindo D, Demartines N, Clavien PA. Classification of surgical complications: a new proposal with evaluation in a cohort of 6336 patients and results of a survey. Ann Surg 2004; 240(2): 205-13.
[http://dx.doi.org/10.1097/01.sla.0000133083.54934.ae] [PMID: 15273542]

[39]　Shao T, Qiu W, Yang W. Anatomical variations of the recurrent laryngeal nerve in Chinese patients: a prospective study of 2,404 patients. Sci Rep 2016; 6: 25475.
[http://dx.doi.org/10.1038/srep25475] [PMID: 27146369]

[40]　Cernea CR, Hojaij FC, De Carlucci D Jr, *et al.* Recurrent laryngeal nerve: a plexus rather than a nerve? Arch Otolaryngol Head Neck Surg 2009; 135(11): 1098-102.
[http://dx.doi.org/10.1001/archoto.2009.151] [PMID: 19917921]

[41]　Jung A, Schramm J. How to reduce recurrent laryngeal nerve palsy in anterior cervical spine surgery: a prospective observational study. Neurosurgery 2010; 67(1): 10-5.
[http://dx.doi.org/10.1227/01.NEU.0000370203.26164.24] [PMID: 20559087]

[42]　Kulekci M, Batioglu-Karaaltin A, Saatci O, Uzun I. Relationship between the branches of the recurrent laryngeal nerve and the inferior thyroid artery. Ann Otol Rhinol Laryngol 2012; 121(10): 650-6.
[http://dx.doi.org/10.1177/000348941212101005] [PMID: 23130539]

[43]　Dankbaar JW, Pameijer FA. Vocal cord paralysis: anatomy, imaging and pathology. Insights Imaging 2014; 5(6): 743-51.
[http://dx.doi.org/10.1007/s13244-014-0364-y] [PMID: 25315036]

[44]　Haller JM, Iwanik M, Shen FH. Clinically relevant anatomy of recurrent laryngeal nerve. Spine 2012; 37(2): 97-100.

[http://dx.doi.org/10.1097/BRS.0b013e31821f3e86] [PMID: 21540775]

[45]   Miscusi M, Bellitti A, Peschillo S, Polli FM, Missori P, Delfini R. Does recurrent laryngeal nerve anatomy condition the choice of the side for approaching the anterior cervical spine? J Neurosurg Sci 2007; 51(2): 61-4.
[PMID: 17571036]

[46]   Thomas AM, Fahim DK, Gemechu JM. Anatomical variations of the recurrent laryngeal nerve and implications for injury prevention during surgical procedures of the neck. Diagnostics (Basel) 2020; 10(9): E670.
[http://dx.doi.org/10.3390/diagnostics10090670] [PMID: 32899604]

[47]   Oh LJ, Dibas M, Ghozy S, Mobbs R, Phan K, Faulkner H. Recurrent laryngeal nerve injury following single- and multiple-level anterior cervical discectomy and fusion: a meta-analysis. J Spine Surg 2020; 6(3): 541-8.
[http://dx.doi.org/10.21037/jss-20-508] [PMID: 33102890]

[48]   Fountas KN, Kapsalaki EZ, Nikolakakos LG, *et al.* Anterior cervical discectomy and fusion associated complications. Spine 2007; 32(21): 2310-7.
[http://dx.doi.org/10.1097/BRS.0b013e318154c57e] [PMID: 17906571]

[49]   Kilburg C, Sullivan HG, Mathiason MA. Effect of approach side during anterior cervical discectomy and fusion on the incidence of recurrent laryngeal nerve injury. J Neurosurg Spine 2006; 4(4): 273-7.
[http://dx.doi.org/10.3171/spi.2006.4.4.273] [PMID: 16619672]

[50]   Lied B, Sundseth J, Helseth E. Immediate (0-6 h), early (6-72 h) and late (>72 h) complications after anterior cervical discectomy with fusion for cervical disc degeneration; discharge six hours after operation is feasible. Acta Neurochir (Wien) 2008; 150(2): 111-8.
[http://dx.doi.org/10.1007/s00701-007-1472-y] [PMID: 18066487]

[51]   Nanda A, Sharma M, Sonig A, Ambekar S, Bollam P. Surgical complications of anterior cervical diskectomy and fusion for cervical degenerative disk disease: a single surgeon's experience of 1,576 patients. World Neurosurg 2014; 82(6): 1380-7.
[http://dx.doi.org/10.1016/j.wneu.2013.09.022] [PMID: 24056095]

[52]   Yang Y, Ma L, Hong Y. The application of Zero-profile implant in two-level and single level anterior cervical discectomy and fusion for the treatment of cervical spondylosis: a comparative study. Int J Clin Exp Med 2016; 9: 15667-77.

[53]   Liu KX, Massoud B. Endoscopic anterior cervical discectomy under epidurogram guidance. Surg Technol Int 2010; 20: 373-8.
[PMID: 21082589]

[54]   Ahn Y, Lee SH, Shin SW. Percutaneous endoscopic cervical discectomy: clinical outcome and radiographic changes. Photomed Laser Surg 2005; 23(4): 362-8.
[http://dx.doi.org/10.1089/pho.2005.23.362] [PMID: 16144477]

[55]   Kim CH, Chung CK, Kim HJ, Jahng TA, Kim DG. Early outcome of posterior cervical endoscopic discectomy: an alternative treatment choice for physically/socially active patients. J Korean Med Sci 2009; 24(2): 302-6.
[http://dx.doi.org/10.3346/jkms.2009.24.2.302] [PMID: 19399274]

[56]   Ramírez León JF, Rugeles Ortíz JG, Martínez CR, Alonso Cuéllar GO, Lewandrowski KU. Surgical treatment of cervical radiculopathy using an anterior cervical endoscopic decompression. J Spine Surg 2020; 6 (Suppl. 1): S179-85.
[http://dx.doi.org/10.21037/jss.2019.09.24] [PMID: 32195426]

[57]   Zhang C, Li D, Wang C, Yan X. Cervical endoscopic laminoplasty for cervical myelopathy. Spine 2016; 41 (Suppl. 19): B44-51.
[http://dx.doi.org/10.1097/BRS.0000000000001816] [PMID: 27656783]

[58]   Goh GS, Liow MHL, Ling ZM, *et al.* Severity of preoperative myelopathy symptoms affects patient-

reported outcomes, satisfaction, and return to work after anterior cervical discectomy and fusion for degenerative cervical myelopathy. Spine 2020; 45(10): 649-56.
[http://dx.doi.org/10.1097/BRS.0000000000003354] [PMID: 31809467]

[59]    Antwi P, Grant R, Kuzmik G, Abbed K. "White Cord Syndrome" of acute hemiparesis after posterior cervical decompression and fusion for chronic cervical stenosis. World Neurosurg 2018; 113: 33-6.
[http://dx.doi.org/10.1016/j.wneu.2018.02.026] [PMID: 29452319]

[60]    Carey EM, Foster PC. The activity of 2′,3′-cyclic nucleotide 3′-phosphohydrolase in the corpus callosum, subcortical white matter, and spinal cord in infants dying from sudden infant death syndrome. J Neurochem 1984; 42(4): 924-9.
[http://dx.doi.org/10.1111/j.1471-4159.1984.tb12692.x] [PMID: 6321664]

[61]    Chin KR, Seale J, Cumming V. "White cord syndrome" of acute tetraplegia after anterior cervical decompression and fusion for chronic spinal cord compression: a case report. Case Rep Orthop 2013; 2013: 697918.
[http://dx.doi.org/10.1155/2013/697918] [PMID: 23533882]

[62]    Epstein NE. Reperfusion injury (RPI)/White Cord Syndrome (WCS) due to cervical spine surgery: a diagnosis of exclusion. Surg Neurol Int 2020; 11: 320.
[http://dx.doi.org/10.25259/SNI_555_2020] [PMID: 33093997]

[63]    Jun DS, Baik JM, Lee SK. A case report: white cord syndrome following anterior cervical discectomy and fusion: importance of prompt diagnosis and treatment. BMC Musculoskelet Disord 2020; 21(1): 157.
[http://dx.doi.org/10.1186/s12891-020-3162-3] [PMID: 32164644]

[64]    Kalidindi KKV, Sath S. "White cord syndrome" of acute tetraplegia after posterior cervical decompression and resulting hypoxic brain injury. Asian J Neurosurg 2020; 15(3): 756-8.
[http://dx.doi.org/10.4103/ajns.AJNS_240_20] [PMID: 33145248]

[65]    Liao YX, He SS, He ZM. 'White cord syndrome', a rare but disastrous complication of transient paralysis after posterior cervical decompression for severe cervical spondylotic myelopathy and spinal stenosis: A case report. Exp Ther Med 2020; 20(5): 90.
[http://dx.doi.org/10.3892/etm.2020.9218] [PMID: 32973939]

[66]    Mathkour M, Werner C, Riffle J, et al. Reperfusion "White Cord" syndrome in cervical spondylotic myelopathy: does mean arterial pressure goal make a difference? additional case and literature review. World Neurosurg 2020; 137: 194-9.
[http://dx.doi.org/10.1016/j.wneu.2020.01.062] [PMID: 31954909]

[67]    Papaioannou I, Repantis T, Baikousis A, Korovessis P. Late-onset "white cord syndrome" in an elderly patient after posterior cervical decompression and fusion: a case report. Spinal Cord Ser Cases 2019; 5(1): 28.
[http://dx.doi.org/10.1038/s41394-019-0174-z] [PMID: 31240122]

[68]    Papaioannou I, Repantis T, Baikousis A, Korovessis P. Late-onset "white cord syndrome" in an elderly patient after posterior cervical decompression and fusion: a case report. Spinal Cord Ser Cases 2019; 5: 28.
[http://dx.doi.org/10.1038/s41394-019-0174-z] [PMID: 31240122]

[69]    Sepulveda F, Carballo L, Carnevale M, Yañez P. White cord syndrome in a pediatric patient: A case report and review. Radiol Case Rep 2020; 15(11): 2343-7.
[http://dx.doi.org/10.1016/j.radcr.2020.08.047] [PMID: 32994838]

[70]    Vinodh VP, Rajapathy SK, Sellamuthu P, Kandasamy R. White cord syndrome: A devastating complication of spinal decompression surgery. Surg Neurol Int 2018; 9: 136.
[http://dx.doi.org/10.4103/sni.sni_96_18] [PMID: 30090668]

[71]    Haufe SM, Mork AR. Complications associated with cervical endoscopic discectomy with the holmium laser. J Clin Laser Med Surg 2004; 22(1): 57-8.
[http://dx.doi.org/10.1089/104454704773660985] [PMID: 15117488]

[72]    Ahn Y, Moon KS, Kang BU, Hur SM, Kim JD. Laser-assisted posterior cervical foraminotomy and discectomy for lateral and foraminal cervical disc herniation. Photomed Laser Surg 2012; 30(9): 510-5.
[http://dx.doi.org/10.1089/pho.2012.3246] [PMID: 22793668]

[73]    Jeon HC, Kim CS, Kim SC, *et al.* Posterior cervical microscopic foraminotomy and discectomy with laser for unilateral radiculopathy. Chonnam Med J 2015; 51(3): 129-34.
[http://dx.doi.org/10.4068/cmj.2015.51.3.129] [PMID: 26730364]

[74]    Siebert W. Percutaneous laser discectomy of cervical discs: preliminary clinical results. J Clin Laser Med Surg 1995; 13(3): 205-7.
[http://dx.doi.org/10.1089/clm.1995.13.205] [PMID: 10150647]

[75]    Chiu JC, Clifford TJ, Greenspan M, Richley RC, Lohman G, Sison RB. Percutaneous microdecompressive endoscopic cervical discectomy with laser thermodiskoplasty. Mt Sinai J Med 2000; 67(4): 278-82.
[PMID: 11021777]

[76]    Bracken MB, Holford TR. Neurological and functional status 1 year after acute spinal cord injury: estimates of functional recovery in National Acute Spinal Cord Injury Study II from results modeled in National Acute Spinal Cord Injury Study III. J Neurosurg 2002; 96(3) (Suppl.): 259-66.
[PMID: 11990832]

[77]    Miekisiak G, Kloc W, Janusz W, Kaczmarczyk J, Latka D, Zarzycki D. Current use of methylprednisolone for acute spinal cord injury in Poland: survey study. Eur J Orthop Surg Traumatol 2014; 24 (Suppl. 1): S269-73.
[http://dx.doi.org/10.1007/s00590-014-1422-3] [PMID: 24496913]

[78]    Evaniew N, Noonan VK, Fallah N, *et al.* RHSCIR Network. Methylprednisolone for the treatment of patients with acute spinal cord injuries: a propensity score-matched cohort study from a canadian multi-center spinal cord injury registry. J Neurotrauma 2015; 32(21): 1674-83.
[http://dx.doi.org/10.1089/neu.2015.3963] [PMID: 26065706]

[79]    Teles AR, Cabrera J, Riew KD, Falavigna A. Steroid use for acute spinal cord injury in latin america: a potentially dangerous practice guided by fear of lawsuit. World Neurosurg 2016; 88: 342-9.
[http://dx.doi.org/10.1016/j.wneu.2015.12.045] [PMID: 26732969]

[80]    Liu Z, Yang Y, He L, *et al.* High-dose methylprednisolone for acute traumatic spinal cord injury: A meta-analysis. Neurology 2019; 93(9): e841-50.
[http://dx.doi.org/10.1212/WNL.0000000000007998] [PMID: 31358617]

# SUBJECT INDEX